Geriatric Interdisciplinary Team Training

Eugenia L. Siegler, MD, FACP, received her AB from Princeton University and her MD from Johns Hopkins. After finishing her internship, residency, and chief residency in Internal Medicine at Bellevue and New York University Hospitals, she completed a fellowship in Geriatric and General Internal Medicine at the University of Pennsylvania. Formerly on the faculty of the University of Pennsylvania, she is now Chief of Geriatrics at The Brooklyn Hospital Center, Associate Professor of Clinical Medicine in the New York University School of Medicine, and Clinical Associate Professor of Nursing in the New York University Division of Nursing. She serves as a consultant to the John A. Hartford Foundation Geriatric Interdisciplinary Team Training Resource Center.

Kathryn Hyer, DrPA, MPP, is the Project Director for the Geriatric Interdisciplinary Team Training Program's Resource Center at New York University. Prior to assuming the Project Director's role, Dr. Hyer worked as a program consultant for the John A. Hartford Foundation to develop their Geriatric Interdisciplinary Team Training Program. She has held senior level policy and administrative positions in government and not-for-profit health care agencies in both Arizona and New York. Dr. Hyer received her undergraduate degree from Boston College, her master's in Public Policy from the Kennedy School of Government at Harvard, and her Doctorate in Public Administration from Arizona State University. Her dissertation on risk adjustment for Medicare's capitation rates received AHCPR funding.

Terry Fulmer, RN, PhD, FAAN, is Professor of Nursing at New York University Division of Nursing, Director of New York University Division of Nursing Center for Nursing Research, and co-Director of The John A. Hartford Foundation Institute for the Advancement of Geriatric Nursing Practice. She is also an Adjunct Professor at the Columbia University College of Physicians and Surgeons in the Department of Medical Informatics, and Director of the Columbia University–New York Geriatric Education Center. She has served as the Chair of the Clinical Medicine Section of the Gerontological Society of America. She received her bachelor's degree from Skidmore College and her master's and doctoral degrees from Boston College. Dr. Fulmer has been elected to Fellowships in the American Academy of Nursing, the Gerontological Society of America, and the New York Academy of Medicine. Most recently, she was honored by the New York State Nurses Association with the Distinguished Nurse Researcher Award.

Mathy Mezey, EdD, RN, FAAN, received her undergraduate and graduate education at Columbia University. She worked as a public health nurse and on medical and surgical units at Jacobi Hospital, an acute care facility of the New York City Health and Hospitals Corporation. Dr. Mezey taught at Lehman College of the City University of New York. For 10 years she was a professor at the University of Pennsylvania School of Nursing where she directed the geriatric nurse practitioner program and was Director of the Robert Wood Johnson Foundation Teaching Nursing Home Program. Since 1991 she has been the Independence Foundation Professor of Nursing Education at New York University. Her current research and writing focus is on ethical decision making about life-sustaining treatment. Dr. Mezey is exploring decision making by spouses of patients with Alzheimer's disease and preparing guidelines to assist in decisions related to the transfer of patients between nursing homes and hospitals. In September 1996, Dr. Mezey assumed the position of Director of the John A. Hartford Foundation Institute for the Advancement of Geriatric Nursing Practice.

Geriatric Interdisciplinary Team Training

Eugenia L. Siegler
Kathryn Hyer
Terry Fulmer
Mathy Mezey

Editors

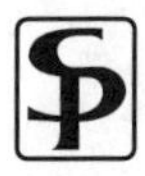 Springer Publishing Company

Springer Publishing Company, Inc.
536 Broadway
New York, NY 10012-3955

Cover design by Janet Joachim
Acquisitions Editor: Ruth Chasek
Production Editor: Pamela Lankas

98 99 00 01 02 / 5 4 3 2 1

Library of Congress Cataloging-in-Publication-Data

Geriatric interdisciplinary team training / [edited by] Eugenia L.
  Siegler . . . [et al.].
     p.   cm.
  Includes bibliographical references and index.
  ISBN 0-8261-1210-2 (hard cover)
  1. Geriatrics. 2. Health care teams—Training. 3. Aged—Medical
care. I. Siegler, Eugenia L.
  [DNLM: 1. Geriatrics—education. 2. Inservice Training—methods.
3. Patient Care Team—organization & administration. 4. Models,
Organizational. WT 18 G3691 1998]
RC952.5.G4432   1998
362.1'9897—dc21
DNLM/DLC
for Library of Congress   98-10334
                                               CIP

Printed in the United States of America

Contents

PART 4   ORGANIZING TEAM TRAINING IN DIFFERENT SITES AND SETTINGS

APPENDIXES

Foreword

Essential to any discussion of interdisciplinary health care is an understanding of the fundamental difference between interdisciplinary and multidisciplinary approaches. Health care has traditionally been *multidisciplinary,* with resources of several disciplines applied sequentially. For instance, in the care of hospitalized patients, the prevailing approach has been for a physician to see a patient on rounds and write a note, often legibly, in the patient's record. The nurse also documents the treatments administered and patient's progress in the record. In many cases, a social worker interviews the patient separately and records the findings and recommendations. Consultants, either from medical specialties or allied health areas, such as physical or occupational therapy, also see the patient and record their findings and recommendations in the record. A medical record evolves in which a comprehensive management plan for the patients is developed sequentially.

An *interdisciplinary* approach recognizes that many clinical problems outstrip the tools of individual disciplines and entails several health care providers simultaneously and cooperatively evaluating the patient and developing a joint plan of action.

Interdisciplinary teams are becoming common in many aspects of medicine, including cardiac and cancer care, major organ transplantation, and in patients with end-stage renal disease who are on chronic dialysis. But nowhere in health care is this strategy more common or more effective than in the care of multiply impaired older patients. In the United States, interdisciplinary care has been most advanced in the hospitals, ambulatory care sites, and long-term care facilities of the Department of Veterans Affairs, which has supported geriatric interdisciplinary teams and their training for well over a decade.

Despite the valuable experience of the Department of Veterans Affairs and several major academic medical centers, our current knowledge regarding the most effective and efficient organization of interdisciplinary teams and their proper training is rudimentary. This lack of readiness notwithstanding, interdisciplinary care is burgeoning. This growth is fueled by the development of integrated systems of care, which link patients through various levels of care, including hospitals, rehabilitation programs, ambulatory care sites, and home care, and by rapid expansion in the involvement of nonphysician health care providers in managed care settings.

With these considerations in mind, The John A. Hartford Foundation, well recognized for its leadership in fostering innovation in geriatric research, education, and care, has made a $10-million commitment to a national, multicenter Geriatric Interdisciplinary

Team Training Program. This effort aims to enhance substantially our understanding of the critical factors that lead to the success of interdisciplinary care and the training of interdisciplinary team members. The Program began in 1995 with identification of 13 sites across the United States judged to have the attitudes, experience, and resources essential to plan a major initiative in interdisciplinary team training. After thorough evaluation of the plans developed by the sites, the Hartford Foundation recently made eight major awards to individual medical centers and regional health systems to implement the most promising of these training plans. The programs selected represent a broad array of approaches in varied clinical and financing environments, and the experience from these models will yield valuable information that can be generalized across the country. In addition to its obvious expected benefits to geriatric care, the tight cooperation intrinsic to these models promises to enhance integration in the emerging health care systems.

This volume represents an important part of this historic Hartford Foundation initiative. By bringing together the experiences and perspectives of the leadership of the various model sites, the initiative's innovative Resource Center, and the Foundation's sophisticated staff, this book provides a robust analysis of the critical issues relevant to the next phase of geriatric interdisciplinary team training in the United States. It is a critical resource for policy analysts and provides practical advice for health care providers in a variety of areas, including identification of care and training sites, approaches to reconciling competing interests of disciplines, strategies for enhancing partnerships between academic institutions and health care resources outside the medical center, curriculum design, and the assessment of training efficacy.

The field of geriatrics is indebted to the Hartford Foundation for yet another important innovation. We look forward to the advances in knowledge that the Geriatric Interdisciplinary Team Training initiative will yield.

JOHN W. ROWE, MD

Preface

This book describes work in progress. All of its contributors have years of administrative or clinical experience in the care of the elderly. What we have asked them to struggle with, and now describe in this book, is how to train health care personnel to work in geriatric teams.

The John A. Hartford Foundation has underwritten this task, first by supporting 13 sites to spend a year contemplating, piloting, and planning Geriatric Interdisciplinary Team Training (GITT), and then by funding eight of these sites to implement their programs. The Foundation has also funded a Resource Center to promote synergy, provide technical assistance, and collect core data.

Although the lessons of the implementation programs are years away, the site personnel already have a great deal to share. They have done so at two meetings (one in January 1996, and another in April 1997) sponsored by the GITT Resource Center. Those meetings are the inspiration for this book.

This book is for those who are contemplating GITT. We have two goals: (a) To describe the components of GITT and suggest potential solutions to the problems one is most likely to encounter while designing and implementing it, and (b) to expose readers to the wide variety of GITT projects that the Hartford Foundation has sponsored. Because we wanted the book to be practical, we have organized by both topic and site, offering authors the opportunity to describe both the basic principles and experiences of the sites.

In addition, we have invited two experts in team training and consultants to the Hartford GITT program, Ruth Ann Tsukuda and Madeline Schmitt, to write chapters. We are grateful for the expertise and perspective that they bring to the book.

We hope that our readers find this book a useful primer for GITT. We think that it reflects the creativity and energy that its contributors have invested in GITT, and we hope that such enthusiasm is infectious.

ELS
KH
TF
MDM

Contributors

Christine K. Cassel, MD
Chairman and Professor
Henry L. Schwartz Department of Geriatrics
    and Adult Development
The Mount Sinai Medical Center
New York, NY 10029

Joann Castle, MA
Project Manager, Great Lakes GITT
Henry Ford Health System
Center for Health System Studies
Detroit, MI 48202

Richard Della Penna, MD
Regional Coordinator, Elder Health Care
Dept. of Continuing Care Services
Southern California Permanente Medical
    Group
San Diego, CA 92120

Denis A. Evans, MD
Professor, Departments of Internal Medicine
    and Neurosciences
Director, Rush Institute of Healthy Aging
Rush University
Rush-Presbyterian-St. Luke's Medical Center
Chicago, IL 60612

Judy Farness, MSN
Geriatric Medicine Associates
Baylor College of Medicine
Houston, TX 77030

Vaunette Fay, PhD, RNC
Associate Professor
University of Texas School of Nursing
Houston, TX

Janet C. Frank, DrPH
Asst. Director, Academic Programs
Multi-campus Program in Geriatrics/
    Gerontology
University of California at Los Angeles,
    Department of Medicine
Los Angeles, CA 90095

Mary S. Gleason, MSN, RNC
Director of Education,
Harris County Hospital District Geriatric
    Program
Ben Taub General Hospital
Houston, TX 77004

Lois Halstead, RN, PhD
Associate Dean, College of Nursing,
    Rush University
Rush-Presbyterian-St. Luke's Medical
    Center
Chicago, IL 60612

Judith L. Howe, PhD
Co-Director, Mount Sinai GITT
    Partnership
Assistant Professor
Henry L. Schwartz Department of Geriatrics
    and Adult Development
The Mount Sinai Medical Center
New York, NY 10029

Rebecca Hunter, MEd
Research Associate
Program on Aging
University of North Carolina at Chapel Hill,
    School of Medicine
Chapel Hill, NC 27599

Jerry C. Johnson, MD
Associate Professor of Medicine
Director Multicultural Programs, Institute
  on Aging
Director, Center of Excellence on Minority
  Health
University of Pennsylvania Health System
Ralston-Penn Center
Philadelphia, PA 19104-6006

Susan Kornblatt, MA
Project Director
On Lok GITT
On Lok, Inc.
San Francisco, CA 94109

Ernestine Kotthoff-Burrell, MS, RN, CS
Project Director
University of Colorado GITT
University of Colorado Health Sciences
  Center
Denver, CO 80262

Stan Lapidos, MS
Rush GITT Coordinator
Rush Institute for Healthy Aging
Rush University
Rush-Presbyterian-St. Luke's Medical Center
Chicago, IL 60612

Sue Levkoff, MSW, ScD
Associate Professor
Department of Social Medicine
Harvard Medical School
Boston, MA 02115

David A. Lindeman, PhD
Associate Professor, Departments of Internal
  Medicine and Neurosciences
Rush Institute for Healthy Aging
Rush University
Rush-Presbyterian-St. Luke's Medical Center
Chicago, IL 60612

Elizabeth R. Mackenzie, PhD
Institute on Aging
University of Pennsylvania Health System
Ralston-Penn Center
Philadelphia, PA 19104-6006

Shirley M. Moore, PhD, RN
Great Lakes GITT
Associate Professor of Nursing
Case Western Reserve University
Cleveland, OH 44106

Kate O'Malley, RN, MS, GNP
Director
On Lok Senior Health Services
San Francisco, CA 94109

Eric Pfeiffer, MD
Professor of Psychiatry and Director,
  Suncoast Gerontology Center
University of South Florida College of Medicine
Tampa, FL

John W. Rowe, MD
President
The Mount Sinai Medical Center
New York, NY 10029-6574

Patricia Rush, MD, MBA
Director, Section of Geriatric Medicine
Co-Director, Rush Institute for Healthy Aging
Rush University
Rush-Presbyterian-St. Luke's Medical Center
Chicago, IL

Roberta G. Sands, PhD, ACSW
Associate Professor of Social Work
University of Pennsylvania School of Social
  Work
Philadelphia, PA 19104

Madeline H. Schmitt, RN, PhD, FAAN
Professor and Coordinator, Doctoral Program
University of Rochester Medical Center
School of Nursing
Rochester, NY 14642

Ann Schneider, MSW
Division Manager, Patient Services
  and Marketing
Kelsey-Seybold Clinic
Houston, TX

Nancy L. Smith, RN, CS, PhD
School of Nursing
University of Colorado Health Sciences Center
Denver, CO 80262

Carol Van Steenberg, MSS
Planning and Program Development
    Consultant
On Lok, Inc.
San Francisco, CA 94109

Neville E. Strumpf, PhD, RN, C, FAAN
Associate Professor and Doris Schwartz Term
    Professor
Director, Gerontological Nurse Practitioner
    Program and
Center for Gerontologic Nursing Science
School of Nursing
University of Pennsylvania
Philadelphia, PA 19104-6096

Ruth Ann Tsukuda, RN, MPH
Director
Interdisciplinary Team Training Program
Portland VA Medical Center
Portland, OR 97207

Maria L. Vezina, EdD, RN
Director, Nursing Education
The Mount Sinai Hospital
New York, NY 10029

Eben A. Weitzman, PhD
Assistant Professor in Dispute Resolution
Graduate Programs in Dispute Resolution
University of Massachusetts, Boston
Boston, MA 02125

Patricia Flynn Weitzman, PhD
Research Associate
Division on Aging
Harvard Medical School
Boston, MA 02115

Nancy L. Wilson, LMSW
Assistant Professor of Medicine
Huffington Center on Aging
Baylor College of Medicine
Houston, TX

PART 1

Background

The John A. Hartford Foundation Geriatric Interdisciplinary Team Training Program

Kathryn Hyer

In June 1994, when The John A. Hartford Foundation of New York City began to assess grant-making opportunities in interdisciplinary clinical team training, many experts in geriatrics asked, "Why does the Hartford Foundation want to prepare health care trainees to be members of teams when health care institutions are firing clinicians, administrators are requiring that more patients be seen in less time, and clinicians find team meetings a waste of time?" This skepticism about the effectiveness and efficiency of teams was an important consideration in planning the Geriatric Interdisciplinary Team Training (GITT) Program.

From the outset, GITT was designed to create training models that would reflect the needs of the changing health care system. The Foundation trustees believed that the need for integrated health care teams and new modes of training was linked to (a) the unprecedented growth in the number and proportion of the elderly whose complex care required the skill of several disciplines; (b) the belief that frail older people benefited from care delivered by an interdisciplinary team; (c) the need for health professions' training to shift from inpatient to ambulatory and community-based care and to teach coordination of care over time and place; and (d) the growth in managed care capitated financing, which was expected to develop efficient ways to deliver care.

Between 1980 and 1995, the John A. Hartford Foundation made awards of over $58 million in their Aging and Health program to train more physicians to care for the elderly and to create integrated medical and social service models designed to improve care to vulnerable and frail older people. Nonetheless, by the mid-1990s, the Foundation trustees were poised to expand their funding to nonphysicians and to create a program that built on the findings from their service programs. It was clear that physicians, nurses, social workers, and others involved in health care each defined their role so independently of one another that they rendered care as if services for the same patient were completely unrelated. This multidisciplinary approach to care has been compared to "parallel play of children—noninteractive and nonintersecting activity" (Clark, 1993).

The trustees believed health care professionals needed to learn how to create interdisciplinary care plans—plans of care that integrated the various disciplines' work and were centered on the patients' needs. This form of teamwork, interdisciplinary care, has been defined as a "special form of interactional interdependence between health care providers who merge different but complementary skills in the service of patients and in the solution of their health problems" (Tsukuda, 1990). Recognizing the growth in sophisticated telecommunications and in-home medical monitoring, the trustees believed that teaching trainees to create interdisciplinary care plans would become a necessity if older people were to receive quality geriatric care. Hence, the trustees initially sought to create a program to enhance the team-building skills of gerontologically competent professionals through GITT. In reality, many of the projects funded used the money to enhance or reinforce gerontologic training for the health care professionals enrolled in the program.

STRUCTURE OF THE GITT PROGRAM

Advisors

When the trustees approved the establishment of funds to explore the feasibility of an interdisciplinary training program in June 1994, they also approved a group of advisors, Mathy Mezey, RN, EdD, FAAN, Independence Professor of Nursing Education at New York University; Risa Lavizzo-Mourey, MD, MBA, University of Pennsylvania School of Medicine; and W. June Simmons, MSW, CEO, Visiting Nurse Association of Los Angeles, to guide the development of any proposal. To create the background papers and develop a potential grant-making strategy, the trustees also approved funds to hire a program consultant (the author of this chapter) to work with the Foundation program staff and advisors.

Goals

The program's four goals were:

1. Improve the responsiveness of academic institutions to the educational and training needs of health care providers by establishing partnerships between academic training centers and health care providers. The trustees assumed funded team training programs would be efficient and effective because the program built its clinical component on real world providers of primary care to older people. It was assumed that teams operating in nonsubsidized settings would be efficient. However, because the clinical providers were not required to be training centers, academic-clinical partnerships were an explicit goal of the program. To be competitive, applicants had to include major managed care programs in the local geographic area. In fact, in the letter of invitation to apply for GITT, applicants "were among a select group possessing the capacity to create the partnerships that we seek." They were also told "this initiative is designed to facilitate the creation of partnerships between health care providers and graduate health professions educational programs to prepare for the service imperatives of the next century—geriatrics and interdisciplinary care."

2. Develop well-tested curriculum for geriatric interdisciplinary team training. Based on the work of team experts (Clark, 1994; Drinka & Bay, 1991; Tsukuda, 1990), the letter of invitation stated that experiential learning was required. Trainees, the letter stated, "would be expected to receive both didactic instruction in team building" as well as "observing and participating in team-delivered care." From the outset, GITT sought to create opportunities to train multiple health profession students together in a participative model. Students were expected to receive explicit instruction on their roles as team members and how those roles relate to other team members, the patient, and the family (Toner, Miller, & Burland, 1994). Students would be expected to learn to provide integrated care and to operate as members of a clinical team providing primary care to older people. Although it outlined the methodologic approach, the Foundation did not anticipate or describe any one model of training.

3. Create a cadre of well-trained professionals competent in geriatrics and interdisciplinary team skills. Academic programs invited to participate were identified as having "large numbers of advanced practice nurses, masters level social workers, and medical residents in primary care, all of whom are well-trained in gerontology." Thus, the program initially assumed that GITT would provide "value added"—an intensive interdisciplinary team training clinical experience—for geriatrically sophisticated trainees. As the program has evolved, it has become apparent that although the funded projects emphasize gerontological training, the level and numbers of gerontologically trained clinicians is so tiny that GITT has become a vehicle to enhance the gerontologic training as well as interdisciplinary team skills for most professionals.

4. Test staff development training models for practicing health professionals. Although GITT was designed to create models of team training primarily for health professions programs, it was always a goal to encourage GITT-type training models appropriate for staff development. Recognizing the importance of training professionals already in practice, the Foundation explicitly encouraged provider organizations competing for GITT funding to include this as part of their program.

COMPONENTS OF THE PROGRAM

The Foundation's GITT initiative was designed with two phases: a planning phase and an implementation phase. Thirty potential sites were invited to compete for 12 planning grants of $100,000 each. Ultimately, the quality of the planning applications encouraged the trustees to fund 13 planning proposals, which were approved in December 1995. Similarly, although the initial letter of invitation stated that "up to seven" of the 12 planning grants were expected to receive implementation grants of $750,000 over 3 years, the success of the planning projects resulted in the ultimate funding of nine planning year sites to become full implementation programs. Table 1.1 lists the names of the institutions receiving planning and implementation grants under the GITT initiatives and the principal investigators at each site.

In addition to the planning and implementation projects, the trustees created a Resource Center (RC) at New York University's Division of Nursing. Terry Fulmer, RN, PhD, FAAN and Mathy Mezey, both nationally recognized experts in gerontologic nurs-

TABLE 1.1 Geriatric Interdisciplinary Team Training (GITT) Grantees

	Planning Projects		
Organization	Principal investigators	City	State
Baylor College of Medicine	Robert Luchi, MD, Nancy Wilson, LMSW	Houston	TX
Harvard Medical School	Barbara Berkman, DSW, Sue Levkoff, ScD	Boston	MA
*Henry Ford Health System	Nancy Whitelaw, PhD	Detroit	MI
Kaiser Permanente, Southern California Medical Group	Richard Della Penna, MD	Los Angeles	CA
Mount Sinai Medical Center	Christine Cassel, MD	New York	NY
On Lok, Inc.	Jennie Chin Hansen, RN, MS	San Francisco	CA
Rush-Presbyterian-St. Luke's Medical Center	Denis Evans, MD	Chicago	IL
*University Hospitals Health System	M. Orry Jacobs	Cleveland	OH
University of Colorado Health Sciences Center	Dennis Jahnigen, MD	Denver	CO
University of Minnesota	Robert Kane, MD	Minneapolis	MN
University of North Carolina at Chapel Hill	Mark Williams, MD	Chapel Hill	NC
University of Pennsylvania	Neville Strumpf, RN, PhD	Philadelphia	PA
University of South Florida	Eric Pfeiffer, MD	Tampa	FL

* Sites merged and are now referred to as The Great Lakes GITT.
Bold type indicates implemented sites.

ing, received $1.5 million over 4 years to be the principal investigators of the RC. The RC's goals are to (a) provide technical assistance to sites and the Foundation, (b) serve as a clearinghouse for curriculum and practicum training information, (c) increase the communication and synergy among the participating sites, (d) ensure the development of core measures, and (e) create dissemination strategies to ensure that the lessons learned from the program are well publicized.

To track the evolution of the program, including the institutional changes that might have occurred as a result of the partnerships, the Foundation awarded $1.3 million in March 1997 to David Reuben, MD, and Janet Frank, DPH, from the University of California at Los Angeles Multicampus Division of Geriatric Medicine. The evaluation, to be conducted over 3 years, will include an analysis of the process and structures that are necessary to develop and sustain GITT. The evaluators will visit each funded project at least three times to track the changes over the 3 years of implementation. They will interview both the academic and the clinical partners involved in GITT.

PARTICIPATING DISCIPLINES

Although the Foundation recognized that many health professionals might benefit from interdisciplinary training, the program design demanded identification of a few key dis-

ciplines. Geriatric experts believe that the core team working with medically complicated elderly people consists of a physician, nurse, and social worker (Rubenstein, Siu,
& Weiland, 1989). This core group generally assesses the needs of elders and their families and, depending on these needs, may call in others for consultation or services.
Thus, advanced practice nurses, social workers, and medical residents from primary
care programs were the initial targets for GITT. Eventually, as Table 1.2 demonstrates,
the implementation sites recommended training in 17 different disciplines.

The level of trainee appropriate for GITT training was also an important consideration. Although in the mid-1990s geriatric training was becoming more common in
undergraduate curricula, the advisors argued that geriatric specialization began at the
master's-degree level. Furthermore, the experience of other training programs reinforced the importance of focusing on graduate-level students because trainees needed to
be competent and confident in their own discipline before being able to contribute to a
team's goals. Ultimately, GITT was designed to be part of a masters level student's
clinical experience. Although undergraduate students are permitted in the program, the
emphasis is on graduate-level trainees.

PLANNING-YEAR EXPERIENCES

Participation in GITT required more than writing an implementation grant. The cost
included a substantial investment in political capital by the principal investigators, finely
honed administrative and organizational skills, and the ability to raise some money for
implementation. The Hartford Foundation criteria for evaluating implementation proposals included (a) the quality of the partnership between and among the participating
clinical and academic entities, (b) evidence that the elements of a successful training
program were in place (space, administrative support, trainees, and so forth), (c) time-
tables for reinforcing university-wide and discipline-specific team training, (d) creation
of systems change at academic and practicum settings, and (e) incorporation of additional financial or in-kind support of a minimum 25% match of the total cost.

By all accounts the most important cost was the investment of political capital by the
principal investigators. Although creating new programs is always risky and difficult,
GITT is a particularly complex program, and the possibility of failure was high. From
the beginning, there was a 50% chance of success because only half of the planning
sites were expected to receive funding. Given the difficulty of creating change, even a
willingness to participate in the planning year remains an enduring testimony to the
commitment of the planning year principal investigators to geriatrics training and improving the clinical care for older people. Without such a commitment, the cost would have
been untenable.

The planning year was arduous and actually compressed into 6 months. Planning-year
grantees received funds in December 1995, but implementation proposals were due on
July 1, 1996, with site visits scheduled during the summer of 1996. At the site visit, the
principal investigators were expected to demonstrate the viability and practicality of
the project. Thus, by mid-1996, projects were expected to have (a) created a working
relationship with a major managed care clinical partner, (b) negotiated most of the details

TABLE 1.2 Percentage of Students by Discipline Projected to Complete GITT (1997–1999)

Project	Baylor	Great Lakes	Harvard	Kaiser	*Mt. Sinai	On Lok	Rush	Univ. Colorado	Univ. Minnesota	Univ. North Carolina	Univ. Pennsylvania	Univ. South Florida
Geographic Location	SW	MidW	NE	W	NE	W	MidW	W	MidW	S	NE	S
Proposed Disciplines												
Advance practice nursing	28	32	12	18	34	10	16	6	20	10	34	35
Medical residents	40	27	40	44	48	49	25	69	60	36	34	16
Social work	4	28	7	17	18	10	10	9	10	10	26	15
Audiology							5					
Dental								7				
Dietetic interns			14									
Ethics							1					
MBA/health administration							4			6	7	
Law								4				
Nutrition		4					5					
Occupational therapy			7			13	14					
Pastoral counselors							2					12
Pharmacy	14	6	4	16			7	5	11	33		8
Physical therapy			7			18	6			5		
Physician assistant	13	2										
Psychology	1											8
Public health interns				6								7
Speech language pathology			7				3					
Total number of trainees	854	157	347	463	262	347	364	202	178	239	307	153

* Does not include students trained in less intensive model.

on structuring the clinical and didactic components of the team-training, (c) identified the pool of trainees, (d) secured preceptors for new off-site practicum settings, and (e) created a credible management and decision-making structure.

The Foundation's philosophy is that the most successful projects leverage Foundation dollars with local money for work that would have been accomplished regardless of the Foundation's investment. In this way, the trustees believe they are merely enhancing or expediting the implementation of important programs. In an effort to gauge the commitment of the institution and ensure a higher probability of long-term sustainability, the Foundation required a minimum of 25% contribution from the institution. Although all projects had soft money contributions such as contributed time, space, and equipment, most also raised cash contributions, especially from local foundations. The Hartford Foundation's Senior Project Officer explicitly discussed the quality of the 25% match, and there was no doubt about the importance of raising funds to supplement the actual cash contribution of the Foundation.

With the funding of the implementation grants, GITT has proved to be a substantially different team-training program from earlier programs. The 1-year planning process, as will be evident by reading the experiences contained in this book, allowed sites to share experiences and to help each other with the many complexities that plague creating interdisciplinary programs. These sites were able to track and monitor the steps required to create GITT. Although sites were competitive, they were also cooperative. As one principal investigator said during the planning year, "Initially I thought to be successful with GITT, we'd have to have a creative or different approach to interdisciplinary team training, and that sharing such an idea would be preposterous. In the end, I realized that GITT was a logistics nightmare, and that actually obtaining agreements among all the competing forces might be all that we'd really need to get funded."

GITT builds on the success of previous programs, and it is poised to be responsive to the demands of a changing health care system. The characteristics that make GITT unique are its scope, its focus on primary geriatric care, its emphasis on systems change through partnerships, the quality and quantity of managed care placements, and the commitment of projects to collect cross-site common core measures.

SCOPE OF GITT

Over the 3 years of implementation funds, GITT is expected to train 2,633 student trainees and 173 practicing health professionals in geriatric interdisciplinary team training. On average, each GITT site will develop a training model and train 300 students in GITT. The principal investigators from the two large provider organizations, Henry Ford Health Systems and On Lok, Inc., explicitly designed GITT models for staff practitioners in addition to their student trainee models. As indicated in Table 1.2, 17 different disciplines are participating in GITT. Although about 75% of the trainees represent the required disciplines, the remaining 25% comprise an interesting array of health care clinicians such as therapists, dentists, and pharmacists and nonclinical trainees such as health care administrators and lawyers. The ability of GITT to develop nonclinical models of team training and to sensitize nonclinicians, particularly health care managers, about older people's need for interdisciplinary geriatric care may be among the most important legacies of GITT.

The scope also includes the diversity of the projects receiving funding. They include major academic training centers that are geographically distributed across the county. Also represented are some of the largest not-for-profit health care systems, such as Henry Ford Health System and Rush Health System of Chicago. On Lok, the original community-based capitated program for frail indigent older people and the model for the federally funded Program for All-Inclusive Care for the Elderly (PACE), is another funded project.

Experience in creating training programs across sites seems to be an important marker for success in GITT. Six of the eight funded implementation projects were Geriatric Education Centers (GECs) or were part of a GEC network. GECs have had a mission of training and educating practicing clinicians to understand the health care needs of older people. Most have created multidisciplinary programs and have created models of training for large geographic areas.

FOCUS ON PRIMARY GERIATRIC CARE

Although most of the research on the effectiveness of geriatric teams focuses on inpatient geriatric assessment teams, from the outset GITT concentrated on primary care teams. The planning year proposal asked projects "to demonstrate excellent comprehensive geriatric care for a broad range of community living elders."

Every project includes major primary care programs treating large numbers of older people in multiple settings, especially outpatient geriatric care. Primary care teams may concentrate efforts on frail elderly or seek to identify a group most likely to benefit from an interdisciplinary team. The variety of settings is also illustrative of the changing health care system. While inpatient units are included in some of the proposals, home care settings are a practicum setting for every funded GITT. Similarly, hospice or palliative care providers are included in seven of the eight projects. Adult day care, assisted living centers, and other long-term care settings are also included. Even some preventive outreach programs are also included as GITT clinical settings.

SYSTEMS CHANGE THROUGH PARTNERSHIPS

GITT is complex. It represents an array of partnerships and agreements across the country. Academically, it fosters agreements to train clinicians in 26 different academic programs within 18 distinct institutions. At some universities, preparing for GITT was the first time deans representing medicine, nursing, and social work had ever worked together. Certainly in cities where certain academic health centers do not have social workers, it may have been the first time that those institutional representatives had met to plan a curriculum that would be taught across institutions. Agreeing on schedules for training, payment, credit, and who can precept "our" trainees were major logistic issues confronted by every GITT.

On the clinical side, GITT represents 42 providers across the continuum of care. These providers are large not-for-profit or major national for-profit managed care corporations. These sites had to agree to moderate their clinical service goals to assume the important role of training clinicians. The balance between clinical time and teaching time is a tension that has implications far beyond GITT; GITT sites may be able to contribute to the debate because projects are quite self-conscious about the expectations of providers versus academic institutions.

An explicit goal of GITT is creating system change by fostering communication between academic training centers and the providers who employ graduates of those training centers. The partnerships created by GITT may be merely short-term agreements between parties for clinical placements over GITT's short life, or they may signify more fundamental change. The University of Colorado, for example, created a list of competencies for trainees by discipline in an effort to encourage clinical settings to allow trainees to treat patients. This set of competencies has become the standard for clinical centers to assess the impact of the GITT training and the value of GITT. All GITT planning and implementation sites reported that GITT forced a dialogue that was overdue.

MANAGED CARE PLACEMENTS

GITT supporters had always envisioned team training placements in managed care settings. As indicated earlier, the trustees expected that market forces would ensure efficient teams. Discussions with major insurers revealed that actuaries and program developers were uncertain of the needs of Medicare beneficiaries, and that training clinicians was expensive. Although some managed care organizations were leery of the cost involved in training, others were eager to create a relationship with the local university to enhance their image with local older people.

Every GITT project has at least one major managed care provider in the local market. Most have multiple partners, some of whom are competitors. The specifics of the managed care placements are described in chapter 11, but it is important to note that the GITT program expects to explore how various managed care entities use teams and how the teams vary to meet the needs of the elderly and the organization.

COMMITMENT TO CORE MEASURES

Chapter 10 provides the details on the core measures that will be collected for GITT. Although the eight training projects employ distinctly different approaches to didactic and practicum team training, each project collects a common set of data. Each trainee will be assessed at baseline and after the GITT experience to measure change that can be attributed to the training. We anticipate that change scores will be aggregated by discipline, recognizing that each discipline may have different amounts of exposure to the training program by virtue of scheduling restrictions.

We are creating new measures of geriatric team knowledge to assess the effectiveness of training. We ask trainees to state one overarching or dominant issue that the team must address. Focusing on the patient and where the team needs to target its work should increase the effectiveness of treatment as well as training.

This commitment to capturing the effect of GITT training is an important component of the overall GITT program that will help create new measures of team knowledge and should dramatically advance our understanding of teams, team functioning, and interdisciplinary training. Never before in geriatric team training have such an illustrious group of clinicians and scholars joined together to capture what constitutes geriatric team knowledge and effective team behavior.

GITT represents a new generation of team training. The Foundation expects it will produce models that will be replicable in many settings for many different providers. The ultimate test of GITT will be its longevity; we hope that the practice and education models it fosters will be used throughout the country to help prepare the next generation of clinicians.

REFERENCES

Clark, P. (1994) Learning on interdisciplinary gerontological teams: Instructional concepts and methods. *Educational Gerontology, 20,* 349–364.

Drinka, T., & Ray, R. O. (1991). Perceptions of upper-level trainees in an interdisciplinary geriatrics practicum: Implications for curriculum development. *Gerontology & Geriatrics Education, 12,* 47–59.

Rubenstein, L. Z., Siu, A. L., & Weiland, D. (1989). Comprehensive geriatric assessment: Toward understanding its efficacy. *Aging, 1,* 87–98.

Toner, J., Miller, P., & Burland, B. (1994). Conceptual, theoretical and practical approaches to the development of interdisciplinary teams: A transactional model. *Educational Gerontology, 20,* 53–69.

Tsukuda, R. A. (1990). Interdisciplinary collaboration: Teamwork in geriatrics. In C. K. Cassel, D. E. Riesenberg, L. B. Sorensen, & J. R. Walsh (Eds). *Geriatric medicine* (2nd ed.), pp. 668–675. New York: Springer-Verlag.

CHAPTER 2

Why Teams?

Eric Pfeiffer

WHY TEAMS IN GENERAL?

Anyone who has ever seen a team—a team of horses, a theatrical troupe, a scientific team, a family, a sports team—has to be impressed with the energy, synergy, choreography, motion, and emotion generated by teams. Teams are in themselves striking achievements. And they can produce striking achievements, achievements that no individual alone could produce. Moreover, they may be achievements produced with grace and elegance.

When Are Teams Needed?

We don't need teams for everything. Many human endeavors lend themselves perfectly to individual effort. Teams are needed when we seek to address complex problems, problems for which any single skill or art would be incapable of giving a full measure of response. Two can be a team; or 20. Mother and father engaged in upbringing of the young can be a team, whether the young be human beings or animals. Thus, teams are not even a uniquely human achievement. In fact, teams are older than recorded time, and there is nothing new about the concept or its various forms of implementation. So what is all the fuss about now?

It is beyond the scope of this chapter to discuss all the reasons why teams are particularly relevant to us late in the 1990s, other than that we are facing some extraordinarily complex challenges as we enter the next century. Perhaps it is based on the notion that all of us together are smarter than any one of us, a humbling, as well as a comforting, notion.

A Definition of Teams

Katzenbach and Smith (1994) offer the following definition of a team: "A team is a small number of people with complementary skills who are committed to a common purpose, performance goals, and approach for which they hold themselves mutually accountable" (p. 45).

Every word in this definition is important. For teams to function best, a small number of people, generally between 2 and 20, is thought to be optimal. Larger numbers make the process too cumbersome and tend to exclude participation by all members. The term "complementary skills" defines why there must be a team. A mere collection of like-minded or similarly skilled individuals does not result in a team. In health care in particular, diagnostic, evaluative, restorative, financial, ethical, and many other skills may be needed to implement a health care program for individuals or for whole populations. Complementary perspectives as well as complementary skills are critical to the concept of "team."

Also, most experts in the area of team performance emphasize the need for clearly defined purpose, goal, and approaches to the team tasks. This will not happen by itself. The need for clear-cut goals must be emphasized by team leaders and made clear to all team participants. Until everyone on the team is clear about purpose and approach, we do not have a team. This may require some training if team members are new to team participation. But the work of the team will not begin until members agree on these issues.

The phrase "holding themselves mutually accountable" emphasizes that responsibility for performance rests with every team member and cannot be delegated to a team leader or any single individual on the team. Throughout this volume there will be many discussions and illustrations that will test and probably affirm the definition of teams cited here.

The Nature of Teams

Even the simplest team, a team of two—husband and wife, boss and secretary, boxer and trainer—is based on the assumption that members of a team bring to the task for which the team exists differing skills, perspectives, experiences, and propensities. To take the team of boxer and trainer, one boxes, the other trains. As the task for which the team exists becomes more complex, more and more players may contribute more and more skills, perspectives, and experiences.

The Nurture of Teams

Chopra (1994), writing from an entirely different perspective, characterizes the cells in the human body as a huge, well-functioning team. "Every cell gives to and supports every other cell, and in turn is nourished by every other cell" (p. 106). On well-functioning teams, every member respects and cherishes every other member of the team, and is in turn respected and cherished by every other member of the team. Such nourishment can take many forms: being appreciated, recognized, valued, utilized, praised, and so forth. There are many ways team members can support each other: by affirming a common philosophy and common goals, and by sharing experiences within and outside the team with one another. Inasmuch as all team members are mutually accountable for the productivity of a team, it is in everyone's interest to keep every team member strong and contributing. Thus, when colleagues are encountering difficulties, team members can also be particularly helpful by showing concern, comforting them, and helping to seek out solutions to their problems.

Stages of Team Development

Teams must be formed, developed, grown, fine-tuned, and modified for a specific purpose. This opens the whole issue of the natural life of teams and how team members can be trained. Tuckman (1965) in a much-quoted work identified four stages of team development:

- Forming
- Storming
- Norming
- Performing

In the *forming* stage, the team members get acquainted. They test each other out; trust is still at a very low level. Members are tentative but open to experiencing the new process. They seek clarification of the team's purpose and the methods it will use.

During the next stage, described as the *storming* stage, team members explore their values and may encounter significant conflicts. They may compete with one another for attention or control, and they may assert their traditional roles, rather than assuming newly expected roles. In this process, members begin to recognize their differences more overtly, a process necessary for later collaborative efforts.

As teams continue to interact, some of the conflicts will subside, and the team now enters the *norming* stage. The team members have by now agreed on a common set of goals and a common set of values. They begin to undertake the work of the team.

It is shortly after this that the team enters the *performing* stage. Their enthusiasm catches fire. A real sense of we develops. Team members begin to strongly support one another, and they receive feedback that the team is really working. In this phase the team will achieve its greatest accomplishments.

Teams can achieve spectacular results beyond anything a loosely organized group of individuals can achieve. The literature on teams suggests that this occurs only when there is a well-functioning team coupled with a high level of commitment to a cause. Most teams will produce acceptable results, and outstanding achievements are probably serendipitous to some degree.

Drawbacks of Teams

It is easy to think of drawbacks to teams. They are personnel intensive. They require adjustments on the part of every team member. Conflicts may occur as people of diverse backgrounds and skills attempt to work toward a common goal. Lack of experience on teams, lack of leadership, and lack of clear goal definition are some of the common bugaboos that interfere with successful team functioning. Teams should not be begun by a group of people who lack at least some members experienced in teamwork.

Causes of Team Failure

Inexperience, lack of leadership, lack of training, lack of a clear set of goals, and lack of commitment are some of the most common causes of team failure. Individuals who suffer from a great deal of psychopathology can also destroy a team. In my opinion, it is important not to dwell on the many things that can derail teams, but rather to empha-size the few necessary characteristics of teams contained in our definition.

Teams as Tools for Quality Improvement

A relatively novel use of teams, advocated by Juran (1995) and other management experts, has been as a tool for continuous quality improvement. An alertness to team performance will of necessity result in desire to improve team performance. Once a team identifies areas in which it needs to improve, it can immediately go to work on implementing the needed changes, without resorting to outside or higher authority.

WHY INTERDISCIPLINARY TEAMS?

Multidisciplinary versus Interdisciplinary Teams

For several decades now it has been recognized that professionals from multiple disciplines can all help determine the type of treatment program provided for older persons. This has generally been referred to as a multidisciplinary approach. In the multidisciplinary approach, each discipline provides vital information toward decision making about the patient's care. But in general, only one person, such as a physician or nurse case manager, makes the treatment decisions. Although the multidisciplinary approach is clearly superior to input from only a single health professional or a single discipline, receiving input from a variety of disciplines is merely the first step. The second is combining that input into a common decision-making process. Hence, the birth of the interdisciplinary team.

The Interdisciplinary Team as Decision Maker

The transformation of a multidisciplinary team into an interdisciplinary one begins with an appreciation of the contributions of various disciplines toward health care decisions. A true interdisciplinary team is in fact the logical clinical decision maker, in which all of the team members, including the patient and family caregivers, have important, even critical, input into the care plan.

Furthermore, the interdisciplinary team as decision maker acts not just once, at the inception of the process, but in a continuing way, as treatments alter the status of the patient, or further illness or other changes in circumstances occur. Clearly, such an assertion that this process can work and is in fact better than standard approaches to patient care remains to be demonstrated. For the time being, the concept appears sound, but we have yet do determine when and where an interdisciplinary team approach to health care decisions is optimal.

WHY TEAMS IN GERIATRICS?

One of the major ways in which the practice of geriatric medicine differs from medical care of other age groups is that it deals with a more complex set of health care problems— multiple illnesses, multiple disabilities, multiple medications, multiple procedures, and multiple disciplines brought to bear on one problem.

Some Basic Principles of Working with Older Patients

Even in geriatrics, not every older person needs care by a team. A single internist for the patient's general medical care, an ophthalmologist for the patient with cataracts, an orthopedic surgeon for the fracture sustained while skiing may be sufficient. On the other hand, the health care needs of older persons are rarely so simple (Pfeiffer, 1985):

1. Older patients are responsive to treatment, but diagnostic, treatment, and rehabilitative techniques may require modification to meet the special circumstances of older persons.
2. Older patients require the input of multiple disciplines, including those related to physical health, mental health, social circumstances, economics, self-care capacity, and the environment.
3. Comprehensive assessment, along the lines mentioned in the second principle, must precede any intervention.
4. Older patients require care management, or case management, services. Based on the need for multiple types of intervention, a care coordinator must take responsibility for organizing the care plan of an individual. This can be a person, such as a social worker, or nurse, or a family member, or it can be an interdisciplinary team.
5. Family members are critically important in gathering information about the patient, determining the priorities for treatment, and carrying out the agreed-on treatment plan.
6. Care of the elderly requires special training in gerontology and geriatrics. Such training is most effective when carried out in an interdisciplinary setting.
7. Elderly patients are teachable. We can teach them to play active roles in the management of their own illnesses.
8. Older patients themselves can serve as effective teachers of those working on health care teams. From a certain perspective, they are uniquely qualified to determine what matters most to them.

Apart from the eight basic principles previously listed, there are a number of other principles that I feel serve as the underpinnings for employing teams in the care of geriatric patients. These include:

9. When you've met one older person, you've not met them all. This principle speaks to the enormous variation in the elderly, both experientially and physiologically; only a highly individualized approach to the older patient can be successful.
10. Working in the field of geriatrics is very rewarding. It may even be addictive. Feedback from patients and families is the reward that keeps people working in this field.
11. The long life experiences of older individuals qualify them to be considered living documents of history. Further, it is impossible to treat older individuals properly without understanding their life histories.

12. There is no elderly individual for whom we cannot do something. In particular, it is almost always possible to improve functioning in an older individual (Burton, Cairl, Keller, & Pfeiffer, 1983). At worst, we can at least provide empathic understanding for the person's life situation.

Types of Teams in Geriatrics

There are a number of purposes for which teams may be employed in geriatric health care. These can include the following:

Clinical or Case Management Teams

These are teams designed to make case management decisions concerning clinical problems in elderly patients. Typically they include at a minimum a physician, a nurse, and a social worker. Common additional team members include dietitians, pharmacists, rehabilitation therapists (including occupational, physical, and speech therapy), and pastoral counselors. The patient and an appropriate family member may also be included in the treatment decision-making team for reasons already discussed. The purpose of these teams is to gather and integrate all information relevant to the specific clinical situation and to reach a decision regarding how and by whom the treatment decisions are to be implemented. Multiple cases may be reviewed at a single team session. This team meets on a regular basis to assess and reassess patients under its responsibility.

Administrative Teams in Geriatrics

These are teams charged with making administrative decisions about services, finances, personnel, public relations, and other aspects related to management of a health care organization. Team members typically include administrators, clinicians, and financial experts. These teams discuss not individual patients, but the categories of patients to be served and the services to be provided. Again, a return to our basic definition of teams as a small number of individuals with complementary skills . . . is in order here.

Training Teams for Health Professionals

These are teams designed specifically to educate health professionals in geriatrics and in the team process. They share some elements with clinical teams, yet unlike clinical teams they contain academic faculty, clinical preceptors, and trainees from a variety of health care disciplines similar to those described under clinical teams. These teams allow trainees to observe and participate in the team process as it relates to geriatric patients. In busy clinical sites, a team may have both clinical and training goals.

Drawbacks of Teams in Geriatrics

It has been said that geriatric teams are too costly, requiring input from multiple disciplines for a single patient or a single care decision. No sophisticated studies of the cost-effectiveness of teams have yet been published. Most commonly, teams have been used for individuals for whom health care costs are already extremely high—individuals who are heavy users of health care services; those with excess disabilities; those who are noncompliant with treatment recommendations; and those with factors such as social isolation or economic deprivation, complicating an otherwise relatively simple health care problem. It is assumed that care would be even costlier, and less beneficial, without the insights of several appropriate disciplines. For instance, if depression complicating a physical illness is not discovered and treated, it may interfere with treatment and delay recovery (Yesavage, 1993). Clearly, the cost issue must be addressed in further studies.

A second assertion against teams in geriatrics is that they cannot be made to work in all situations, for a variety of reasons. These include interprofessional rivalries, unwillingness to change, unwillingness to empower patients to participate in decisions concerning their own health care, lack of team training, and many others. The scarcity of well-functioning models in geriatrics also makes it difficult to establish such teams.

Finally, it must be allowed that geriatric teams require a great deal of work, change of roles and behaviors, changes in prerogatives, new learning, and much more. As professionals in health care already feel overworked, this can be cited as another drawback to teams in geriatrics.

CONCLUSIONS

Creating and maintaining a good team require hard work. The effort is worthwhile; a good team has so much to offer its members and the patients and clients that it serves. This is the philosophy that underlies the Geriatric Interdisciplinary Team Training Program. The following chapters describe the challenges of the GITT Program—training professionals to be part of a good geriatric team.

REFERENCES

Burton, B., Cairl, R., Keller, D., & Pfeiffer, E. (1983). *Functional assessment inventory: A training manual.* Tampa, FL: Suncoast Gerontology Center.

Chopra, D. (1994). *The seven spiritual laws of success.* San Rafael, CA: Amber-Allen Publishing and New World Library.

Juran, J. M. (1995). *Managerial breakthrough: The classic book on management performance* (rev. ed.). New York: McGraw-Hill.

Katzenbach, J. R., & Smith, D. K. (1994). *The wisdom of teams.* New York: Harper Business.

Pfeiffer, E. (1985). Some basic principles of working with older patients. *Journal of the American Geriatrics Society, 33,* 44–47.

Tuckman, B. W. (1965). Developmental sequences in small groups. *Psychological Bulletin, 63,* 384–399.

Yesavage, J. (1993). Differential diagnosis between depression and dementia. *American Journal of Medicine, 94,* 23–28.

CHAPTER 3

A Perspective on Health Care Teams and Team Training

Ruth Ann Tsukuda

Health care teams, which have waxed and waned in popularity, recently have generated renewed interest that parallels the increased attention to teams in business. In the last 30 years, over 3,500 citations related to health care teams have appeared in the literature (Tsukuda, 1996). Although references to health care teams abound, it is difficult to trace the origins of health care teams, and only four articles contain thorough descriptions of their history (Baldwin, 1996; Brown, 1982; Ryan, 1996; Schmitt, 1994). The purpose of this chapter is not to duplicate the works of other team historians. Instead, what follows is an effort to highlight the most influential literature on health care teams and on efforts to educate students in the concepts and practice of health care teams.

DEFINITIONS

In reviewing the literature on health care teams, one of the striking findings is the complexity of language describing them. Over the years, many authors have attempted to differentiate among various types of teams, and the lexicon of team types seems almost overwhelming: unidisciplinary, intradisciplinary, multidisciplinary, interdisciplinary, interprofessional, and transdisciplinary. For purpose of this historical review, I make no distinction among these team types. Instead, the definition of team work proffered by Brill nicely describes the key components of an effective team. She states:

> Team work is that work which is done by a group of people who possess individual expertise, who are responsible for making individual decisions, who hold a common purpose, and who meet together to communicate, share and consolidate knowledge, from which plans are made, future decisions are influenced and action determined. (Brill, 1976, p. xvi)

This definition captures the essence of team work involving more than one discipline without using confusing language. How many disciplines should be involved depends on the kinds of skills and expertise that are necessary to address the needs of the clients being served. Because the literature makes clear distinctions between dyadic and multidisciplinary teams, I have limited my discussion to those health care groups composed of representatives from more than two disciplines, recognizing that excellent examples of creative team work may be excluded.

A comprehensive review of the literature reveals that it is difficult to separate the experience of teams whose purpose is to deliver health care services from those focusing on education. Largely, the health care team experience is an amalgam of teams that do both. Education may take the form of new learning for health professionals as they begin to practice in this new structure, or the team may serve as a primary site for the clinical education of students.

HEALTH CARE TEAMS IN THE 20TH CENTURY

The Early Years

One of the earliest references to team work during the 20th century is credited to Richard Cabot (Brown, 1982). In 1915, Cabot wrote about "team work of the doctor, educator, and social worker" (Cabot, 1915). A few years later in an address presented to the Yorkville Medical Society in New York City, Barker (1922) suggested that general practitioners must work in cooperation with medical specialists, surgeons, other consultants, and laboratory workers as they focus on diagnostic plans for individual patients. From Barker's perspective, team work in the clinic involved consideration of the efforts of medical specialists and general practitioners to provide a general diagnostic approach that would "diagnose the patient as a whole, with full consideration of all the somatic, psychic and social elements concerned" (Barker, 1922, p. 776). Through this approach, the team was able to provide integrated diagnostic plans, with the general practitioner serving as the primary care provider. Thus, an early application of the team approach was to improve relationships between the general practitioner and the specialist.

Rogers (1932) articulated a slightly different early picture of the team in a presentation to a convention of national nursing organizations. She advocated interdependence of professional groups within the hospital that included nursing, administrative staff, medicine, dietetics, research, x-ray, and laboratory, with a focus on the welfare of the patient. She delineated numerous occasions where cooperation between the medical and nursing staff was necessary throughout the hospital experience, and described the roles and relationships of health professionals as a "game." Clearly, this is the first reference to make use of a sports analogy as a metaphor for team work!

Post–World War II

The focus on the patient continued as Martin Cherkasky (1949) developed the Montefiore Hospital Home Health Care Program. Cherkasky's beliefs about patients defined his approach to their care. He said, "When we think about a patient, we should think about him not only as an organic and spiritual whole but also as a whole in society" (p.163). He saw the patient as a part of a family and acknowledged social factors as a contributor in disease. Cherkasky advocated for new approaches to care, including social services, home evaluations, and family interventions. Stating that it was no longer enough to provide medical care in a clinical setting, he suggested that comprehensive health care should be taken to the patient's home. Such a revolutionary approach demanded an expanded repertoire of services, including the patient's physician, subspecialists such as orthopedists, ophthalmologists, and surgeons, as well as social services, occupational therapists and physical therapists, nursing homes, transportation, medication, and equipment. Cherkasky is usually credited as the originator of the concept of health care teams; his efforts, however, address the services provided by the team rather than the team itself.

To receive services by the home health care team, patients had to be medically and socially eligible. Eligibility was determined by a series of patient, family, and home assessments. The intent of the program was to take services normally provided in the hospital to the home. Therefore, medical services were available around the clock 7 days per week, with specialized services, including medical procedures, conducted in the home. To support the needs of medically and socially complex patients, a variety of additional services were necessary. The Visiting Nurse Association provided nursing services, including case finding, evaluations of the home, nursing care, and patient education. But in what was clearly a very progressive program, other support was also available. Social services provided a link between the hospital and the home by providing continuing care throughout the course of the illness. Medications and rehabilitation services were provided in the home. Housekeeping services were available and transportation to the hospital by ambulance was available when it was impractical to deliver a service in the home. Cherkasky (1949) described the benefits of the home health care program as providing individualized care in the comfort of the patient's home and less expensively than in the hospital.

Without a doubt, Cherkasky's innovative foray into home care was ahead of the times. Although we have complete descriptions of the scope of services provided by health professions and support personnel, we know little about the relationships that existed or the process of team care. Yet, Cherkasky's work is usually cited as the first major team effort.

George Silver continued these pioneering efforts at Montefiore in the 1950s. Silver (1958), acknowledging the passing of the general practitioner, attempted to develop a new format for the provision of medical services. He proposed a new type of family medical practice. His effort, the Family Health Maintenance and Demonstration Program, was designed to "determine what services can reasonably be added to a comprehensive medical program which would result in favorably influencing the health of the families concerned" (p.33). In this effort, 150 average families who were members of both the Health Insurance Plan of Greater New York and the Montefiore Medical Group were selected at random. In perhaps the first documented reference to a health care team, Silver states, "Preventive and medical services are provided by a 'health team' composed of a physician trained in internal medicine, a psychiatric social worker, and a public health nurse" (p.33). A pediatrician provided care for children.

In this article, Silver provides one of the first descriptions of team process. The health care team operates "by dividing responsibility, delineating individual roles, and accepting each other's professional competence" (p.33). Each discipline on the team had defined roles and responsibilities; in some areas, such as disease prevention, it was recognized that responsibilities would overlap.

The Montefiore Demonstration Program was unique because it described the routine functioning of a team. Individual team members saw families either at home or in the medical office. Team members also had access to the family record. Later the team met to discuss findings and develop a family plan. The team discussed the plan with the families, and individual team members had the responsibility to follow through with the plan. Others joined the team as their expertise was needed. Routine team conferences ensured that the team members exchanged relevant information and shared new developments.

Team activities expanded beyond the actual practice of the team as team members participated in joint educational efforts. The Demonstration Program team valued interaction as essential. Silver stated, "Every contact is an opportunity to tap the knowledge and skills of all members of the team because the intercommunication of the team members leads to exchange of skills and interests" (p. 34).

Silver describes several opportunities for a team approach. He saw the team as a way to address the changing demands of medical education. Forces such as declining hospital populations, increasing outpatient workload, and increased medical coverage were affecting education. He suggested that learning within a health care team might provide an "easier and more rewarding" way to learn how to provide medical care and practice preventive medicine.

One of the most interesting aspects of the Demonstration Program was that it was part of a group practice with prepayment. Although actual cost information related to the project is not available, Silver stated that the experiment increased the cost of health care very little. He predicted that a 10 or 15% increase in the cost of health insurance would be necessary to provide all the services described. He concluded that the health team replaces the advantages of the services that in earlier times were provided by a general practitioner and were still deemed essential for comprehensive care.

During the World War II period, literature on psychiatric teams began to appear. Ryan (1996) describes the actions of the International Congress on Mental Health as being a key factor in the emergence of interdisciplinary approaches. It called for mental health practice to expand beyond medicine, described the need for principles about cooperative practice, advocated increased training, and suggested that leadership should not lie within one discipline. Membership on these early psychiatric teams typically consisted of a psychiatrist, a psychiatric social worker, and a psychologist.

One of the earliest efforts in psychiatry is attributed to orthopsychiatry and child guidance; there was considerable disagreement, however, about how extensive team care should be. It seemed appropriate to involve a variety of team members in the assessment and intake process, but their involvement in therapeutic activities remained controversial. Despite conflicts and difficulties in implementation, the movement supporting team work in traditional institutional mental health settings continued to grow (Caudill & Roberts, 1951; Williams, 1959).

According to Ryan, interest in team work in mental health peaked in the 1960s. The movement of psychiatric care from the hospital to the community threatened traditional roles and relationships among team members, and the process of care in the new model offered new challenges. Most noticeably, the friction between treatment and social activism and conflicting values about roles, power, and leadership resulted in decreased interest in team care (Ryan, 1996).

The field of rehabilitation has offered a more positive experience with team work. Rehabilitation teams typically have managed patients with disabilities (Caldwell, 1959; Patterson, 1959) and offered a process to address the total person with multiple needs (Wagner, 1977). Traditionally, rehabilitation professionals have accepted teamwork, recognizing that no single person or discipline possesses the knowledge and skills to meet the needs of persons with multiple problems. However, despite this recognition, Wagner suggested that teams in rehabilitation are most successful when directed toward care planning and case review. It should be noted that similar language will resurface later as the literature on geriatric health care teams appears.

These early efforts in teamwork laid the groundwork for a surge of activity during the decades of the 1960s and 1970s. An explosion of literature documents the burgeoning interest in teamwork, both for health care services and education.

The Period of Social Change (1960s and 1970s)

Perhaps reflecting the turbulence of the 1960s and early 1970s, the literature on teams in health care also seemed different from what had appeared previously. Whereas prior to this, finding literature on teams required careful searching, it now appeared everywhere. Building on earlier themes, the literature focused on themes involving comprehensive care and community-based models for providing such care. In a dramatic shift, team interest seemed to leave the hospital behind and sought new roots in community experiments. The literature also emphasized health professions education, in addition to the continued focus on practice. Authors such as Baldwin (1996), Brown (1982), and Hermary (1991) relate much of this interest to the involvement of the federal government in increasing funding for health and social programs during the Johnson administration. In particular, the Office of Economic Opportunity (OEO) funded many innovative programs that provided primary community-based health care using a health care team. The most well known of these community health centers included Columbia Point in Boston, Mound Bayou in rural Mississippi, Watts in Los Angeles, Mile Square in Chicago, Gouverneur in New York City, and Denver (Beloff & Korper, 1972; Beloff & Willet, 1968; Cowen & Sbarbaro, 1972; Kindig, 1975; Lashoff, 1968; Light & Brown, 1967).

One project, the Dr. Martin Luther King, Jr. (MLK) Health Center in the Bronx, warrants special attention. Created in 1966 under the direction of Dr. Harold Wise and supported by Montefiore, the Center received funding from OEO. The Center was a complex organization with multiple programs, including health careers training, community development around health and environmental issues, research and evaluation concerning special medicine, and the delivery of health care using a team structure. Health services were provided by eight care teams, whose membership included an internist, pediatrician, several nurse practitioners, and several family health workers (Wise, 1972). Each team provided comprehensive primary health care services to approximately 3,500 patients (Kindig, 1975).

Perhaps the most well known of all early community team development efforts, MLK's experience is documented in *Making Health Teams Work,* a classic resource for understanding team development (Wise, Beckhard, Rubin, & Kyte, 1974). *Making Health Teams Work* outlines an intervention to improve team effectiveness by consultants from the Massachusetts Institute of Technology in collaboration with the teams at MLK and addresses team issues such as goal-setting, roles, decision-making, problem-solving, leadership, and conflict (Beckhard, 1972; Rubin & Beckhard, 1972). This effort evolved into self-directed learning modules that teams could use to guide their own team development activities. While no longer in print, these modules served for many years as a primary source for assisting newly created teams as they developed a structured process for the delivery of team care and began to address the inevitable challenges of practice in new relationships with other providers.

Another example of an extensive team effort was the Family Health Care Project at the Yale–New Haven Medical Center. It was an experiment to develop a system of care that addressed the gap between patient needs and fragmented resources (Beloff & Willet, 1968). The goals were to evaluate the ability to provide comprehensive family health care service to a medically indigent, inner-city, urban population while assessing the usefulness of the team model for teaching medical students. The designated health care team consisted of a physician, public health nurse, and health aides, in addition to consultants (such as social workers, psychiatrists, and dietitians).

This experiment demonstrated that even with structures such as formalized procedures for intake and assessment, a shared family record, an implementation plan, and regular team conferences, putting health professionals together in a group does not ensure a team. In fact, the team required approximately 1 year's experience before it could work together effectively. Even then, consultant team members had difficulty accepting this new model of care. They continued to expect a more traditional approach; confused about team goals, they slowed the team's progress. As the team developed, members spent significant time in role definition (something they valued highly), but the actual team in practice was the real teacher about teams.

Experience in this Family Health Care Project stressed the need for careful team planning, including the definition of team roles, the establishment of goals, the importance of team orientation, and the value of effective communication. The need for compatible and competent team members was paramount (Beloff & Willet, 1968, p. 79).

The Denver Department of Health and Hospitals (Cowen & Sbarbaro, 1972) created another innovation in the delivery of health care service in 1966 when it decentralized its citywide health program to provide family-centered team care to 100,000 medically indigent patients (p.164). This large-scale reorganization effort involved 28 different clinics providing a wide variety of services. Known as the Denver Neighborhood Health Initiative, this program was designed to demonstrate that (a) combining public health, mental health, and physical health services and providing coordination could address the needs of an urban indigent population; (b) a unified program could efficiently use the skills of scarce health professionals; and (c) the program would be an acceptable change from the traditional city hospital approach, which often alienated impoverished patients (Cowen & Sbarbaro, 1972, p. 157).

In the Denver experience, most of the unresolved patient problems were social or economic or related to multiple chronic diseases, rather than acute illness, necessitating a family approach to care with an emphasis on health and social factors; familiarity with community resources was essential. Team care, as initially conceived, was not equipped to meet the needs of this population. Thus, in a new approach, the social worker, in conjunction with a community health aide, became the backbone of the team. The neighborhood aide became the central point for communication with the family, and in what might be one of the earliest descriptions of the role of case management (although it was not labeled as such), the social worker would call on the resources of a "flexible" team defined by the specific problems or needs of the family.

Despite the growing interest in health care teams and considerable attention to the successful efforts of specific programs, these initiatives were not problem-free. The literature addresses some of these problems (Beloff & Korper, 1992; Wise, 1972), but Banta and Fox (1972) focused their attention on the problems experienced by one effort, Columbia Point Health Center, the country's first OEO-sponsored neighborhood health center, located in Boston.

Banta and Fox identified the role dilemmas and strains experienced by each of the professional groups—medicine, nursing, and social work—working at Columbia Point. They found that "high motivations to work as a member of an interdisciplinary health team in a poverty setting is a necessary, but not a sufficient condition for such a collaborative effort" (p. 697). Based on interviews of the staff working at Columbia Point, they identified many problems. These included the following:

- Lack of consensus regarding the project's goals
- Physical environment of the center, which was described as depressing
- Unmet expectations for the center that members of the community held
- Conflict over the role of community health workers
- Poor staff morale
- The actual demands of the center's work
- Inadequate definition of roles
- Lack of team orientation
- Strain between the registered nurses and social workers
- Lack of physician commitment.

What could have been done to improve the situation? Suggestions included preliminary work on role definition and role boundaries (Banta & Fox, 1972, p. 721), recognizing the need for team meetings, and attention to team development. Team consultants joined the team later to address these strategies.

THE PERIOD OF SPECIFIC DISEASES
AND DEFINED POPULATIONS

Beginning in the late 1970s, team initiatives began to change the clinical emphasis from primary care and community-based, comprehensive, family-centered care to one more focused on the needs of specific populations. The health care team continued as a strong foundation for the delivery of rehabilitative services (Diller, 1990; Keith, 1991; Wagner, 1977) and remains so now. In addition, articles addressing such diverse topics as family planning (Fairweather & Law, 1978), dialysis (Lowe & Herranan, 1978), child abuse (Gallmeier & Bonner, 1992), hospice (Eng, 1993), surgical care (McHugh et al., 1996), and oncology (Itano, Williams, Deaton, & Oishi, 1991) began appearing in the health care team literature. Today, the literature on health care teams seems even more diverse. It addresses not only the needs of specified population groups, but also has expanded across the continuum of health care services including acute, critical, ambulatory, long term, and community care. Although health care literature abounds with information about teams, in recent years, the geriatric population has received the most attention. This increased attention to adults over 65 perhaps reflects their growing numbers, increased visibility, and political activism. Although interest in this population was growing in many sectors—health, social services, housing, and economics to name a few—perhaps no other organizational effort was more extensive than that developed by the Department of Veterans Affairs (VA).

In response to the changing demographics of the population served by its multifaceted health care delivery system, the VA mounted a multidimensional effort involving the creation of specific research, education, and clinical programs that targeted the needs of this rapidly growing segment of the veteran population. Specialized programs such as the Geriatric Research Education and Clinical Centers (GRECCs) were one of the earliest efforts. Following the GRECC Program were: (a) the Geriatric Fellowship, a program to provide advanced training for physicians, (b) the development of geriatric assessment services, (c) expansion of nursing home and other long term care services, and (d) the creation of the Interdisciplinary Team Training Program in Geriatrics (ITTG).

A unique aspect of the VA's efforts was a commitment to a team approach for the delivery of health care services irrespective of the focus of care. Consequently, all of its clinical programs had a health care team to provide care. Although the composition of the teams varied based on the needs of the patients and the setting for service delivery, a common basic structure for clinical services was a team comprised at a minimum of physician, nurse, and social worker. More often than not, other professionals supplemented the basic teams to address the complex needs of patients. These disciplines included pharmacy, psychology, dietetics, occupational therapy, and physical therapy. In many settings, attention to the needs of this specific population offered an opportunity for innovative treatment approaches to adult day health care services, psychiatric services, case management, and comprehensive geriatric assessment. In each case, a team of health professionals learned to work in conjunction with other disciplines, providing a vast array of physical, social, emotional, and environmental approaches to care and serving as a clinical base for education about health care teams.

INTERDISCIPLINARY EDUCATION

The literature on interdisciplinary education and team work is abundant and confusing. It is very difficult to separate the experience of programs designed to promote interdisciplinary education and team work from those programs designed to deliver actual clinical services using a team of providers. In reality they are often the same endeavors. Innovative clinical sites have become desirable places for students in a variety of health professions to learn about teams. At the same time, creative educational programs have developed new clinical services or helped to change the means by which care was provided in previously existing health care organizations. Furthermore, it is difficult to distinguish the specific contributions of key players because private and publicly supported efforts are frequently interconnected and provide a collaborative approach to the development of innovative programs. Furthermore, the literature does not follow a neat chronologic path; perhaps most frustrating are the many actors who have not infrequently changed the names of their programs. It is, however, accurate to say that students, faculty, universities, free-standing community health centers, federal and state programs, and private foundations have supported team education.

In one of the earliest articles on interdisciplinary professional education, Dana and Sheps (1968) described the challenges of developing these opportunities for students in the health professions. They suggested that many forces were promoting interdependence in health care, including the expanding knowledge base in science, changing clinical practice, public policy, and the availability of funding. The authors suggested that in response to changing demands in health services, members of the health professions, ". . . must learn to work together, and must link up effectively through the optimum use of their skills in the maintenance of the public trust and in the interest of the public good" (p. 37). They stressed that the intent of interdisciplinary training was not to make the disciplines think alike, but instead to allow them to act together. Thus, an opportunity for new forms of educational programs existed 30 years ago.

However, providing students with the knowledge and skills to work together is no simple task. For many educational pioneers, working together—participating as a member of a health care team—was the most appropriate entry into this unmarked territory. Thus, early team education was clinically based.

Once again, the OEO was a major player, this time in the creation of team-oriented learning experiences for students. In cooperation with the Children's Bureau and other federal agencies, community-based programs developed learning opportunities for students. The Student Health Organization, in projects in Chicago and Southern California, provided clinical experiences for trainees from various professional backgrounds to work together as a team in existing community health centers. Duncan and Kempe (1968) reported that students from social work, dentistry, nursing, and medicine were able to increase their understanding and appreciation of the different professions by working together in a common experience.

The role of the federal government as a sponsor of interdisciplinary and team education efforts over the last 30 years has been significant (Baldwin, 1996). In addition to those programs funded through the vast social initiative, The War on Poverty, many other endeavors are worthy of mention. The Comprehensive Health Manpower Training Act of 1971 authorized the Health Manpower Education Initiative Awards (HMEIA), which awarded funding on a competitive basis to programs providing interdisciplinary education in primary care (Baldwin, 1996). Initial funding was awarded to the University of Hawaii (Takamura, Bermosk, & Stringfellow, 1978) and to the American Medical Student Association (AMSA), which contracted with universities to develop interdisciplinary team training programs (Baldwin, 1996). AMSA and its predecessor, the Student American Medical Association, are especially noteworthy because their activities evolved from medical student dissatisfaction with the lack of community experience and contact with other students in the health sciences. Their efforts included the development of team-based summer experiences for students from multiple disciplines (Carlton, 1977) and supported the creation of many interdisciplinary educational experiences (Kindig, 1975). AMSA subcontracted with universities to increase the availability of interdisciplinary education opportunities.

From 1975 to 1978, HMEIA provided funding to seven medical schools and universities to develop interdisciplinary team training programs. These included the University of Nevada, Michigan State University, the University of North Carolina, the University of Washington, the University of Utah, and the University of California at San Francisco (Baldwin, 1996). These efforts used a variety of approaches to address the desire for interdisciplinary education. Some devoted energy toward the development of clinical experiences and some developed academically based programs, whereas others used a combined approach. The breadth of effort included single and multiple courses, comprehensive interdisciplinary programs, and the development of clinical practices. Unfortunately, many of these activities were dependent on external funding, and as federal priorities changed in 1980 and funding ceased, so did many of these innovative early efforts in interdisciplinary education.

Beginning in the early 1970s, the literature on teamwork took a new direction, reflecting the increased interest and activity in the education of students in the health professions. The disciplines of medicine, nursing, and social work all contributed to this growing body of knowledge. For example, the University of Wisconsin Family Health Service offered students an opportunity to participate in a comprehensive community-based team that included nurses, social workers, physicians, and family health counselors to deliver a comprehensive array of health services to children (Aradine & Hansen, 1970). This program was based on the assumption that students needed practical experience in real life situations, where the demands for service and education were both seen as necessary goals.

Addressing the learning needs of the same three disciplines, the University of Miami (Florida) developed a clinical experience for students early in their professional education (Tanner & Soulary, 1972). These students—first-year medical, sophomore nursing, and first-year social work students—participated in a clinical experience to reduce barriers to effective teamwork. The three disciplines became a team and delivered clinical services to families under the supervision of preceptors. Like their predecessors in interdisciplinary education, students reported that they gained an appreciation of other disciplines through working together; not surprisingly, problems arose because of the differing levels of knowledge and clinical experience of the three disciplines.

Although these programs ceased when external funding ended, they made a rich contribution to the accumulation of knowledge about interdisciplinary education. Dozens of articles appeared in the literature addressing both clinical practice and interdisciplinary education.

The interprofessional and intercollegiate program, Community Health Organization Program for Students (CHOPS) in Louisville, Kentucky was created in 1972 through sponsorship by SAMA (Discher, 1974). Its approach stressed participation by students in community-based primary care teams in a variety of urban and rural communities. In 1974, the University of Alabama was selected by the Institute for Health Team Development as one of several institutions to participate in a 2-year program for training faculty health care teams. Other participating universities included: University of California, San Francisco; Michigan State University, East Lansing; University of North Carolina, Chapel Hill; and the University of Washington, Seattle (Bottom et al., 1976). These initiatives were charged with creating model teams and educational resources through the development of curriculum to support the educational mission.

The Institute for Health Team Development deserves a word of explanation. The Institute, located at the Montefiore Hospital and Medical Center, was funded by the Robert Wood Johnson Foundation in the mid-1970s to promote training for students in the health sciences to deliver primary care within the context of a health care team. The Institute's mission was evaluation of team efforts, development of curriculum, and development of clinical team training sites (Wise, 1972).

In two separate articles, Harris (Harris, 1978; Harris, Saunders, & Zasorin-Connors, 1978) outlines the experience of Virginia Commonwealth University in the development of interdisciplinary community-based educational activities. These contributions describe the benefits of interdisciplinary clinical education while acknowledging the many challenges in establishing such complex programs.

Federal support for the development of model programs was also available through the Division of Allied Health Professions during the 1970s. In one such effort, Mazur, Beeston, and Yerxa (1979) describe the experience of Rancho Los Amigos Hospital's experimental interdisciplinary clinical education program. It provided comprehensive health care services for profoundly disabled people, allowing them to leave the institution and return to community living. Participating students represented the disciplines of medicine, nursing, occupational therapy, physical therapy, and social work and were engaged actively in the delivery of rehabilitation services.

Federal funding for interdisciplinary education has been sporadic but sustained. Programs such as the Area Health Education Centers (AHECs) have promoted interdisciplinary efforts through continuing education. In many instances, AHECs have become the home for activities supported by the Interdisciplinary Training for Health Care in Rural Areas grants, one of several initiatives of the Bureau of Health Professions of the Health Resources and Services Administration (HRSA). These grants have enabled students not only to learn about team practice, but also to gain experience in the delivery of health care services in rural communities throughout the United States. The Bureau, through its support of Geriatric Education Centers, has also advanced the understanding and appreciation of interdisciplinary education. Within the last 2 years, HRSA has published two documents *(A National Agenda for Geriatric Education: White Papers and Forum Report)* that outline the state of geriatric education in our changing health care environment and provide policy recommendations to prepare the workforce to meet the needs of an aging population. Interdisciplinary education was targeted as one of the important areas making a contribution in this effort (HRSA, 1995, 1996).

In recent efforts, the Bureau has promoted the concepts of interdisciplinary education and teamwork through collaborative projects to foster improvements in the quality of health care education. Building on a strong commitment to team work across disciplines, these new efforts are also addressing the challenge of promoting collaboration among agencies that share a common purpose or serve a common population.

No federal agency has maintained as great a sustained commitment to interdisciplinary education as the VA. In 1979, the Office of Academic Affairs launched its first interdisciplinary education effort with the initiation of the ITTG. ITTG was conceived as a clinically based educational program for VA employees and affiliated students from three or more health professions. Using didactic, experiential, and clinical instructions, it fosters interactive problem-solving and teamwork and promotes an understanding of the roles and contributions of many varied disciplines in the delivery of health care services. The goals of the program are as follows:

- Develop a cadre of health professionals with the knowledge and competencies required to provide interdisciplinary team care to meet the wide spectrum of health care and service needs of aging veterans
- Provide leadership in interdisciplinary education and training and the team approach to care throughout the health care system and other VA medical centers
- Provide role models and team care, patient care, and discipline-specific skills for students in medical and associated health professions.

Sites for the ITTG were chosen by a competitive process. Initially, two programs were funded, and after 4 years the program reached its target of 12 established sites. Financial support provided to each program included salary for a program coordinator, stipends for trainees, and approximately $10,000 per year to support educational efforts. Disciplines eligible to receive financial support for trainees included nursing, social work, psychology, speech pathology, audiology, optometry, occupational therapy, pharmacy, and podiatry.

The ITTG curriculum focuses on geriatrics and team work. It addresses discipline-specific learning needs as well as content common to the multiple professions involved in providing geriatric care. Students in ITTG have chosen the VA as the site for required clinical rotations and participate in the program from 3 to 12 months for as much as 40 hours per week. At the completion of their educational program, many of these students have chosen to practice in geriatric settings where team skills are an essential component. In its 18 years, ITTG has provided team-based clinical training to thousands of health professional students.

In addition to this significant contribution to basic clinical training in geriatrics, ITTG has provided team training to practicing health professionals throughout the VA system and in the larger health care community. The contributions to the promotion of team delivery models extends far beyond the field of geriatrics and has influenced all aspects of the VA's vast system of care. Within the last few years, the ITTG changed its name to the Interdisciplinary Team Training Program (ITTP), reflecting a broadening of its mission from geriatrics to other important health care services, such as primary care. As the ITTG/ITTP has developed over the years, one of its major contributions has been for staff to serve as consultants to enhance and expand team care throughout the VA. It is probably not an exaggeration to suggest that all of the 172 institutions comprising the VA health system have had some degree of exposure to team care through the work of this program. Through its multiple levels of educational programs, its provision of direct patient care services, and its contribution to the team care and interdisciplinary education knowledge base, the influence of this program should not be underestimated.

Finally, I will comment on another significant development in teamwork beginning in the 1980s and continuing to the present. That development is the phenomenal growth in literature related to geriatric teams and interdisciplinary geriatric education programs. Some of this growth can be attributed to the work of the ITTP and consultants working with this program, but many other individuals and programs have made significant contributions to this knowledge base. A cursory review of recent geriatric publications yields articles on topics such as consultation teams, team approaches to geriatric case management, assessment teams, educational teams, community-based teams, acute care teams, rural geriatric teams, and even maladaptive teams. And this just scratches the surface!

As the 1990s draw to a close, it is exciting to see the growing interest centered around team care. Clinical programs whose roots reach back to the 1970s are thriving, providing team care in community-based health centers. Education initiatives continue to develop new opportunities and programs. Teams have enjoyed new recognition as the model for improving the delivery of care in diverse settings, including intensive care, adult day care, hospice, and a variety of acute care settings. This new level of respect and recognition is reflected in a growing body of literature that is providing a more sophisticated knowledge base about teams and interdisciplinary education and making significant contributions to understanding of team practices.

WHAT HAVE WE LEARNED?

I really wanted to entitle this chapter, "Everything Old Is New Again," but was dissuaded. Although this may stretch the truth a bit, it makes a significant point. The concepts of teamwork and interdisciplinary education are not new. Their rich and interesting history is reviewed superficially here; we have much to learn from those who went before us. I find it interesting that some of the earliest models for health care teams were developed in managed care programs and were community based more than 40 years ago. Language has changed over the years; we have gone from client-centered holistic care to comprehensive patient-centered care. When examined closely, these terms look very much alike, however, and the entire focus has remained the improvement of services to the individual by a team of providers with differing yet complementary skills. Throughout the literature on health care teams, certain themes remain consistent, even if scientific evidence to support these claims is scarce. These consistent themes include:

- Team care improves the quality of care
- Successful teams must be developed—they do not just happen
- Team work is difficult, requiring active learning and practice of specific knowledge and skills
- Team development takes time
- Teams need administrative and financial support to succeed
- Team education must take place at all levels.

For me, the most important thing that I have learned concerns the educational process for students. I believe that to be truly meaningful to students, team education must be based in some aspect of clinical practice. Classroom exposure to team concepts needs reinforcement by experiences, with well-functioning, effective teams delivering relevant services to real people. It is this clinically based team practice that helps to develop life-long team skills. Moreover, these skills are relevant far beyond the immediate team practice to all levels of interaction within the complex health care environment.

CONCLUSION: GAZING INTO THE CRYSTAL BALL

The future of team work in health care seems bright. New initiatives are targeting managed care, and others are addressing continuous improvement, education, and reorganization of the traditional practice into team practice for health care delivery.

But still I worry. Will teams fall out of favor? Are we becoming so familiar with the use of the word "team" that we automatically assume we practice teamwork effectively? Will we continue to believe that as sophisticated health care providers we are highly skilled team members and forgo additional training as superfluous?

In the same vein, words such as "coordination," "collaboration," and "consensus" are used so commonly that we assume that their meaning is understood, and that our behavior reflects them. If only this were true! It is fortunate that support for these basic concepts is being expressed in new ways. The continuous improvement movement (as applied in health care) reinforces concepts basic to teamwork and stresses interdisciplinary efforts and interdependency. Its efforts have brought new audiences to the benefits of teams and an understanding of the process of teamwork.

One very important issue continues as a concern. Whether team care is cost effective is a question that has been asked many times in the past; this issue will receive more scrutiny in the future. Unfortunately, only scant literature addresses the topic, and the question remains unanswered. Team care may or may not be more expensive than usual and customary care, but false assumptions about the cost of team care may unfairly influence decisions to implement change. We need good evidence about cost effectiveness to make rational decisions about the organization of care in the future.

As we look ahead, it is reasonable to expect that health professionals will work together more and more. Communications technology will allow virtual team meetings for those who are involved in a client's care but geographically separated from each other. The potential for rapid access to new data will enhance the team's ability to share information and make decisions. However, this virtual team or team meeting should not be seen as a replacement for the face-to-face encounters that address both formal and informal care needs. The team of the future will not be judged on the quality of its team meetings, but instead on its effectiveness in delivering high quality appropriate services. Thus, the connectedness and commitment team members feel to commonly understood and shared goals will remain paramount.

Others have also gazed into this crystal ball, and the Pew Commission summarizes the need for team work in an emerging system that emphasizes increased accountability. In their words, health practitioners will:

Function in new health care settings and interdisciplinary team arrangements designed to meet the primary health care needs of the public and emphasize high quality, cost-effective, integrated services and respond to increasing levels of public, governmental and third party participation in the direction of the health care system. (Pew Commission, 1994, p. 18)

Health professionals will continue to advocate for quality services; the team remains an effective means to deliver such services. Although not all of us recognize it now, each day we are drawn more and more into interdependent relationships with our colleagues.

REFERENCES

Aradine, C. R., & Hansen, M. F. (1970). Interdisciplinary teamwork in family health care. *Nursing Clinics of North America, 5,* 211–222.

Baldwin, Jr., D. C. (1996). Some historical notes on interdisciplinary and interprofessional education and practice in health care in the USA. *Journal of Interprofessional Care, 10,* 173–187.

Banta, H., & Fox, R. C. (1972). Role strains of a health care team in a poverty community. *Social Science and Medicine, 6,* 697–722.

Barker, L. (1922). The specialist and the general practitioner in relationship to teamwork in general practice. *Journal of the American Medical Association, 78,* 773–779.

Beckhard, R. (1972). Organizational issues in the team delivery of comprehensive health care. *Milbank Memorial Fund Quarterly, 50,* 287–316.

Beloff, J. S., & Korper, M. (1972). The health team model and medical care utilization. *Journal of the American Medical Association, 219,* 359–366.

Beloff, J. S., & Willet, M. (1968). Yale studies in family health care. *Journal of the American Medical Association, 205*(10), 73–79.

Bottom, P. A., Bottom, W. D., Buckingham, J. L., DiMicco, W. A. P., Elledge, C. D., Setzer, F. B., Sherrill, R. G., & Thompson, R. W. (1976). Alabama interdisciplinary health team development program: interdisciplinary team health care at UAB. *Alabama Journal of Medical Science, 13,* 370–372.

Brill, N. (1976). *Teamwork: Working together in the human services.* Philadelphia: Lippincott.

Brown, T. B. (1982). An historical view of health care teams. In G. J. Agich (Ed.), *Social responsibility in health care* (pp. 3–21). Dordrecht, The Netherlands: Reidel.

Cabot, R. (1915). *Social service and the art of healing.* New York: Moffat, Yard and Company.

Caldwell, B. (1959). Role similarity on the rehabilitation team. *Journal of Rehabilitation, 25,* 11–13.

Carlton, W. (1977). The health team training model: A teaching-learning approach in community health. *Health Education Monographs, 5,* 62–74.

Caudill, W. A., & Roberts, B. (1951). Pitfalls in the organization of interdisciplinary research. *Human Organization, 10,* 12–15.

Cherkasky, M. (1949). The Montefiore hospital home care program. *American Journal of Public Health and the Nations Health, 39,* 163–166.

Cowen, D. L., & Sbarbaro, J. A. (1972). Family-centered health care—A viable reality? *Medical Care, 10,* 164–172.

Dana, B., & Sheps, C. (1968). Trends and issues in interprofessional education: Pride, prejudice, and progress. *Journal of Education for Social Work, 4,* 35–41.

Diller, L. (1990). Fostering the interdisciplinary team, fostering research in a society in transition. *Archives of Physical Medicine and Rehabilitation, 71,* 275–278.

Discher, M. (1974). Building a health team with participation training. *Journal of Continuing Education in Nursing, 5,* 14–18.

Duncan, B., & Kempe, C. H. (1968). Joint education of medical students and allied health personnel. *American Journal of Diseases of Children, 116,* 499–504.

Eng, M. A. (1993). The hospice interdisciplinary team: A synergistic approach to the care of dying patients and their families. *Holistic Nurse Practitioner, 7,* 49–56.

Fairweather, D. V. I., & Law, B. (1978). Multidisciplinary training in family planning. *Medical Education, 12,* 205–208.

Gallmeier, T. M., & Bonner, B. L. (1992). University-based interdisciplinary training in child abuse and neglect. *Child Abuse & Neglect, 16,* 513–521.

Harris, J. L. (1978). Interdisciplinary health education: A case study of fact and fancy. *Journal of Community Health, 3,* 357–368.

Harris, J. L., Saunders, D. N., & Zasorin-Connors, J. (1978). A training program for interprofessional health care teams. *Health and Social Work, 3(2),* 36–52.

Health Resources and Services Administration. (1995). *A national agenda for geriatric education: White papers.* Washington, DC: USDHHS, Health Resources and Services Administration, Bureau of Health Professions.

Health Resources and Services Administration. (1996). *A national agenda for geriatric education: Forum report.* Washington, DC: USDHHS, Health Resources and Services Administration, Bureau of Health Professions.

Hermary, M. (1991). An analysis of the "team" concept in the health care literature (Master's thesis, McGill University, 1991). *U.M.I. Dissertation Abstracts.*

Itano, J. K., Williams, J., Deaton, M. D., & Oishi, N. (1991). Impact of a student interdisciplinary oncology team project. *Journal of Cancer Education, 6,* 219–226.

Keith, R. A. (1991). The comprehensive treatment team in rehabilitation. *Archives of Physical Medicine and Rehabilitation, 72,* 269–274.

Kindig, D. A. (1975). Interdisciplinary education for primary health care team delivery. *Journal of Medical Education, 50* (12), 97–110.

Lashoff, J. (1968). The health care team in the mile square area, Chicago. *Bulletin of the New York Academy of Medicine, 44,* 1363–1369.

Light, H. L., & Brown, N. J. (1967). The Gouverneur Health Services Program: A historical view. *Milbank Memorial Fund Quarterly, 45,* 375–390.

Lowe, J., & Herranen, M. (1978). Conflict in teamwork. *Social Work in Health Care, 3,* 323–330.

McHugh, M., West, P., Assatly, C., Duprat, L., Howard, L., Niloff, J., Waldo, K., Wandel, J., & Clifford, J. (1996). Establishing an interdisciplinary patient care team. Collaboration at the bedside and beyond. *Journal of Nursing Administration, 26(4),* 21–27.

Mazur, H., Beeston, J., & Yerxa, E. (1979). Clinical interdisciplinary health team care: An educational experiment. *Journal of Medical Education, 54,* 703–713.

Patterson, C. H. (1959). Is the team concept obsolete? *Journal of Rehabilitation, 25,* 11–13.

Pew Health Professions Commission. (1994). *Primary care workforce 2000: Federal policy paper.* San Francisco: Pew Health Professions Commission.

Rogers, D. (1932). Teamwork within the hospital. *American Journal of Nursing, 32,* 657–659.

Rubin, I., & Beckhard, R. (1972). Factors influencing the effectiveness of health teams. *Milbank Memorial Fund Quarterly, 50,* 317–335.

Ryan, D. P. (1996). A history of teamwork in mental health and its implication for teamwork training in gerontology. *Educational Gerontology, 22,* 411–431.

Schmitt, M. (1994). USA: Focus on interprofessional practice, education and research. *Journal of Interprofessional Care, 8(1),* 9–18.

Silver, G. A. (1958). Beyond general practice: The healthy team. *Yale Journal of Biology and Medicine, 31,* 29–39.

Szasz, G. (1970). Education for the health team. *Canadian Journal of Public Health, 61,* 386–390.

Takamura, J., Bermosk, L., & Stringfellow, L. (1978). *Health team development program report.* Honolulu, HI: School of Medicine, University of Hawaii.

Tanner, L. A., & Soulary, E. J. (1972). Interprofessional student health teams. *Nursing Outlook, 20,* 111–115.

Tsukuda, R. A. (1996). *A comprehensive analysis of interdisciplinary health care teams: Using information synthesis.* Paper presented at the Eighteenth Interdisciplinary Health Care Teams Conference, Minneapolis, MN.

Wagner, R. (1977, March). Rehabilitation team practice. *Rehabilitation Counseling Bulletin.* 206–217.

Williams, G. (1959). Problems in the team treatment of adults in state mental hospitals. *American Journal of Orthopsychiatry, 29,* 95–99.

Williams, T. F. (1986). Geriatrics: the fruition of the clinician reconsidered. *Gerontologist, 26,* 345–349.

Wise, H. (1972). The primary-care health team. *Archives of Internal Medicine, 130,* 438–444.

Wise, H., Beckhard, R., Rubin, I., & Kyte, A. (1974). *Making health teams work.* Cambridge, MA: Ballinger.

Setting Up a Team Training Program

CHAPTER 4

Recruiting Students for GITT

Shirley M. Moore

Recent reports by the Bureau of Health Professions (1993) and the Pew Health Professions Commission (1991; Grant, Finocchio, & The California Primary Care Consortium, 1995) point to a critical gap between the education of health professionals provided now and the preparation needed for the future. In particular, few nurses, physicians, and social workers are trained to lead and participate in interdisciplinary teams in the provision of geriatric health care. Although the geriatric disciplines have recognized interdependence to some degree, recent changes in health care reimbursement, such as capitation, have resulted in redesigned systems that benefit from a team approach. Health professions education has changed more slowly than health care practice, creating a gap between what is taught and what is needed. Health professionals graduate without sufficient opportunity to learn how to work together across disciplines to deliver and improve health care (Headrick et al., 1996).

The John A. Hartford Foundation (1995) and the Institute for Healthcare Improvement (Headrick et al., 1996) have funded recent demonstration projects that develop partnerships between academic and practice sites to design and test models of interdisciplinary team training for health professions students. The Hartford project, the focus of this book, funds new approaches to geriatric interdisciplinary team training (GITT) for medical residents, nurse practitioner students, and social work students. The Institute for Healthcare Improvement (IHI) is a nonprofit organization committed to fostering integrated and collaborative efforts to improve healthcare systems. Since 1994, the IHI has funded four demonstration project sites (Cleveland, Pennsylvania, South Carolina, and Washington, DC) to develop a model curriculum on continuous quality improvement for students in medicine, nursing, and management. The interdisciplinary teams trained in both the GITT and IHI projects also include health professions students in pharmacy, dentistry, physical therapy, and occupational therapy.

Crucial to geriatric team training programs is the effective recruitment of students from different disciplines, but this creates numerous challenges; some of these challenges are generic to any type of interdisciplinary training experience, some are specific to geriatric training, and others are unique to team training. In this chapter, I will describe: (a) management of the logistics of interdisciplinary learning that affect student recruitment, and (b) approaches to increasing student interest in geriatric team training.

RECRUITING STUDENTS FOR INTERDISCIPLINARY LEARNING

Students do not want to be inconvenienced. They recognize that interdisciplinary educational experiences will present logistic problems, and they want reassurances that these problems are resolved before signing up for a course. For example, physical architecture of the buildings and schools in universities is designed for separation of the disciplines, rather than interaction. Usually professional students within the same university share little or no common physical space; they have limited association with each other during their training programs. For students of the various schools to engage in combined educational experiences, the "outside" students must gain access to buildings they don't often use (Moore et al., 1996). Faculty should expect to expend considerable amounts of time and energy to ensure that all students have access to classroom and library resources within particular buildings.

Transcending physical access problems is essential to successful recruitment of students for interdisciplinary learning. One approach to overcoming these architectural barriers is to institute interdisciplinary student interest groups or programs without walls that address common needs and interests of health professions students. Examples of such interest groups are the Interdisciplinary Connection at the University of North Carolina and the Nursing and Medical Students' Alliance at Case Western Reserve University. Members of these groups receive e-mail and flyers to keep informed of programming, services, research opportunities, and network gatherings. For this reason, these groups provide excellent communication avenues to recruit students interested in interdisciplinary learning experiences. At Case Western Reserve University, the interdisciplinary student organization is an informal program run by the students themselves, without staff support from the university. At the University of North Carolina, the interdisciplinary network is supported with staff services from the health sciences schools. Further information about how these interdisciplinary structural platforms function can be obtained by contacting the deans' offices of the professional programs at the universities.

Difficulty in course scheduling can present a logistical nightmare when attempting to recruit students from different disciplines for interdisciplinary learning experiences. If students from different universities come together for interdisciplinary learning, each university has its own academic calendar; even within the same university, multiple academic calendars may be in use. Junior and senior medical students and medical residents often change rotations monthly, having no real academic calendar at all. Finding common class meeting times that fit the schedules of students across disciplines requires great creativity. One approach to this dilemma is the design of learning modules or cycles (thus working outside the semester or quarter concept of scheduling) that use only the common or overlap time of the different schedules.

In the Cleveland IHI interdisciplinary project, student evaluations clearly reflected their preference to participate in a course that falls within the time frame of their usual program of study. To accommodate students on both semester and quarter systems in this project, the interdisciplinary course began 3 weeks into the semester to coincide with the beginning of the quarter, thereby using the common time of both universities' schedules. In addition, each of the different spring breaks of the respective schools was honored. Student evaluations indicated that these kinds of accommodations were an incentive for them to participate in what was considered an experimental course in their curriculum.

Finding a time of day that is convenient for students of different disciplines is another logistic factor that affects student recruitment for interdisciplinary learning. Daytime clinical practica of the nursing students and graduate social work students make it difficult to schedule interdisciplinary classes during the day, whereas medical residents/students say that their fatigue at the end of the day makes it difficult for them to participate in evening classes. Offering the interdisciplinary course from 5 P.M. to 7 P.M. may provide a compromise. In the IHI Project, this late afternoon schedule encouraged students to move from the course to dinner and develop friendships outside of class. In the On Lok community-based interdisciplinary project in San Francisco (Eng, 1987), early evening dinners provided as part of the program were a successful incentive.

Student expectations for a course may be very discipline specific. Elective courses in medical schools are frequently offered as opportunities for students to explore an area of interest and rarely require excessive class preparation or formal testing. In the IHI project, nursing students requested more extensive bibliographies and the opportunity to have readings in advance of the course so that they could get a jump on the class assignments, whereas medical students requested that the amount of required reading be kept to a minimum. Such differences among student expectations necessitated both individual and group faculty-student discussions about learning in new types of modes that differed significantly from those to which they had been socialized in their professional education.

Students in academic programs may perceive interdisciplinary courses as risky; they need assurances that they will obtain traditional credits toward their program of study. Flexible grading options, such as both pass/fail and letter grades, optional readings and projects, and flexible number of credits for the course are additional strategies to manage student expectations. Medical school electives often are graded pass/fail; attending physicians evaluate knowledge, attitudes, and skills of medical residents monthly on a scale of 1 through 9 using a form based on American Board of Internal Medicine guidelines. In contrast, nursing and social work students expect formal tests for student evaluation and a final letter grade. In the Great Lakes GITT project of the Hartford initiative, students from two academic institutions representing at least two disciplines each have different grading options that were negotiated individually with faculty in their respective academic departments. Advertising these kinds of course flexibilities can enhance recruitment of students for interdisciplinary team training.

An appropriately balanced number of students from each discipline is necessary to design interdisciplinary learning experiences that reflect authentic clinical care environments. It is often demoralizing for a student to serve as sole representative of a discipline in an interdisciplinary course. Moreover, a student who serves as the sole representative of a discipline in a course may lose the opportunity to learn how to separate personal from disciplinary opinions. The right balance of students is based on the goals of the course, the patient population, clinical experiences involved, practitioner/mentor availability, and faculty resources. Policies that specify a closed enrollment based on permission of the faculty are one way of controlling the mix of students in interdisciplinary courses. Targeted recruitment strategies, such as altered grading options, personal contact by project faculty, and public announcements made in other courses may be necessary for hard-to-recruit student groups.

Medical students and medical residents are traditionally difficult to recruit; their educational programs are often inflexible and based on models of education that do not consider interdisciplinary training an essential skill. Fortunately, today many medical students and residents are interested in interdisciplinary learning, and all demonstration sites in the IHI project found that this was a strong motivator for student enrollment; students cited the opportunity to participate in an interdisciplinary experience as often as an interest in continuous improvement as a reason for taking the course. In addition, the presence of multiple interdisciplinary courses in the curriculum helps stimulate interest in interdisciplinary learning. In the Cleveland IHI project, students who completed the course on continuous improvement were inquiring about how get into the Great Lakes GITT Project course.

Clinical practica present special logistic challenges when trying to coordinate the academic and clinical schedules (clinics don't close for school holidays, clinics are not open in the evenings when working students want to do their course requirements). Partnerships between academic institutions and clinical agencies, such as those recommended in the GITT project, provide mechanisms for dialogue between field placement and classroom faculty. This dialogue provides the opportunity to design clinical learning environments that meet the needs of clinical and academic agencies by identifying what both want and need. Many of the GITT project sites are negotiating clinical training settings for teams of interdisciplinary students and avoiding discipline-specific planning.

Making an interdisciplinary course required is another strategy that eases student recruitment. This decision mandates consideration of faculty commitment and resources and student demand and interest in such courses. In some of the GITT projects, geriatric team training is a required part of the programs in schools of nursing and social work, but not for medical residents.

Top-level administrative support may be critical to waive traditional curriculum approaches and overcome logistic and scheduling issues during the testing of new curricula. It is important to start small to minimize administrative issues (such as, who gets tuition dollars; how to get official course numbers from curriculum committees). In the IHI Project, building the course through a series of pilot projects permitted the faculty to proceed with course development without having to work out all the administrative issues in advance (Moore et al., 1996).

Getting students involved early in course planning is an important approach to overcoming logistic barriers affecting student recruitment. In both the GITT and IHI projects, student input was critical in working out the logistics of the interdisciplinary learning experiences; they knew each program's curriculum and its requirements and limitations better than anyone. Including students on planning committees for program design and recruitment assistance can spur student interest and motivate the faculty as well. For example, in the IHI and the GITT projects, early recruitment and discussions with students accelerated faculty planning and decisions about the curriculum. Finally, the faculty's commitment to a shared vision of innovative education and respect for the varied expertise represented in the different disciplines can be helpful in overcoming many of the logistic and convenience barriers to interdisciplinary education. Table 4.1 displays a summary of the strategies designed to recruit students for interdisciplinary learning.

INCREASING STUDENT INTEREST IN GERIATRIC TEAM TRAINING

A major challenge to the successful recruitment of students for GITT is the lack of popularity of both geriatrics and team training. Despite the large numbers of elderly patients that receive care in internal medicine, family practice, and many specialties (such as neurology and orthopedics), not all students and faculty are interested in geriatrics. The resistance to specialty training in geriatrics comes from several sources, including discomfort with the elderly, lack of time in the curriculum, financial considerations, and scarcity of adequately prepared faculty in geriatrics.

One strategy to sidestep resistance to geriatrics training is to design a geriatrics component as a subspecialty within existing fields, such as primary care practitioner, adult nurse practitioner, family nurse practitioner, or family social worker. A subspecialization certificate in geriatrics can be given to students who participate in the programs. Students also appreciate enriched learning experiences such as research opportunities and access to special populations. They find a geriatrics course more attractive if they can obtain course credit for participating in the program or if it fulfills course requirements in their respective curricula.

Creating opportunities for students to explore the specialty of geriatrics early in their professional training also enhances interest in geriatrics training. These introductions to the elderly can be part of current required courses, independent study opportunities, or short study modules. The GITT projects provide several models of such specialized programs.

Personal contact methods of recruitment are useful, such as recruitment luncheons and short lectures by experts on topics such as team accountability and decision-making and including patients as members of teams. Less personal approaches to marketing team training to students include the use of specially designed flyers, newsletters, faculty meetings, and open letters to students.

Financial incentives also attract students to geriatrics coursework. Sources of support include research moneys and institutional training grants that offer faculty and student tuition support for geriatric specialty training. Training grants sometimes contain funds that can be used for student incentives, such as payment for participation, tuition support, or the development of exemplary student status options. The On Lok community-based interdisciplinary program in San Francisco has used these kinds of incentives; paying students to attend the training sessions on interdisciplinary teams was a successful recruitment strategy.

The Advisory Panel on Health Professions Education and Managed Care for the Pew Health Professions Commission has recommended that health professions programs develop interdisciplinary teaching and learning experiences that teach the knowledge, skills, and values needed for effective teamwork (Tresolin, 1995). Other reports have

TABLE 4.1   Strategies to Reduce Logistic Problems Associated with Recruiting Students for Interdisciplinary Learning

1. Provide students with easy access to the buildings of all disciplines involved.
2. Develop interdisciplinary student interest groups.
3. Develop modular learning units outside the traditional semester or quarter system.
4. Offer individualized, flexible grading options.
5. Consider late afternoon scheduling for didactic classes.
6. Involve students early in the planning stages of designing interdisciplinary activities.
7. Recruit students using personal, faculty-to-student contact.
8. Create partnerships between academic and clinical agencies that are committed to interdisciplinary learning for health professions students.
9. Obtain administrative support to waive traditional curriculum approaches while pilot testing new curriculum models.

shown that recent health professions graduates and young practitioners report discomfort with their knowledge and skills for work in health care teams. New medical graduates, in particular, have been described as not prepared to work in team care that is required for managed care organizations (Council on Graduate Medical Education, 1994; Group Health Association, 1993). In general, the knowledge and skills that health professionals learn in their training programs have been discipline specific and have not included knowledge of other related disciplines, such as management or organizational behavior. In most cases, health professions students have had little training in team skills, such as how to run a meeting, balance group process and product, support group decision making, and manage conflict.

In the IHI project, we found that many of the health professions students did not know the key terms for searching the literature to learn more about team work. Indeed, it was necessary to convince the students that a body of empirical literature existed about team work, and that the skills required for team work were not just "common sense." This understanding about the "science" in team work was enlightening to most of the health professions students, who then were more open to learning the knowledge and skills related to team work in a focused, structured way. A resource center that contains recent literature and training material on team work in health care can be useful to familiarize students with this subject matter. Easy access to a set of resources, such as articles and books devoted to team skills, will provide students with information about the types of journals that report research addressing team work and promote informal discussions about the more controversial issues of team work in health care.

Exposing students to geriatric team care provided in managed care environments may be one of the most useful ways to increase students' interest in team approaches to geriatric care. Students want realistic training experiences with transferable skills related to future employment. Managed care organizations often use a collaborative practice delivery system that creates an environment in which interdisciplinary team training can be modeled and encouraged. Managed care programs for the elderly are designed to provide a comprehensive, integrated response to the health care and related needs of the enrollees.

Educating students early about future trends in health care can increase their interest in geriatric team training. National reports, such as those cited above from the Bureau of Health Professions (1995) and Pew Charitable Trusts (Grant et al., 1995) enable students to understand national trends in health care manpower needs. Expert practitioners and future employers can offer seminars about the kind of geriatric team training that is needed and expected of future health professionals. Information provided in these ways can convince students that expertise in interdisciplinary team care of the elderly will set them apart from other applicants in job interviews.

Faculty charisma can accomplish wonders when marketing this training. Faculty provide students with the values and commitment to geriatric team training. Needless to say, institutions must create a critical mass of interested faculty who will champion the cause. Faculty must create an environment that supports the attitudes and perceptions they wish their students to hold (provision of a team care delivery approach to geriatric care). Traditionally, the medical discipline has placed little emphasis on team training in geriatric training programs, suggesting that team skills are not highly valued by the faculty or are not considered a set of skills that are appropriate to learn in a training program. Faculty comfort level in team training may be a problem; faculty often have not received formal team training themselves.

Interdisciplinary faculty teams that model team skills can serve to reinforce the values of geriatric teamwork (see chapter 5). Matching trainees with faculty mentors who provide ongoing encouragement and guidance to help them make the most of available interdisciplinary opportunities can be an important influence on student interest in geriatric team care. It is important to choose committed faculty who are willing to try new approaches to surmount all the barriers. Faculty must be prepared to invest time, try different strategies, learn, and revise. They must learn to suspend their discipline-specific ideas about education and to search for creative solutions together. Conceptualizing each training effort as a pilot study, faculty are more likely to give something new a try.

Creating a critical mass of interested students can be one of the best recruitment methods. Word of mouth or testimony from past students enhances credibility and enthusiasm among the next cohort of students about good experiences in geriatric team training. Public recognition of students who participate in geriatrics training, such as nominating them for awards to be given at graduation, is another way to enhance students' interest.

When recruiting students for participation in national demonstration projects, tell them what they will be joining. In the Great Lakes GITT Project, the recruitment flyers list it as a national demonstration project and an opportunity for students to be involved in designing and testing professional education for the future. Table 4.2 provides a summary of approaches to increase student interest in GITT.

SUMMARY

Students participate in geriatric interdisciplinary team training for different reasons, and it is important to design strategies to involve them and appeal to their different motivations. Recruiting students for GITT entails applying multiple strategies aimed at specific issues associated with student recruitment. One set of strategies addresses the logistic problems students associate with interdisciplinary learning. Student recruitment can be

TABLE 4.2   Strategies to Increase Student Interest in Geriatric Team Training

1. Create geriatric subspecialties within other specialties (primary care, internal medicine, adult nurse practitioner).
2. Offer a subspecialization certificate in geriatrics.
3. Create a critical mass of faculty to champion the team approach to geriatric care and serve as mentors to students.
4. Obtain student financial assistance through the acquisition of geriatric training grants.
5. Have clinical agency partners/future employers talk with students early in their education about desired competencies of future health care professionals.
6. Teach students how to market their geriatric teamwork specialty training.
7. Provide a resource center of reference material about teamwork.
8. Expose students to team models of clinical care provided in managed care environments.
9. Nominate students who participate for special awards at graduation.

enhanced if interdisciplinary learning experiences are designed to accommodate the diverse scheduling needs, grading requirements, and learning-style preferences of the different disciplinary student groups. Another set of recruitment strategies is aimed at increasing student interest in geriatric team training. Student motivation to study geriatrics can be fostered by offering flexible options for exploration of the subspecialty of geriatrics and facilitating contact with faculty mentors who champion the cause. Exposing students to managed care delivery systems, faculty modeling, and sensitization to future trends in health care manpower needs can also increase student interest in team training.

Curricular innovations require flexibility in existing systems and experimentation with new ideas. Students are usually highly motivated to engage in designing and testing new models of care, and inviting student participation is the role of both faculty and practitioners alike. Although working across multiple agencies and disciplines is challenging, partnerships between academic and clinical practice agencies that view the tension of the idealism of the academic world and the realism of practice sites as positive can be effective in changing and improving health care. Students will participate in and enjoy education programs that are responsive to their needs.

REFERENCES

Bureau of Health Professions. (1993). *An Agenda for Health Professions Reform.* Washington, DC: US Department of Health and Human Services, Public Health Service, Health Resources and Services Administration.

Bureau of Health Professions. (1995). *A national agenda for geriatric education: White papers.* Washington, DC: US Department of Health and Human Services, Public Health Service, Health Resources and Services Administration.

Council on Graduate Medical Education. (1994). *Recommendations to improve access to health care through physician workforce reform.* Rockville, MD: US Department of Health & Human Services, Health Resources and Services Administration.

Council on Graduate Medical Education. (1995). *6th Report on managed health care: The physician workforce and medical education.* Rockville, MD: US Department of Health and Human Services, Health Resources and Services Administration.

Eng, C. (1987). Multidisciplinary approach to medical care: The On Lok model. *Clinical Report on Aging, 1*(6), 9–11.

Grant, R. W., Finocchio, L. J., & the California Primary Care Consortium Subcommittee on Interdisciplinary Collaboration. (1995). *Interdisciplinary collaborative teams in primary care: A model curriculum and resource guide.* San Francisco: Pew Health Professions Commission.

Group Health Association of America. (1993). *The recruitment experience of health maintenance organizations for primary care physicians.* Rockville, MD: Health Resources Services Administration.

Headrick, L. A., Knapp, M., Neuhauser, D., Gelmon, S., Norman, L., Quinn, D. & Baker, R. (1996). Working from upstream to improve health care: The IHI Interdisciplinary Professional Education Collaborative. *Joint Commission Journal of Quality Improvement, 22,* 149–164.

John A. Hartford Foundation. (1995). Internal document.

Moore, S., Headrick, L., Alemi, F., Flowers, D., Hekelman, F., Neuhauser, D., & Novotny, J. (1996). Using learning cycles to build an interdisciplinary curriculum in quality improvement for health professions students in Cleveland. *Joint Commission Journal on Quality Improvement, 22,* 165–171.

Pew Health Professions Commission. (1991). *Healthy America: Practitioners for 2005.* San Francisco: Pew Charitable Trusts.

Tresolin, C. P (1995). *Health professions education and managed care: Challenges and necessary responses (report of The Advisory Panel on Health Professions Education and Managed Care for The Pew Health Professions Commission).* San Francisco: Center for the Health Professions.

CHAPTER 5

Selecting and Preparing Team Training Educators

Elizabeth R. Mackenzie, Neville E. Strumpf, Jerry C. Johnson, and Roberta Sands

Health policy analysts, educators, and clinicians continue to call for greater emphasis on team training for health professionals, especially those caring for older adults (Grant, Finocchio, & the California Primary Care Consortium Subcommittee on Interdisciplinary Collaboration, 1995; Pew Health Professions Commission, 1995a). As we make the transition to integrated managed care systems, case management and careful usage of resources necessitate interdisciplinary team care (Klein, 1995). Although geriatrics has recognized the benefits of team care for many years and has incorporated it more than many specialties, professional schools in most academic institutions have nevertheless devoted little of their curricula to training for collaborative care (Grant et al., 1995).

Team training programs are only as good as the educators who provide the training. Therefore, a crucial component of a program of GITT is the selection and preparation of participating educators (faculty, clinical educators, or other preceptors). This chapter describes the challenges and issues of preparing educators for effective interdisciplinary team training. These include:

- Identification of appropriate teams and clinical educators
- Gaining commitment (buy-in) for interdisciplinary team training by all educators
- Overcoming institutional barriers to educating health professionals in collaborative care.

We will use experiences from a planning year at the University of Pennsylvania and other GITT sites around the country to highlight these common issues.

BACKGROUND

Virtually nothing has been written on the topic of selecting and preparing educators for team teaching and training. Few faculty or clinical educators receive formal education in teamwork themselves. Nor have many had experience teaching about team skills;

most educators are trained to teach in a discipline-specific style. Depending on the institution, trainers may be faculty only, clinical preceptors only, or faculty-preceptors. Because not every clinical preceptor has a faculty appointment, commitment to teaching per se may vary considerably depending on the institutional context. The very distinctions made between faculty and preceptors (or clinical educators) reflect institutional norms that generally do not support team-training initiatives. In fact, the nomenclature is indicative of the very barriers faced in creating well functioning teams and in designing effective team training programs. For this reason, we will use the term educators or trainers (rather than faculty and clinical preceptors).

Team training in general requires thinking less of academic disciplines (or institutional roles) and more of team building, team skills, team identity, and collaboration. A brief overview of existing material on team training reveals several themes as described below.

Trainers Transcending Their Own Disciplines

An effective training program in collaborative care requires trainers who are able to transcend their own disciplines at conceptual and institutional levels (Gurland, 1994). Overcoming institutional and conceptual barriers among the disciplines is a major part of establishing a team-training initiative, and participating faculty and preceptors must be committed to this goal. An essential step is the formation of core curricula that extend traditional boundaries of the disciplines involved, along with recruitment of faculty who are committed to and capable of delivering interdisciplinary education (Baldwin & Baldwin et al., 1995; Browne et al., 1995; Kahn, Davis, Wartman, Wilson, & Kahn, 1995).

One approach to overcoming disciplinary boundaries is the formulation of course work that integrates perspectives from many disciplines, such as content in health care ethics. Browne et al. (1995) describe such an offering at the University of British Columbia for medical and senior nursing students. Facilitators are specially trained to deliver the material and are drawn from medicine, nursing, pharmacy, rehabilitation medicine, social work, law, philosophy, and pastoral care. Prior to the course, facilitators undergo a 3-hour tutor-training session, essentially a crash course in ethics by experienced ethicists, accompanied by presentations of techniques and tools for the facilitation of an ethics seminar. The format for the 12-week course included lectures, seminar, and student team presentations with content on ethical decision making, patient autonomy and informed consent, professional autonomy, interdisciplinary relations and decision making, confidentiality, effectiveness of treatments, decisions to treat or not to treat, and allocation of resources.

Need for Case-Based Learning

Case-based learning is crucial to interdisciplinary team training, as real situations, rather than theoretic examples, better emphasize the necessity and value of an interdisciplinary approach to patient care (Anderson et al., 1994; Gilmore & Schall, 1996; Irby, 1994). Cases may be drawn from record reviews or the current caseload of the clinical team. Although case-based learning is common in health professions education, team training faculty must be familiar with this educational form and adept at its application.

They can learn how to use the case method by observing skilled teachers (Irby, 1994) or using such resources as *Interdisciplinary Collaborative Teams in Primary Care—A Resource Guide* (Grant et al., 1995).

Using Experiential Learning

In the classroom, the best approach to imparting an in-depth understanding of team dynamics is through experiential learning (Headrick, Norman, Gelmon, & Knapp, 1995), rather than lecture or seminar formats typically found in academic settings. Role modeling (Baldwin & Baldwin, 1978), role clarification (Lister, 1982), and role-playing and simulation (Kues et al., 1992) are all useful techniques for creating an interactive educational experience. Educators involved in a team training program need leadership skills in these kinds of exercises and may also need training in experiential teaching and gaming prior to initiation of the program.

Importance of Relationship-Centered Care

Teachers of collaborative care must appreciate the importance of patient-centered care (Coles, 1995) and interpersonal communication (Myers, 1994) or relationship-centered care (Tresolini & the Pew-Fetzer Task Force, 1994). Knowledge of relationship-centered care is vitally important for caregivers, patients, and families and is essential to understanding and responding to psychosocial influences on health and disease (Tresolini et al., 1994). The Pew Health Professions Commission gives the following recommendations for education in relationship-centered care:

- Recruit faculty based on commitment to mission and diversity across health professions
- Provide faculty development and continuing education programs to promote the understanding and practice of relationship-centered care
- Identify and recognize faculty who are interested in patient-centered care
- Provide training for current and future academic leaders who can promote visionary team teaching across disciplines and professions.

The Commission also suggests identifying barriers related to interdisciplinary practice and education and names possible barriers as class and salary differences, hierarchical administrative structures, leadership issues, and traditions of authoritarianism (Tresolini et al., 1994).

Facing the Challenge of Managed Care

With the arrival of managed care systems, collaborative care teams take on a new significance and are faced with new challenges (Grant et al., 1995; Headrick, Neuhauser, Schwab, & Stevens, 1995). Participating team educators should understand the interplay between team care and managed care and the importance of collaborative practice in a managed care environment (Pew Health Professions Commission, 1995a). A focus on the team as provider appears (in theory, at least) to be part of a larger paradigm shift toward community-based care, preventive and chronic care, cost awareness, and managed primary care (Pew Health Professions Commission, 1995b). In this model, teamwork is essential to the tenets of managed care, namely, efficiency, cost-effectiveness, and quality. All educators involved in team training—a rapidly growing group—must appreciate the larger context in which team care is delivered and practiced.

IDENTIFYING TEAM EDUCATORS

A natural place to begin an interdisciplinary team training program is to examine existing models, frameworks, systems, and individual teams already engaged in and committed to collaborative practice and teaching. To prepare for GITT, planners sought geriatric care teams known to excel in collaborative clinical care. They also looked for teams already serving as a training ground for students/residents, and those with experience in a capitated system (i.e., managed care). Obviously, selected teams and sites must also serve a diversity of patient populations and provide a continuum of care (such as hospital, long-term care, assisted living, rehabilitation, geriatric assessment). The team's degree of cultural competency must also be taken into consideration when choosing team educators. Are they familiar with concepts of patient-centered care? Do they exhibit an awareness of ethnogeriatrics? Educator teams that do not possess these competencies should either be excluded from interdisciplinary training programs or retrained.

Whenever possible, identify educators already functioning as a team; how well does the team function as a whole? Choosing trainers has less to do with specific individuals than with exemplary teams having (at the very least) representatives from medicine, nursing, and social work who are experienced practitioners and team members and who have supervised students in the past.

The University of Pennsylvania planning year group—based on the preceding criteria—ultimately identified six clinical sites and their teams of educators as appropriate locations for geriatric interdisciplinary team training. These are typical of an array of sites nationally where interdisciplinary team training takes place.

The Nurse-Dominated Team

Our example of a nurse-dominated team is an academic practice operated by the School of Nursing as a Comprehensive Outpatient Rehabilitation Facility. The team consists of nurse practitioners, a geropsychiatric clinical nurse specialist, physical and occupational therapists, speech and language pathologist, social worker, geriatrician, and physiatrist. This team is strongly patient centered and focused on time-limited, intensive rehabilitation of elders (Evans, Yurkow, & Siegler, 1995). The Practice Director, a gerontologic nurse practitioner, provides leadership and direction for the team without suppressing the contributions of other members.

The Nurse–Physician Team

The nurse–physician team is composed of geriatricians, two nurse practitioners, and one social worker. This particular team, part of services provided by the Division of

Geriatric Medicine within the University of Pennsylvania Health System, delivers community-based care in the patient's home (a team without walls) and relies heavily on shared roles and informal mechanisms of communication and clinical management.

The Physician-Dominated Team

This team has nine physicians, one nurse, two nurse practitioners, and one social worker. It is a Comprehensive Geriatric Evaluation Program, providing interdisciplinary assessment and primary care for older adults. Patients are assigned to a physician and interact with other team members as appropriate.

The Social Work-Dominated Team

This team practices in a setting for assisted living located on a campus offering other levels of acute and skilled nursing home care. The team consists of an administrator, assistant administrator, social worker, physicians, nurse manager, and an activity coordinator. The team involves physicians as medical problems arise, but for the most part, social workers manage day-to-day care for these community-dwelling elders experiencing functional losses.

The Consensus Model Team

This team practices in a 240-bed extended-care facility, where each of four units has its own team led by the nurse practitioner, in consultation with the medical director. In general, this type of team provides roles for a wide range of team members, including nurses, social workers, dietary staff, and recreational aides. Team leaders make considerable effort to include the entire team in decision making.

The Evolving Team

These kinds of teams are useful for training, inasmuch as they reflect common real world situations and can help trainees learn to negotiate in a complex institutional structure. An example is an newly formed Acute Care of the Elderly unit, with recently assembled team members currently organizing themselves to deliver interdisciplinary care.

The search for exemplary teams will uncover many styles. Assuming commitment to the overall philosophy of GITT, any one of the teams can be an effective instrument for teaching collaborative practices to trainees.

GAINING COMMITMENT FOR GERIATRIC INTERDISCIPLINARY TEAM TRAINING

Having identified (and selected) teams and trainers for a team training program based on their clinical, academic, or team expertise, the next step is to gain sufficient commitment to the process and program. Buy-in is an essential. To ensure a high level of support for this (or any) program, the authors recommend approaching the educators (who have been identified using the above criteria) about participation in designing the team training program.

Planning meetings, in addition to building commitment to the program among educator teams, can serve several other important functions: facilitating the exchange of information between each site and the planning group, further familiarizing sites with the interdisciplinary team training initiative, and helping the planning group devise an interdisciplinary team training model appropriate to all sites on both conceptual and logistic levels. One strategy for shaping the planning meeting process is to ask team members to complete a questionnaire in advance of the planning meetings. Respondents should be prepared to discuss topics such as the definition of an interdisciplinary team, implementation of patient-centered team care, benefits and differences compared to other models of care, roles and functions of team members, types of precepting currently taking place at their site, priorities for students, and attention to diversity and cultural competence.

Moving any interdisciplinary team training initiative forward necessitates a series of discussions about the team's capacity for educating students from core disciplines, current team function, number of clinicians available to serve as team educators, team commitment, and ability to be part of the overall academic training, as well as any anticipated barriers to implementing the training program at each site. This process of surveys and discussions allows each team member to reflect on and articulate experiences with their teams, an important activity that is often ignored in the face of inevitable time pressures. The process of making the implicit explicit is an important first step in preparing the clinical teams to serve as team educators, and is also a good segue to the train-the-trainers segment of the overall program.

An important part of the planning process is to assess how much (and what kind of) preparation the educator teams think they need. This can vary considerably, depending on the training activities the team already performs. GITT planners may find that the clinical educators believe that they need little or no preparation to begin a GITT program, especially at academic health centers where clinicians already serve as preceptors. In this case, it is advisable to honor the educators' perceptions of their competencies, while pinpointing areas in which additional training and preparation could be beneficial. On the other hand, sites with no formal educational systems in place may have considerable gaps in preparation, and GITT planners may be called on to offer a comprehensive, nuts and bolts train the trainer program. In any case, the program should be tailored to the needs of the clinical educators. These needs can best be assessed through the planning meeting process.

OVERCOMING INSTITUTIONAL BARRIERS

At every potential training site, GITT planners will undoubtedly face institutional barriers to implementation. One of the greatest barriers to team training programs is differences among the cultures and philosophies of the academic disciplines involved (Evans, 1994). Although these differences are probably most apparent at academic health centers, they exist elsewhere because all clinicians receive much of their training in discipline-specific programs. A different type of barrier may be encountered at managed care sites. Despite a theoretical commitment to team care, capitated payment mechanisms are not team focused, rendering the managed care environment simultaneously proteam and antiteam. Planners must identify all such potential hurdles early in the planning process, assess them honestly, and address them appropriately.

The disciplines of nursing, social work, and medicine all have unique characteristics that create distinct cultures. Dress codes, jargon, schedules, salaries, and a host of other attributes mark each discipline as distinct. Furthermore, a societal hierarchy places medicine first, and nursing, social work, and other disciplines in competition for second place. Because society as a whole typically values the work done by men more than that performed by women (especially female caregivers) and also values the natural sciences more than the social sciences, we end up with a hierarchy of medicine first, and others, often labeled as paraprofessionals or nonphysician providers, as second, third, or fourth. Team training programs, including train-the-trainer components, must take these power dynamics into consideration when evaluating possible barriers to implementation. For example, is there any covert animosity or competition between physicians and nurses or social workers and nurses? How do members of the teams from other fields (such as physical therapy, occupational therapy, psychology, and so forth) participate in these dynamics? Are clinical educators aware of (and articulate about) the status factors that may influence team care?

Even after securing high-level administrative commitment to interdisciplinary training, individual clinical educators may need additional preparation in the interdisciplinary perspective (Strumpf & Whitney, 1994). How comfortable are nurses with training medical residents? Will medical residents understand and respect the skills and expert knowledge of the social worker? What is the relationship of interdisciplinary work to the educator's discipline-specific career? Planning meetings can effectively address some of these issues; other problems will require more sophisticated approaches, such as gaming techniques formulated in the field of organizational development.

The discipline-based power differentials and variations in philosophic perspectives may be the most important faced by a GITT planning group. Planners must establish a frank and open dialogue about status and discipline-specific perspectives as part of team educator preparations. One possible ice breaker is to ask participants in the planning meetings why they think geriatric interdisciplinary team training has been slow to take root in academic environments, and what steps are necessary to create a more interdisciplinary friendly milieu.

Less controversial factors can emerge as annoying obstacles to team training. Scheduling issues are a perennial problem for interdisciplinary training. Schools of social work, medicine, and nursing usually create their schedules without consulting one another, which can leaving the GITT planning group with the temporal equivalent of a Rubik's cube. Social work field placements, medical residencies, and so forth are all of varying lengths, and adapting calendars shaped by customary clinical preceptorships for each discipline to an interdisciplinary framework is likely to be a challenge at any site. Enlisting the help of educators to solve this problem will encourage buy in, and can serve as a form of trainer preparation, inasmuch as it enhances an interdisciplinary perspective, that is, helps everyone think team rather than discipline.

Both logistic and cultural barriers to team training initiatives should be discussed openly and frankly as part of the preparation of clinician educators (Health Resources and Services Administration, 1996). The more honest the dialogue, the more effective the solutions.

TRAINING THE TRAINERS

For institutions such as ours, where clinical practices already serve as an educational laboratory for trainees from a variety of disciplines—ranging from social work to geropsychiatry to medicine—the main challenge is preparation of trainers to teach specifically about team work, rather than to be good preceptors. The clinical teams chosen by our planning year group were already heavily committed to training medical residents and other advanced students (such as social work, nursing, physical therapy). Many individual students had already attended team meetings, participated on team rounds, and observed team communication in the clinical setting. What remained, in terms of training the trainers, was to assist clinical preceptors in assessing their performance as a team, introducing the concept of Teams Training Teams, and utilizing tools derived from organizational development. In other words, our goal was to raise team training skills to a more sophisticated level of expertise. Obviously, when planning a GITT initiative at a nonteaching clinical site (such as On Lok), the challenges are different (see chapter 12). But from the perspective of an academic health center, the primary focus is likely be on improving (rather than establishing) interdisciplinary team training.

Many advances in team building and team skills have come from an organizational development perspective, beginning with Dr. Elton Mayo's work in the 1930s and 1940s, continuing through the Tavistock experiments in the 1950s, the training-group concept of the 1960s and 1970s, and finally the advent of Continuous Quality Improvement in the 1970s and 1980s. Most of the innovations in our understanding of work team dynamics occurred in corporate management and industrial psychology (Mears, 1994). Thus, it is not surprising that the shift to managed care has created an increased interest in management approaches, collaboration, and team work groups for the health professions (Headrick, Neuhauser, Schwab, & Stevens, 1995). For these reasons, one effective approach to training team educators how to teach others about delivering care in teams is to include organizational development methods and theory in train-the-trainer components of the program (Mears, 1994). Likely sources for such expertise are management consulting firms, business schools, and health management training programs.

We facilitated the inclusion of organizational development perspectives by contracting with a university-affiliated management consulting firm, The Center for Applied Research. This training-the-trainers component ensured exposure to organizational development theories of team development and gave GITT educators the opportunity for self assessment and reflection. Facilitators from CFAR encouraged workshop participants to consider their own beliefs about collaborative team care. Questions included:

1. Think back to when you first found yourself in a team context. What do you think are the two or three critical insights or concepts for people who are just beginning to grasp the power and the challenge of being effective in team settings?
2. If you were on a task force to design a curriculum for the month-long rotation, what two or three key skills or concepts do you think would be most important to cover?
3. As you look to the future of geriatric health care in terms of payment systems, what two or three external forces are increasing the incentives for team work? What two or three forces do you think are inhibiting the growth of team delivery systems?
4. The teams you will train will consist of students from medicine, social work, and nursing. Based on your experience, what are the three or four issues these three disciplines have the most difficulty dealing with openly and honestly? What are the key stereotypes each has of the other?
5. From the vantage point of patients and cost-effectiveness, what do you think are the two or three greatest benefits of effective team work?
6. Generally, there is a great gap between the rhetoric about teams and the reality. For your specific team, what are the two or three areas in which people have the greatest difficulty walking their talk?

This process involves team member interaction and honest reflection on strengths and weaknesses of the team. An exercise in reflection and frank communication helps team members (and soon-to-be team educators) shape and articulate the real issues and challenges that trainees confront when delivering collaborative care.

The second half of our training workshop involves group problem-solving through analysis of critical incidents. First, participants analyze critical incidents thematically. For example, one recurring theme might be conflict that is displaced, mediated, or diffused by a third party; another might be dilemmas of authority and leadership. Through this exercise, teams realize that their dilemmas fit into a broader picture, and they are increasingly able to teach trainees about the intricacies of team dynamics. The next steps in this particular workshop are to solve problems collaboratively, enact, role play, and role-switch. Each exercise helps the incipient team educator to ask, "How do I know what I know?" (about delivering collaborative care), and "How can I best teach others the same?" Train-the-trainers workshops should raise the following issues:

- What are team dynamics from a systems point of view?
- How is the whole team dynamic responsible for the actions of individuals?
- Is there something about the team that forces an individual into a particular role or action?
- Are there some conflicts that appear to be individual personality conflicts, but which, in fact, are systemic issue conflicts?
- Inasmuch as we create and maintain systems through our actions, are there patterns of behavior that we can change through performing different actions?

Having asked and answered these questions for themselves, team members are in a much better position to educate others in team building and team skills.

Participants can complete a short questionnaire to evaluate the workshop. Responses can be used to design future workshops on team work and team building and to facilitate the imparting of these skills to future trainers. It is our sense that such workshops would be a necessary and ongoing process in a GITT Project.

CONCLUSIONS

Academic institutions must redesign the training of health professionals to prepare for practice in integrated systems of care. Nowhere is this more important than in caring for frail older adults. Team training must be considered a necessary part of any educational initiative that aims to teach health professionals geriatrics skills. The authors developed a model of team training, one that is attuned to services mainly affiliated with the University of Pennsylvania and to the needs of elders living in Philadelphia. This model may be fully or partially transferable to other health systems and academic institutions in other cities. Certainly, the approach and philosophy can be employed in any setting.

The following is a list of important elements to consider when selecting and preparing faculty and clinical preceptors to become team trainers:

- Educators should display a commitment to transcending the boundaries of academic disciplines and learning how to practice relationship-centered and culturally competent care.
- Educators must be exposed to the application of concepts and methods in team training from the field of organizational development (e.g., Continuous Quality Improvement, Responsibility Charting, and so forth).
- Educators should have an awareness of the role of collaborative care within integrated health care systems and of the payer perspective in general.
- Educators must be trained in experiential, interactive classroom experiences (role playing, gaming, and so forth).
- Educators must be proficient in case-based learning and oriented toward problem solving.
- Educators must be ready to go beyond one-to-one discipline-specific training and engage in team-to-team preceptorships.

As primary, relationship-centered, preventive care gains a larger role in the overall delivery of geriatric health services, team training will become more important in the future of health professions education. Team educators who assume educational leadership for collaborative care may be called on to exhibit team-building competencies (as distinct from teamwork competencies for practitioners). One way to begin shaping team-building competencies is to promote these strengths and qualities in geriatrics educators who excel in team skills and in teaching others how to engage in teamwork. In this way, GITT initiatives could make a significant contribution by helping educators in the health professions provide relevant teaching and learning for geriatric trainees charged with caring for older adults in the next century.

Acknowledgments

The authors would like to thank Risa Lavizzo-Mourey, MD, MBA; Mario Moussa, Ph.D., Center for Applied Research; Robin Goldberg-Glen, Ph.D., MSW; and Cati Coe, M.A. for their contributions to the program or this chapter.

REFERENCES

Anderson, L. A., Persky, N. W., Whall, A. L., Campbell, R., Algase, D. L., Gillis, G. L., & Halter, J. B. (1994). Interdisciplinary team training in geriatrics: Reaching out to small and medium-size communities. *Gerontologist, 34,* 833–838.

Baldwin, D. C., & Baldwin, M. A. (1978). Interdisciplinary education and health team training: A model for learning and service. In A. D. Hunt & L. E. Weeks (Eds.). *Medical education since 1960: Marching to a different drummer* (pp. 201–203). East Lansing, MI: Michigan State University Foundation.

Browne, A., Carpenter, C., Cooledge, C., Drover, G., Ericksen, J., Fielding, D., Hill, D., Johnston, J., Segal, S., & Silver, J. (1995). Bridging the professions: An integrated and interdisciplinary approach to teaching health care ethics. *Academic Medicine, 70,* 1002–1005.

Coles, C. (1995). Educating the health care team. *Patient Education and Counseling, 26,* 239–244.

Evans, L. K. (1994). Overcoming institutional challenges to collaborative practice. In E. L. Siegler & F. W. Whitney (Eds.). *Nurse–physician collaboration: Care of adults and the elderly* (pp. 33–42). New York: Springer Publishing Co.

Evans, L. K., Yurkow, J., & Siegler, E. L. (1995). The CARE Program: A nurse-managed collaborative outpatient program to improve function of frail older people. *Journal of the American Geriatrics Society, 43,* 1155–1160.

Gilmore, T. N., & Schall, E. (1996). Staying alive to learning: Integrating enactments with case teaching to develop leaders. *Journal of Policy Analysis and Management, 15*(3), 1–13.

Grant, R. W., Finocchio, L. J., & the California Primary Care Consortium Subcommittee on Interdisciplinary Collaboration. (1995). *Interdisciplinary collaborative teams in primary care: A model curriculum and resource guide.* San Francisco: Pew Health Professions Commission.

Gurland, L. (1994). Attitudes, values, and ideologies as influences on the professional education and practice of those who care for the aged. In D. G. Satin (Ed.). *The clinical care of the aged person: An interdisciplinary perspective* (pp. 159–167). New York: Oxford University Press.

Headrick, L. A., Neuhauser, D., Schwab, P., & Stevens, D. P. (1995). Continuous quality improvement and the education of the generalist physician. *Academic Medicine, 70* (Suppl. 1), S104–109.

Headrick, L. A., Norman, L., Gelmon, S., & Knapp, A. (1995). *Interdisciplinary professional education in the continuous improvement of health care: The state-of-the-art.* Washington, DC: Health Services Resources Administration, Bureau of Health Professions.

Health Resources and Services Administration. (1996). *A national agenda for geriatric education: Forum report.* Washington, DC: USDHHS, Health Resources and Services Administration, Bureau of Health Professions.

Irby, D. M. (1994). Three exemplary models of case-based teaching. *Academic Medicine, 69,* 947–953.

Kahn, N. B. Jr., Davis, A. K., Wartman, S. A., Wilson, M. E., & Kahn, R. H. (1995). The interdisciplinary generalist curriculum project: A national medical school demonstration project. *Academic Medicine, 70* (Suppl. 1), S75–80.

Klein S. (Ed.). (1995). *A national agenda for geriatric education: White papers*. Rockville, MD: Health Resources and Services Administration.

Kues, J. R., Fitzwater, E., Schwartz, P. J., Braun, D. M., Frederick, K. A., & Greengus, L. B. (1992). The development and use of gaming in multidisciplinary geriatric education. *Educational Gerontology, 18*, 27–40.

Lister, L. (1982). Role training for interdisciplinary health teams. *Health and Social Work, 7*, 19–29.

Mears, P. (1994). *Healthcare teams: Building continuous quality improvement*. Delray Beach, FL: St. Lucie Press.

Myers, J. E. (1994). Education and training of aged-care providers. *Disability and Rehabilitation, 16*, 171–180.

Pew Health Professions Commission. (1995a). *Health professions education and managed care: Challenges and necessary responses*. San Francisco: UCSF Center for the Health Professions.

Pew Health Professions Commission. (1995b). *Critical challenges: Revitalizing the health professions for the twenty-first century*. San Francisco: UCSF Center for the Health Professions.

Strumpf, N. E., & Whitney, F. W. (1994). Teaching collaborative skills to nurse practitioner students. In E. L. Siegler & F. W. Whitney (Eds.), *Nurse–physician collaboration: Care of adults and the elderly* (pp. 159–167). New York: Springer Publishing Co.

Tresolini, C. P., & the Pew-Fetzer Task Force. (1994). *Health professions education and relationship-centered care*. San Francisco: Pew Health Professions Commission.

CHAPTER 6

Planning GITT: The Providers

Joann Castle

The Geriatric Interdisciplinary Team Training (GITT) Program offers the opportunity for participating sites to rethink how to provide the best geriatric care for patients and their families while enhancing the satisfaction of clinicians. This chapter examines the development of a training model for geriatric interdisciplinary teams from the perspective of clinicians who are front-line providers of care for geriatric patients. In evaluating the GITT experience, we are learning how to solve the problems clinicians face as they move from the traditional independent practice model to the GITT project, where they must both precept trainees and work in teams to meet the multidimensional needs of an exploding population of frail elderly.

This chapter is divided into three sections. The first section describes factors that motivate clinicians to work in teams. The second considers barriers to program implementation especially relevant to clinicians and offers a progress report on how we are addressing these barriers. The final section summarizes lessons we have learned in the process of establishing teams, and how these issues may affect the establishment of new training sites.

Although this chapter focuses on the Great Lakes GITT, discussions with colleagues in GITT Projects around the country confirm that the themes presented here apply generally. Great Lakes GITT is a collaborative effort of provider organizations and academic affiliates in both Cleveland and Detroit. Participating institutions include the Henry Ford Health System, University Hospitals Health System, Case Western Reserve University, Wayne State University, and the Benjamin Rose Institute. Both health systems are vertically integrated, nonprofit delivery systems with long histories and strong relationships in their respective communities. Clinical settings include family practice and internal medicine clinics, geriatric clinics, retirement community clinics, inpatient units, home care, nursing homes, and a Program for All-Inclusive Care for the Elderly replication site, based on the On Lok model (see chapter 12).

Our initial interest in teamwork developed in response to (a) dissatisfaction voiced by frustrated clinicians who were attempting to address all the medical, functional, and social needs of older patients in traditional practice, and (b) inefficiencies in the continuum of care resulting from poor communication between providers and between providers, patients, and families. Most challenging have been frail patients with some combination of health problems, cognitive dysfunction, functional impairments, and family stresses. Often these patients present with a variety of geriatric syndromes that do not lend themselves to quick resolution with the traditional tools of acute care medicine—medication and surgery.

The increasing prevalence of managed care has also magnified provider stress. These systems place more pressure on the clinician to provide comprehensive and coordinated service—to be the primary care provider and care coordinator, patient educator, patient advocate, and gatekeeper.

FACTORS THAT MOTIVATE PROVIDERS TO WORK IN TEAMS

Over the years, clinicians and administrators have identified patterns of caring for the elderly that limit provider and patient satisfaction. We can think about these issues in three categories: the challenges of caring for frail elderly, patient response to care and treatment recommendations, and clinician response to the work environment (such as provider satisfaction and professional development in the practice setting). As we reviewed these issues, we began to develop strategies for addressing them. We believed from our own experience and the experiences of others that some form of teamwork would help.

The Challenges of Providing Care for Frail Elderly

A single provider cannot treat the multiple, complex problems of frail older patients. Clinicians in geriatrics realize early on what an immense breadth of knowledge is needed to work with this group. Patient needs are complex, and their conditions are often chronic and debilitating. Patients with functional impairments require additional resources to maintain a good quality of life. As a result, clinicians become frustrated with their inability to be all things to all people; they feel personally responsible when there is a poor outcome.

Caring for the frail elderly takes significantly more clinic time. With them, not only is the physical exam slower and more elaborate, but clarifying and sorting out issues for demented patients and communication with family or caregivers also take more time. In complex cases, providers often must consult nutritionists, psychologists, rehabilitation professionals, or pharmacists.

Ad hoc communication is not adequate to manage a complex patient successfully. Clinicians have learned from experience that good support systems are critical to successful outcomes. Yet, all too often, communication breakdowns in large health systems result in gaps in continuity of care and become a major factor in litigation. Both clinicians and patients would benefit from a total patient management plan that is more responsive.

Patient Responses to Care and Treatment Recommendations

The traditional practice model often fails elderly patients. They may have difficulty complying with treatment regimens that they do not understand or are alien to their lifestyle. A patient may be unable to afford medication, may not have transportation to an appointment, or may have limited function and be living alone. In addition, elderly patients can become depressed with their diminishing function and have difficulty complying with treatment.

Patients may express dissatisfaction with the referral process and lack of care coordination, or they may be confused about goals of care. Often families are distant from these issues until there is a crisis, and then differences in culture and belief systems and ethical dilemmas add another level of complexity. It is difficult for clinician, patient, and family to develop trust.

Professional Satisfaction and Development

The care of seniors can be especially frustrating when a clinician's best efforts are not enough to improve the patient's quality of life. Clinicians routinely face adverse outcomes or end-of-life decisions that may be overwhelming. They often become isolated, lacking opportunities for professional development. The limited opportunities for continuing education usually occur off site on conference days, and there is little time for follow-up research or reflection on the material.

Learning to Work Together

Thus, the daily life of providers is often characterized by complex patients, adverse outcomes, ethical decisions, and managing and responding to everyday stresses in the clinic environment. These are key factors that motivate providers to form teams. Teamwork, in the broadest sense, offers potential solutions to all of these challenges.

According to our clinicians, the formation of teams was a natural evolution in geriatric care. These providers reported that teams had developed spontaneously as long as 15 years ago; other teams were more recent creations, but all seemed to emerge as a logical solution to the challenges of geriatric care.

Clinicians believe that teams hold promise. Patient care plans improve with input from medicine, nursing, and social work; teams set patient management goals based on the functional and interpersonal aspects of care. Team members learn from each other, identify weak spots in the care plans, and improve them. Team meetings frequently provide new insights into patient problems. It is not unusual for team members to call patients following a team meeting and share new ideas. With a team approach, members believe that they are able to anticipate issues, set goals, and be more productive. Team care also increases provider availability to patients, and patient satisfaction is a significant reward.

Clinicians believe that the efforts of multiple team members increase the opportunities for satisfactory communication. Improved communication between patients and caregivers contributes to a successful treatment outcome. The interdisciplinary knowledge of the team and the relationships between family and team members facilitate discussion of patient values and preferences during stressful times. Considering patients and their families as contributing members of the team and incorporating their input in the care plan builds understanding, encourages trust, and results in a more successful patient-centered plan.

In sharing the care, clinicians believe that they enhance their practice skills. Team members report that in the course of day-to-day work, the interdisciplinary setting offers an opportunity to go back to their colleagues and evaluate what remains to be done. Teams provide a forum to consult with trusted and supportive colleagues, acknowledge difficulties, learn from the experience, and move ahead.

Given that many of our clinicians were working in teams and believe in the value of team care, what motivated them to participate in GITT? GITT provides an educational structure, with training in a wide variety of collaborative skills and techniques, team concepts, managed care, technical innovations, and competence in geriatrics. GITT provides more opportunity for group interaction, critical and creative thinking, and setting goals for improvement. Clinicians are interested in the structured way that the GITT Demonstration Project improves the work setting. The Great Lakes GITT Project, for example, teaches learning tools to process and analyze day-to-day activities with the goal of improving care.

GITT also provides opportunities to meet people from other areas and other systems who are facing similar challenges. The exchange of ideas is stimulating. Access to experts and learning materials accelerates learning, and team members set aside time to consider how to improve outcomes. In addition, involvement in GITT brings outside consultants to assist in evaluating the project and provides opportunities to publish. All of these benefits motivate our clinicians to work in teams and to participate in GITT.

BARRIERS TO TEAMS

Early implementation of GITT has not occurred without challenges. As the teams formed, and clinicians moved from conventional practice to teamwork, we observed both practice and structural barriers to team functioning. I describe here some of these barriers and how we are addressing them.

Changing Norms of Practice

Working together in the interdisciplinary setting requires a change in norms of practice. Team members must face issues such as egalitarian relationships and the loss of autonomy for physicians, disciplinary and gender biases, and shared responsibility and accountability. These issues are subtle and sometimes personally threatening, because they touch at the deepest levels of practice style.

Defining roles and relationships can be a helpful and nonthreatening format for discussion of disciplinary and interpersonal differences. One pilot team in the Great Lakes program began these discussions using a team assessment tool to evaluate their interactions and then reflected on the results. The team decided to devote 20 minutes at each meeting to ongoing discussion, which lasted a number of weeks and allowed the group to solve specific problems, rather than engage in a quick, shallow review.

In team decision making, each discipline must sacrifice some degree of autonomy for collaborative problem solving to occur (Abramson & Rosenthal, 1995). Physician dominance of the team's decision making can be a difficult issue for members of other health professions. Individual practitioners who have long-term involvement with particular patients and have developed special relationships may at times be reluctant to transfer responsibility for the patient to team care and team decisions. Because they have been socialized to take charge, many physicians may be reluctant or just find it difficult to give up authority. In the course of one team's recent self-assessment, a question in the team assessment tool inquired about the physician's authority to change a decision made by the team, prompting fruitful discussion and conscious reflection on team roles.

Case Study

The primary physician presented a case, explaining that he had been following this patient without input of other team members. According to the physician, the patient had not been seen by a nurse practitioner because each time she presented for care, it was related to a health crisis that required immediate medical management.

> The patient was an 89-year-old woman with congestive heart failure. Based on her prognosis, the patient had already exceeded her life expectancy by 5 years, which the physician perceived had much to do with successful medical management. His specific reason for bringing the case to the team meeting at this time was his frustration over her inpatient management. The patient's condition was deteriorating, and every time the patient had a crisis and went to the emergency room or was hospitalized, providers who did not know the patient chose treatment plans that disrupted the delicate balance of his care. In such a tightly managed treatment plan, the physician felt that the primary provider should have some authority when the patient was evaluated in the emergency room or admitted to the inpatient setting.
>
> The response from the team was not what the physician expected. An initial comment was that this was a team clinic, and this patient did not have the benefit of a team. The response from nursing was a recommendation that the patient be offered the option of hospice care. The physician had difficulty with the suggestion of hospice. He reported that the patient expressed a desire to live and he felt that the proposal of a hospice would be a breach of the patient's right to autonomy. He had checked on the possibility of a heart transplant but the patient was not a candidate. In later discussion with the patient about do not resuscitate orders, the patient was not able to make up her mind and had requested that the physician consider power of attorney so that he could decide how to respond when the situation arose. When the social worker asked about family, the physician reported that there was none.
>
> Team members then began to comment that this patient was trying to make difficult decisions on her own, without the benefit of a team. Further discussion revealed that the patient had a friend and possibly a nephew who had in the past expressed an interest in her condition. The social worker suggested a family or caregiver conference at which the issues could be fully discussed.
>
> The case study is a good example of contrasts between individual and team approaches and the varying perspectives of the disciplines. Ultimately, after the family conference, the patient chose hospice as her care alternative.

As teams set goals and learn to work together, cultural differences among the professions will normally be an asset, but can also act as a barrier to team development. Clark (1995) emphasizes that cultural differences in knowledge and value-related dimensions of professional practice affect our work. Values underlie conflicting and competing communication patterns among health professionals, whose distinct educational experiences lead to different styles of practice and a different logic in approaching the geriatric patient.

Physicians have been trained to approach the treatment plan by ruling out problems and systematically eliminating possibilities. In some cases, physicians, who are oriented to curing illness, may become frustrated or lose interest when a cure cannot be achieved (Kayser-Jones, 1986). Social workers, on the other hand, approach the problem by ruling in problems, looking at the workings of things and the interrelationships in the patient's broader world. Nurses may be more focused on patient preferences or abilities.

Individuals may have different perspectives on life-extending treatment, hospice, or the goals of care. The team approach seems our best option for breaking down these barriers in the professions. Working together in teams creates a broader spectrum of options and greater potential for developing a successful treatment plan. To facilitate positive use of cultural differences, the curriculum of Great Lakes GITT includes sessions on culture and communication issues, examining the cultural values of both the professions and of the patients.

Responsibility and Accountability

Team care also requires a new approach to responsibility and accountability. This change requires individuals to adjust their practice styles. Clinicians report that decision makers who wish to be the center of attention have particular difficulty with shared responsibility; one team has reported reconfiguring its membership because a seasoned professional was not comfortable sharing accountability. Not all individuals may be suited for teams.

Teams require a merging of individual and mutual accountability. In the past, physicians alone have been held accountable for the care of patients. Legally, this remains the case. But in the team setting, each member of the work team feels responsible and is held accountable for the team's performance. All members participate in discussion and decision making.

Team members become more aware of their own accountability when they are dependent on each other's contribution to meet their collective goals. No one can procrastinate or ignore the work to be done because the whole group is dependent on each individual's effort. The team must review its progress regularly and create an incentive for each individual to be responsible to the work of the whole. This is another reason for aggressively protecting team time, as the quality and continuity of patient care may depend on the team's problem-solving and follow-up activities.

Structural Issues

Structural change of the scope envisioned in GITT can occur only when all are committed and cooperative. Although specifics will vary, all sites must confront structural issues such as time, space, risk management, and financing. Clinicians participating in GITT often feel a conflict between expectations of the project, which requires time for team meetings and teaching, and broader organizational priorities for cost cutting and provider productivity. There is no easy solution to these challenges, but administrative support and commitment are crucial (see chapter 12).

Time and Space

As the GITT Project was introduced to providers, their immediate concern was time. Opportunities for team development and continual improvement are central to the learning team, but a team that works on its development is taking that time away from other activities. If clinicians take time from their extremely busy and stressful work day, that investment must in turn provide value to their patients. For this reason, the teams found that using the case method approach was an efficient way to learn: first, to resolve individual patient cases, and second, to grow as a team by analyzing the effectiveness of their collaborative effort.

Faced with the conflict of personal and professional needs and the needs of patients, practitioners find it difficult to take time for themselves, often working through lunch or staying late to accommodate patients. When interrupted during a meeting time for phone calls or patient walk-ins, clinicians will give higher priority to their patients. Several of our teams have reported this to be a problem and are working on approaches such as controlling schedules and routing phone calls to protect team time without short-changing patients.

Finding space for trainee offices, team meetings, and family conferences is frequently difficult. Some GITT clinical settings are converting a single office into multiple work stations for trainees. Team meetings can even be held in the waiting room because patients are not scheduled at those times. Clinicians of different disciplines may share large offices to facilitate efficient use of space and increase cross-discipline communication.

To accomplish our goals and minimize the effect of time, space, and other structural barriers, Great Lakes GITT took a strong position in support of administrative involvement in the program. From the early development of our collaborative work, we felt that the involvement of managers and the management sciences in our project would facilitate GITT, and we invited administrators of target clinics to participate in the central team training program.

Realizing that clinic managers and administrators across clinics and cities would have much in common, administrators arranged a breakout session to focus on their concerns. A faculty member from the business school facilitated the session.

Discussion in the breakout session focused on outcome measures from the clinic and health system perspective. At this session, administrators shared their goals: (a) improve the efficiency of clinical operations, (b) enhance the quality of care, and (c) preserve the financial resources of the parent system. We have tried to organize Great Lakes GITT to help them meet these goals and are using the following tactics to secure administrative involvement:

- Managers are participating as actively as possible with their individual learning teams.
- We are informing managers about evaluation activities, particularly those that relate to patient outcomes.
- We are soliciting input from managers about common measures for evaluation.

- We are developing the computer-based library to support managers' interests in clinical teams and outcome measurement and an electronic conference folder through which managers can participate in dialogues about their role in the program.
- We are establishing a process to respond to administrators' interests in curriculum and program development.

Active involvement and investment in the program allow administrators to address issues of productivity, scheduling, and budget within the context of the program as part of their broader responsibilities for these operational functions.

Risk Management

In some circles, the exploration of team care raises legal questions. Although risk management administrators are often concerned about team care, not all agree that collaborative practice presents more risks than practice by individuals. On one hand, the greater the number of people involved in patient care decisions, the more vulnerable the system. On the other hand, the more clinicians there are who understand what the patient needs and wants, and the more the patient feels attended to, the less likely mistakes will occur. Ultimately, administrators comment that no matter what team members do individually or collectively, when something goes wrong, the institution is responsible.

Experts argue that the key to avoiding risk is good communication (Frankel, 1994). Sharing information is a key element in collaborative practice. Each team member's role in the transmission of information should be clearly understood and clarified in team meetings (Henry Ford Health System, 1995). Teams should investigate and discuss limits and restrictions as they relate to patient care and to individual versus team responsibility. After teams gain experience, they can review their work together, perhaps as a continuous improvement exercise, in an effort to minimize risky behaviors and identify guidelines for proactive risk management.

In addition, in the interdisciplinary model, the patient's role within the collaborative practice environment is becoming better defined. As teams make greater efforts to include patients in team activities, on-going negotiation with patients for the most appropriate course of treatment will keep the team on course and lower risk. The process of soliciting information from and informing patients will avoid misunderstandings and keep the team working in concert with the patient's best interest.

Financing

As the fee-for-service environment erodes, financial incentives are changing. The growth of various models of managed care has contributed to an environment that is more conducive to team care. These new systems are designed to promote the management of resources, but they also permit new flexibility and options for provider organizations to be innovative in designing how care is delivered.

In many ways, the growth of managed care has opened the door to teams; some systems are requiring clinicians to provide care efficiently and at the same time have eliminated the reimbursement limitations that existed under the fee-for-service method. The group practice setting also seems to enhance team development. Team care flows more easily where salaried colleagues work together and share resources under a financial structure that rewards professionals for keeping patients healthy and self-reliant. In independent practice, under a fee-for-service incentive structure, this is more difficult but not impossible; in these settings, teams or their administrators should investigate billing options for team members.

SHAPING CHANGE

Choosing a Team Model

For the demonstration project, each of the GITT sites has developed a unique team training model that best fits its particular circumstances and resources. The training method adopted by Great Lakes GITT is based on the belief that change can best be achieved with a model that first targets geriatric practice sites and then works upstream to effect change in academic institutions. According to Berwick (1996), the best way to change systems is through careful inductive learning by persons who have a deep knowledge of their own work and behavior and who are most intimately involved in the system processes. Similarly, the best way to improve the care of older adults is for those persons most intimately involved in that care to observe and understand the care processes and the relationship between those processes and care outcomes.

Learning Teams

Consistent with our commitment to inductive learning, the Great Lakes GITT Project participants believe that interdisciplinary learning teams provide an effective mix of structure and process for organizing and improving geriatric care. Learning teams (Michaelsen & Black, 1994) are characterized by their focus on learning by improving their process and their product through conscious and continuous cycles of learning together. Great Lakes GITT learning teams, coached by facilitators, use a reflective process and cycles of learning to identify problems or issues, gather relevant data, test solutions in the workplace laboratory, and evaluate results. We believe that this process is effective for finding new solutions to old problems and enabling care systems to be flexible and responsive to changing needs. Conscious cycles of reflection, learning, and doing can accelerate team growth, benefiting both the patient and provider. The model offers a highly structured approach often used in quality improvement models. The process establishes meeting objectives, assigns roles, and rotates leadership and includes a meeting evaluation as a learning tool for continual improvement.

Identifying a Learning Cycle

The theory of learning cycles proposes that there is a circular pattern to change and development that can be viewed in a series of small plan, do, check, and act cycles (Langley, Nolan, & Nolan, 1994) associated with quality improvement. Initially, we found the concept of learning cycles to be vague and difficult to describe to clinicians in our pilot program. Our curriculum plan to teach the method in workshops was met with some resistance. Clinicians who attended the workshop as trainees strongly expressed their feelings that teamwork cannot be learned in a classroom but has to be experienced in the patient care setting. We quickly learned that clinicians do not like to be talked at, and the continuous quality improvement jargon was not helpful. However, clinicians were willing to use a structured process to improve the efficiency of their meetings. Thus, we used this tool as a bridge to the more elusive concept of learning cycles.

After several cycles of meeting evaluations, clarifying objectives, and planning of next agendas, the learning cycle concept unfolded in the team as a group discovery. This realization occurred when the team was making plans to present their experiences at a workshop. As the team developed a storyboard to display their work, members expressed surprise at their accomplishments. They identified the following learning cycles in a team meeting.

As a team they had:

Studied the dynamics of team meetings
Discussed roles and responsibilities in team practice
Performed a team assessment and discussed results
Identified a process determining when to refer patients to social work and when to
    refer to geropsychiatry
Discussed how to prepare the teams to receive students and drafted a new scheduling
    procedure to accommodate team meeting time
Identified the desire to become better preceptors and were pursuing resources to
    achieve that goal.

Thus, within three or four months, the clinician teams became comfortable with the concept of learning cycles and could see how to design and implement these cycles. Chapter 5 describes faculty training in more detail.

Redefining Team Roles and Relationships

The responsibilities of team members must be clearly defined. These may vary for each team or clinic depending on mission, practice styles, or team goals. All team members must discuss and understand their roles and their relationships with each other. Use of a team assessment tool for members to evaluate their team's performance often facilitates discussion. Some sample survey questions (Schmitt, Heinemann, & Farrell, 1994) that one team used were: "My team's basic mission is clear to me," "Members of this team spend considerable time doing things that are not consistent with our main goals," and "Responsibilities for implementing the team's decisions are not always well defined." Respondents answered on a 6-point scale ranging from "strongly disagree" to "strongly agree," setting the stage for discussion.

As the team grows, roles can become more flexible and interchangeable. As teams mature, changes begin to occur in patterns of care delivery. These changes, in turn, require reevaluation of members' roles and duties.

Clinicians agree that it is important to select team members carefully. Members must believe in teams, must want to be team players, and must understand the function of team roles. Individuals must be able to support each other, share a common vision, and have an appreciation of each person's role in making this vision come alive. They must have a respect for others and their contributions. They need not be close friends or socialize together outside the clinic.

Experienced clinicians report that team development is much like individual development, only it occurs in the group setting. Strides forward often occur out of crises or in the context of adversity, for instance, when there is an external threat or a serious problem occurs. At one of our clinics, team development accelerated when everyone banded together to reverse a projected closing of the clinic. At such times, much is usually at stake and goals become crystal clear.

CONCLUSIONS

How These Issues Affect the Establishment of Future Clinical Training Settings

This is a demonstration project that is unfolding and developing as we learn from our experiences. All parties will feel uncertain and anxious. As we move toward a more clearly defined vision of team models, we will encounter clinician apprehensions about changing roles and relationships and tension and conflicts between team members. Those who have not been teachers in the past will be nervous about precepting. Building trust and confidence takes time.

We can best allay clinician fears about teams by helping them to understand the process in the broader context by coaching and supporting, by sharing experiences, and by searching for a broader understanding of the concept of change. GITT staff, in coordination with the Resource Center, can provide information about techniques and communication skills that will help clinicians through the process. Administrators must support the effort and address the structural problems of space, time, and resources to facilitate the work. For providers, the GITT Project will require both personal and organizational change to effect new norms and patterns of practice.

Lessons Learned

We are at the beginning of a 3-year demonstration project, and it is difficult to fully comprehend what we are learning. There are a number of issues that have come to our attention in the clinic setting, including:

1. The change we are proposing is not a surface change. It is far reaching and fundamental. It affects the way clinicians practice and the way administrators organize a clinic. As a consequence, we need to be honest and clear with people about the depth of the change and what we are asking of them.
2. Current patient case loads are large, and the demands on practitioners' time are in conflict with ideal conditions for implementing a training program. We continue to work closely with administrators and clinicians to find the time to build and train teams; we have also been obliged to make adjustments in our program.

3. We live in a world that promotes solitary achievement. Many practitioners have become vested in discipline-specific work and are rightfully proud of their individual accomplishments. Although team care offers advantages, the loss of autonomy or the personal gratification that comes from individual accomplishment may be compromised. This program requires patience.

4. We must struggle to bridge the gap between practitioners and academics that results from the historic separation of our work environments. The academic, theoretic approach must be rooted in the daily practice of health care. Similarly, learning team theory has been essential to the development of practice teams. Theory can provide the conceptual framework that can give greater meaning to spontaneous experiences of complex clinical care.

5. In the course of the GITT experience, we have learned that clinicians can be excited about the concept, its learning environment, and the opportunity to work with and learn from colleagues who share a commitment to improving health care for elderly adults. The committed clinicians are key ambassadors and role models for more reluctant professionals in our delivery systems.

6. It is imperative to involve administrators in the training process and to keep them close to the action. It is within their realm of responsibility to facilitate change; they control the context and evaluate the value of teams in meeting organizational objectives.

SUMMARY

This chapter has considered the views and concerns of providers in the early development of GITT. Providers who live the change experience are struggling to make teamwork come alive in response to the needs of their patients and their personal commitment to collaborate for a better future.

We see that many dynamics are at work: some motivate providers to support this change and others act as barriers. For the clinician, interdisciplinary teamwork is a natural evolution on the one hand, as it brings multiple providers together to meet complex geriatric problems. On the other hand, it demands a change in practice patterns that may not be comfortable or even possible for everyone. It is a transformation in thinking about our work.

The GITT Program has created a learning environment that stimulates new ways of thinking and offers the opportunity to share and reflect on new ideas. The effort links professionals in different locations and different settings and provides a format for moving the work forward in the context of research and evaluation. Such motivations and rewards make it possible for the pioneers to move ahead while grappling with an undeveloped model in a changing context.

Acknowledgments

I wish to thank the following individuals: Orry Jacobs, Executive Vice-President, University Hospitals of Cleveland; Glenn Davis, MD, Vice President for Henry Ford Health

System (HFHS) Academic Affairs and Chief Medical Officer, Suburban Region; Mary Beth Tupper, MD, Division Chief, HFHS Geriatrics and Project Director for the Great Lakes GITT; Alice Early, Nurse Practitioner and Team Leader at the HFHS Center for Seniors; Phyllis Collier, Nurse Practitioner and Team Leader at the Livonia Medical Center's Nurse Managed Clinic; Murray Hunter, MD, HFHS Center for Seniors; Lynda Iras, Administrative Manager at the Center for Senior Independence (PACE); Peter Metropoulis, MD, also at the Center for Senior Independence; and Lauren Somple, Social Worker at the ElderHealth Center. I would also like to thank Donnie Jones for her invaluable technical assistance and Nancy Whitelaw for her constant support and encouragement and her many suggestions to the direction of this work.

REFERENCES

Abramson, J., & Rosenthal, B. (1995). Interdisciplinary and interorganizational collaboration. In R. L. Edwards (Editor-in-chief), *Encyclopedia of social work* (Vol. 19, pp. 1479–1489). Washington, DC: NASW Press.

Berwick, D. (1996). Harvesting knowledge from improvement. *Journal of the American Medical Association, 271,* 877–878.

Clark, P. G. (1995). Quality of life, values, and teamwork in geriatric care: Do we communicate what we mean? *Gerontologist, 35,* 402–411.

Frankel, R. M. (1994). *Communicating with patients* (pp. 1–16). Deerfield, IL: MMI Risk Management Resources, Inc.

Henry Ford Health System (1995). Caveat. *Office of Medical Legal Affairs–Henry Ford Health System, 7*(9/10), 1–3.

Kayser-Jones, J. S. (1986). Distributive justice and the treatment of acute illness in nursing homes. *Social Science in Medicine, 23,* 1279–1286.

Langley, J. G., Nolan, K. M., & Nolan, T. W. (1994). The foundation of improvement. *Quality Progress, 27*(6), 81–86.

Michaelsen, L. K., & Black, R. H. (1994). *Building learning teams: The key to harnessing the power of small groups in higher education.* Oklahoma City, OK: Growth Partners.

Schmitt, M. H., Heinemann, G. D., & Farrell, M. P. (1994). *Interdisciplinary health care teams: Proceedings of the Sixteenth Annual Conference.* Chicago, IL: School of Allied Health Sciences, Indiana University School of Medicine, Indiana University Medical Center.

CHAPTER 7

Using Existing and Emerging Technologies to Promote GITT

Sue Levkoff, Patricia Flynn Weitzman, and Eben A. Weitzman

Educational efforts designed to promote interdisciplinary learning and team building must fulfill two key requirements. One is a flexible curriculum, which allows trainers to customize learning experiences to account for a variety of perspectives and sources of information. The other requirement is inclusion of open-ended, authentic problems that have direct relevance to the trainees (Jones, Rasmussen, & Moffit, 1997). Educators can use existing and emerging technologies to satisfy both of these requirements. These technologies can offer real-life, interactive learning experiences based on up-to-the-minute information, and they can be individualized. They can make rich observational data available to instructors, trainees, and researchers, and they can facilitate communications among large and geographically dispersed teams of providers, teachers, and trainees.

Although it offers enormous advantages, technology is not essential for meeting the requirements of interdisciplinary learning and team building. Skilled instructors have been using customized learning techniques and open-ended, real-life problems in the classroom and clinic well before current technologies were available. Thus, for technology to make a meaningful contribution to geriatric team training, instructors must carefully consider these applications in advance. Simply putting a textbook on the computer does not add anything substantive to the learning experience.

Are there team building and interdisciplinary practice learning activities that can occur more effectively through the use of technology? The survey of tools being used at the various Geriatric Interdisciplinary Team Training (GITT) projects suggests there are. In particular, technology can eliminate distance barriers to group contact, promote complex clinical data collection and analysis, and offer self-paced learning that is especially helpful when trainees have varied educational backgrounds.

Those who seek to create GITT projects must keep in mind that technology can never substitute for face-to-face encounters and interactions. They merely supplement them. Nonetheless, technology can stimulate growth for instructors by allowing them to develop interactive, innovative learning programs by providing easy access to extensive multidisciplinary sources of information. And, by bringing together instructors and trainees at disparate locations, technology can greatly enhance the scope of GITT. Where team training once was not possible because of geographic obstacles, it now is. Rural trainees can become members of teams training in distant cities and vice versa. Similarly, patients in rural areas can access state-of-the-art team care from practitioners in urban centers. The elimination of distance barriers may be technology's most important role in GITT today.

TECHNOLOGIES USED AT GITT SITES

Several of the GITT centers have integrated technology into their training efforts, including computer software, videotape, teleconferencing, and palmtop computers. The rest of this chapter describes how sites have adapted the technology to meet their specific training needs.

Computer Software

Computer software packages are a widely available, relatively low-cost technology that can assist in data management and communication. Desktop and laptop computers are widely available; for a minimal investment of time and money certain software packages can help address the data management and communication needs that arise in GITT.

The Great Lakes GITT project consists of two merged centers, one in Cleveland and one in Detroit. In their efforts to eliminate distance barriers, they use a groupware software program called First Class (Soft Arc, 1997). First Class is knowledge management software designed primarily to facilitate group collaboration. This software serves the following functions:

1. It provides a communication link between programs operating in Detroit and Cleveland. It acts almost as a common classroom for the two centers so that trainees and instructors in Detroit can maintain easy, regular contact with trainees and instructors in Cleveland. Shared public discussions can occur via E-mail.

2. Within each of the two centers, it also aids communication between faculty and project leaders. Thus it helps promote teamwork on the institutional level—between administrators and faculty—that provides a valuable model for trainee teams.

3. As a knowledge management tool, First Class can be used as a repository of extensive information on the care and treatment of the elderly, including case studies, research, and relevant legislation. Trainees can supplement their learning by accessing this information.

4. Finally, and perhaps most importantly, trainees use the software to communicate with other team members about learning experiences. By eliminating the logistic problems often associated with getting a group of team members together in the same place at the same time (especially during harsh Midwestern winters), First Class enables trainees and team members to spend more time sharing ideas with one another.

The Houston GITT project is using hypertext for its clinical learning modules. Hypertext is a form of software that allows the developer to create links between separate pages of information. The user is then freed from progressing through the material linearly; rather each user can create a unique path through the geriatric content via hypertext linkages. The pages of information comprising each module (typically over 100 in Houston's products) contain text, graphics, audio, and video. The computer mouse is used to click on words or icons, resulting in a jump to another page.

The modules have been used in the clinical teaching setting in two different ways. Some instructors distribute a particular module as an adjunct to a clinical experience, such as following a visit to an incontinent patient or as additional orientation to interdisciplinary team roles. Trainees are asked to install the modules on a computer running Microsoft Windows, review the materials, and comment in a later session. The second use for the hypertext modules is to have several trainees review the material independently in a computer learning center. The instructor floats between the trainees and computers, providing individualized assistance to trainees as they work on the module; group discussions can follow. Although this software does not promote group collaborations in the way that First Class does, it facilitates trainee learning by making multidisciplinary information easily available. In this way, hypertext can link sets of discipline-specific data to promote interdisciplinary thinking and can allow each learner to create an individualized path through the material.

As a part of its training curriculum, On Lok's GITT site is using the electronic information system developed by On Lok, Inc. and used by On Lok Senior Health Services. The Case Management Information System (CMIS 1993–1997, On Lok, Inc., San Francisco, CA) is a computerized medical record system that all team members use to record patient progress notes, evaluations, and treatments. Providers can access progress notes and treatment plans from multiple disciplines, and can create and update interdisciplinary care plans and treatments. The CMIS is an effective tool for teaching trainees about the process and outcomes of interdisciplinary care.

Videotapes

Videotapes can enhance geriatric training in a number of ways. The most straightforward is simply to show existing tapes that focus on particular topics, such as clinical assessment, urinary incontinence, and so forth. Instructors can also videotape actual patient-team interactions. This can be helpful in evaluating trainee progress in a particular clinical content area. Videotapes of interactions between team members during a clinical meeting or between trainees and patients are also helpful. They enable trainees to gain valuable insights into group processes when they watch tapes of themselves interacting with other team members during meetings or during patient exams. The tapes can become a valuable training tool in group interaction for future trainees, as well.

Several of the GITT sites have video projects. These include the development of a videotape library of didactic sessions (Rush GITT), geriatric case studies (University of Colorado GITT), and actual patient–clinical team interactions (Houston GITT). Furthermore, On Lok is currently using the PACE (Program for All-Inclusive Care for the Elderly) Assessment Training Tapes for Nurses. This videotape series introduces nurses to issues related to the evaluation of geriatric patients and on the use of PACE Reliability Forms. The tapes also provide an excellent overview of how to conduct functional assessments. Nurse trainees watch the tapes, complete the PACE forms, and are scored on their performance. On Lok is also in the process of developing an interactive CD ROM (expected to be completed by 1998) through which trainees will receive an orientation to On Lok, an introduction to the concepts of interdisciplinary team practice, and exposure to case studies.

Training techniques called the standardized patient teaching method and objective structured clinic exams (OSCE) used by the Mount Sinai and Houston centers, respectively, incorporate videotaping. Both methods rely on actors who simulate the behaviors of actual geriatric patients. The methods involve the presentation of several simulated cases over the course of the training period. Each interdisciplinary team has the opportunity to interview the patient as a group. An instructor helps shape the interview to highlight information on which team members from the different disciplines should focus. Faculty observe interviews via closed circuit television as they take place; the interviews are videotaped, as well. At the end of the training period, all teams come together as one group to discuss the cases. This meeting is also videotaped and observed by faculty.

Although these methods are not heavily technical—both rely mainly on the data provided by human actors in face-to-face interaction—videotaping enhances the process of evaluation of trainees. Also, the videos that result from these two methods can become an educational resource for future trainees.

Video Conferencing

Although the use of groupware software can close distance barriers between team members and program locations, it consists largely of typed messages between individuals, to which others can have later access. Video conferencing is a far more powerful tool to break down geographic barriers because it permits live audio-video transmissions.

Through a unique arrangement with the state of Pennsylvania, the University of Pennsylvania's Delaware Valley Geriatric Education Center uses state-owned video-conferencing equipment for face-to-face communication with their three remote geriatric training sites. Nursing home professionals from the three sites are brought together at the University of Pennsylvania for a kickoff conference to get to know each other in person and begin the process of team building. Then, every other week after their initial face-to-face meeting, all participants continue to meet via video conferencing. The equipment can transmit didactic lectures, videotapes, slides, and documents. Participants scattered throughout the state can view materials simultaneously, then discuss them together afterward.

The University of Pennsylvania's Institute on Aging has a similar set up that allows video conferencing for meetings and consultations with two remote medical centers that are establishing geriatric education centers. Unlike the state-owned system, this configuration does not use a closed system; it runs over public telephone lines, so its capabilities are a bit more limited.

Faculty at the University of North Carolina (UNC) School of Medicine are also using video conferencing to communicate with trainees in rural training sites. This allows, for example, a GITT faculty member to precept a masters-level social work trainee doing fieldwork at a facility in rural North Carolina where there are no local faculty.

A pioneering program in telemedicine, which is based on video-conferencing equipment, links UNC's Program on Aging with two hospitals, a community health clinic, a senior center, and a nursing home in rural areas. Patients in each of the five sites can receive consultations with health care professionals at UNC or one of the other sites. Usually consultation sessions include the patient's primary care provider and family members and sometimes involve a physical exam. By bringing together providers from different parts of the state, telemedicine not only facilitates interdisciplinary geriatric care, but also greatly increases the access of rural seniors to specialized health care services.

Palmtop Personal Computers

Another type of technology that can facilitate interdisciplinary training is that of palmtop personal computers (PCs). These computers are lightweight, portable, and fit in the palm of the hand, hence the name. Harvard Medical School has been working with Hewlett-Packard for over a decade developing and perfecting palmtop PCs for use in medical education. Palmtops were proposed for use at the Harvard GITT site to enhance geriatric education in two ways: (a) as a palmtop PC-based interdisciplinary communication log and (b) as a didactic resource. The logs can be carried around by trainees, allowing them to record both patient notes and perceptions about their interdisciplinary training experiences as they occur. The logs can then be brought to interdisciplinary seminars where trainees discuss their entries. Through palmtop PC-based self-paced interdisciplinary learning modules, trainees can access lectures and training modules developed through the Hartford Primary Care in Geriatrics Initiative Program. Learning through this database can be self-directed, with trainees tapping information relevant to the specific cases on which they would be working.

ADVANTAGES AND DISADVANTAGES OF
THESE TECHNOLOGIES

If management of patient data in a way that helps ensure coordinated treatment among team members is a concern, then technologies like On Lok's CMIS or Harvard's palmtop PC-based interdisciplinary communication log may be suitable tools. All team members keep progress and treatment notes on these systems, and errors resulting from incompatible treatments are less likely to occur. In terms of dollars, a system like CMIS is cheaper, requiring only an investment in data management software and access to the database by team members at their place of work using standard PCs. The drawback of these programs is their lack of flexibility.

On the other hand, the portability of palmtops allows progress notes to be recorded during and immediately following exams, which helps reduce lapses in record keeping and may increase the accuracy of notes. Because this technology is still in its infancy, it is costly and thus probably not a viable option for most GITT projects.

If communication and coordination needs cannot be met simply through a shared database, then groupware software or video conferencing can help. Both eliminate geographic barriers to team treatment. Although video-conferencing equipment is becoming available through more institutions, it is still costly and often time consuming to set up and maintain. However, the use of video conferencing to provide telemedicine can bring geriatric team care to individuals who are otherwise unlikely to ever see a geriatric specialist, let alone access a whole team of them; it also encourages the integration of patient input into treatment. For those reasons, it has enormous potential to enhance the range and quality of geriatric care, particularly for low-income patients living in rural areas. Unfortunately, the cost of the technology can be prohibitive. Alternatively, communication through groupware requires only that team members have access to a computer at work, or preferably, at home. The cost of the groupware program itself is nominal.

If training needs center on evaluation, the standardized patient teaching method or OSCEs are two viable options. They might, however, lack feasibility because of the time and money needed to train actors and the logistics of coordinating the sessions. Furthermore, both methods rely on closed-circuit TV systems. Observation can be accomplished less expensively by having someone videotaping in the room during the patient interviews, but this could distract trainees and potentially affect their behavior, thus weakening it as an evaluative tool.

If expansion of didactic capabilities is a concern, particularly as faculty have less time available for teaching and mentoring, then one may want to create a library of videotaped lectures or case studies. Existing videotaped lecture series such as the PACE Training Tapes for Nurses are available. Videotapes can provide inexpensive solutions to faculty shortages and have the additional advantage of being available for trainees to review when and as frequently as they wish.

Another didactic solution is the use of hypertext. It is more expensive than videotaped lectures because a development team with specialized software is required to first compose the modules. However, not every institution need support hypertext development efforts. The Windows-based modules are quite transportable, and like other GITT centers, Houston makes much of its educational materials available to others. Personal computers are needed to run the modules, but for most institutions, this requirement can be met. Hypertext allows for individualized, dynamic sessions and thus is more consistent with an interdisciplinary approach to learning than videotaped lectures. Table 7.1 summarizes the best uses for these technologies.

FUTURE DIRECTIONS

Future tools relevant to GITT will reflect both adaptation of current applications and emergence of new technologies. For example, the current use of palmtop computers might be extended to coordinate patient care more effectively if they were used to update and access patient records in a centralized CMIS. This strategy would be most effective if live communication links were established between the palmtops and the CMIS, for example, through cellular communications. Caregivers would enter data on the palmtop, hit a send key, and the entries on the palmtops would be uploaded to a

TABLE 7.1 Summary Table of Technologies and Functions

	Data management	Communication	Instruction	Evaluation	Clinical
CMIS	X	X			
Palmtops	X	X			
Groupware		X			
Video conferencing		X			X
OSCE			X	X	
Standardized patient			X	X	
Videotape			X	X	
Hypertext			X		

CMIS, Case Management Information System.
OSCE, Objective Structured Clinic Exams.

central database. In the other direction, when consulting with a patient, a caregiver would be able to use the palmtop to access up-to-the minute information in the CMIS, in online knowledge bases and references, as well as in groupware facilitated discussions. Such applications, while they may sound far-fetched, are realistic and within current reach. There are a variety of newly emerging palmtop technologies for facilitating wireless data transfer, as well as a new breed of cellular phone that combines telephone communications with E-mail and Internet browsing.

The Internet offers a unique opportunity for the sharing of technology. Faculty at the Houston GITT have already set up a Huffington Center on Aging website. They have made geriatric interactive learning modules available to the general public, and over 185,000 visitors have already logged on to the website. (See Table 7.2 for other training modules and resources available through the Internet.) Web sites can also be used to make interactive threaded discussions available. This is much like what the Great Lakes GITT site is doing with groupware, with the added advantage of easier access and possibly lower costs in the long run. The addition of cellular phone technology could make access even easier. If the user must access data fast and on-the-fly, not just when sitting down to read, reflect, and participate in a discussion, a cellular phone and website would make sense.

Unfortunately, these applications generate increased costs, and current applications are out of the financial reach of some GITT sites. There may also be valuable ways to achieve pared-down versions of existing applications using off-the-shelf technologies. For example, there is an application built for Apple's palmtop, the Newton, called Learner Profile (Sunburst Communications, 1997), which is intended for elementary school teachers. It is designed to allow teachers to enter classroom observation and grading data electronically while walking about the classroom. Data can then be uploaded to a PC. The interface and the observation categories appear to be highly customizable, and an enterprising center might well build a customized patient data collection system at a significantly reduced cost using Learner Profile.

Another existing technology that might facilitate training and ongoing decision-making support is the kind of electronic publishing tools represented by software like Folio VIEWS (Folio Corporation, 1997). Folio allows entry of huge texts (such as books, training manuals, references, etc.), fully formatted, into a central infobase. The

TABLE 7.2   Training Modules and Resources Available Through the Internet

Organization	Address	Type of information
American Psychiatric Association	apa.org/rural/homepage.html	Interdisciplinary rural training materials
Great Lakes GITT	weatherhead.cwru.edu/gitt	Geriatric training materials
Huffington Center	www.bcm.tms.edu	GITT modules

program has remarkably powerful search capabilities. Users can access their own personal shadow copies of the text, where they can apply highlighters, pop-up notes for annotations and comments, and their own hypertext links both within and across infobases. Users can define multiple highlighters, give them names and colors, and use them to narrow searches in the future. Any changes users make to their personal shadow versions of the text are not incorporated into the real infobase, unless the project administrator chooses to incorporate them. Folio VIEWS runs well on either an intranet or an Internet server, raising the possibility that it could be combined with the kind of mobile communication strategies discussed above.

There are also a wide range of other software packages that facilitate the systematic and rigorous tracking, management, and analysis of large bodies of qualitative data, such as physicians' notes, textual records, logs, communications and other textual records, or case study materials (Weitzman & Miles, 1995). These programs allow the user to define and apply complex systems of codes or indices to segments of the text; write and store reflective or methodologic memos about text or code-categories, and link these memos to text or codes; and define complex relationships among code-categories and search for text either by keywords, codes, or memo content.

All of these technological tools can be welcome additions to training efforts. Data management, in particular, is typically accomplished more efficiently and with less error using technology. Technology can never replace one-on-one human interaction and mentoring, however. So in considering which, if any, of these tools are appropriate for training efforts, it is important to evaluate what technology can add above and beyond traditional, face-to-face methods. Technology-based didactic materials, while they can help deal with faculty shortages and scheduling issues, might not measure up as favorably to good, old-fashioned low-tech human instructors. The trainee watching a video is likely to be in a more passive mental state, using less cognitive processing, and poorly integrating new information. Less well-integrated information is more likely to be incomplete and harder to recall (Hine, Summers, Tilleczek, & Lewko, 1997). However, if technology allows didactic materials to be presented in a way that is novel or activates multiple senses, then it is more likely to be thoroughly integrated into existing cognitive networks and better recalled. Some of the technologies outlined here accomplish this; multimedia presentations of didactic materials could do so as well.

CONCLUSIONS

Ultimately, in making choices about the use of technology, those planning GITT must evaluate the training needs, examine the financial constraints, and then decide if a certain technologic approach can work better than a low- or no-tech solution. If a large financial investment is involved in acquiring technology, a small-scale trial period of testing the technology (which in some cases can be borrowed from other departments within one's institution) may be an appropriate first step.

REFERENCES

Folio Corporation (1997). *Folio VIEWS personal electronic publishing software: Version 4.1, for the Windows graphical environment.* Provo, UT: Author.

Hine, D. W., Summers, C., Tilleczek, K., & Lewko, J. (1997). Expectancies and mental models as determinants of adolescents' smoking decisions. *Journal of Social Issues, 53,* 35–52.

Jones, B. F., Rasmussen, C. M., & Moffitt, M. C. (Eds.). (1997). *Real-life problem solving: A collaborative approach to interdisciplinary learning.* Washington, DC: American Psychological Association.

Soft Arc (1997). *First class.* Ontario, Canada: Author.

Sunburst Communications (1997). *Learner profile.* Pleasantville, NY: Author.

Weitzman, E. A., & Miles, M. B. (1995). *Computer programs for qualitative data analysis: A software sourcebook.* Thousand Oaks, CA: Sage.

PART 3

Curriculum

CHAPTER 8

Structuring the GITT Didactic Experience

Judith L. Howe, Christine K. Cassel, and Maria L. Vezina

A cornerstone of Geriatric Interdisciplinary Team Training (GITT) is the didactic curriculum. This curriculum must cover three content areas—gerontology/geriatrics, interdisciplinary teamwork, and health care delivery systems. Defining learning objectives for the three core disciplines of social work, advanced practice nursing, and medicine is a challenge because the content must be interesting and relevant to all of the disciplines, while providing unique information for the management and care of the elderly. Another theme that The Mount Sinai Medical Center GITT Partnership introduced was managed care. This emerging trend of health care delivery and reimbursement is crucial for future health care providers to understand because the practice environment is changing from fee-for-service to a more structured and monitored approach to health care.

DIDACTIC CURRICULUM

Although the overall curriculum includes both a clinical practicum and didactic experience, this chapter focuses on the didactic component. The purpose of this didactic component is fourfold:

1. To relay content in gerontology, the interdisciplinary team, and health care systems;
2. To provide a forum for the disciplines to interact with each other and pose discipline-specific and discipline-shared issues for discussion and resolution;
3. To expose learners to faculty from all three disciplines using a team teaching methodology; and
4. To identify other disciplines within the extended team as key to the delivery of quality of care to older persons.

Educational and curricular goals of didactic training differ from site to site, but most include the following:

1. Skills
   - Conflict resolution
   - Team interaction
   - Communication
   - Leadership dynamics
2. Attitudes
   - Respect for older people/awareness of ageism
   - Respect for other disciplines
   - Respect for patient and family input
   - Respect for effective patient management and patient focused care
3. Knowledge
   - Roles and responsibilities of each discipline
   - Role of extended team
   - Group dynamics
   - Common geriatric problems and clinical issues
   - Application of clinical concepts
   - Changing health care environment and its effect on teams

This chapter focuses on the three required disciplines of social work, advanced practice nursing, and medicine. The GITT curriculum aims to introduce new knowledge, reinforce previous knowledge, and stimulate critical thinking within a team structure.

The Mount Sinai Partnership GITT Project has three clinical sites, The Mount Sinai Hospital, Beth Abraham's Comprehensive Care Management Program, and the Jewish Home and Hospital. The four educational partners are the Mount Sinai School of Medicine, New York University's Division of Nursing, Hunter College School of Social Work, and Hunter/Bellevue School of Nursing. The framework for the Mount Sinai GITT didactic component is as follows:

- A 3-hour orientation seminar;
- One-day workshops on teams and applications to geriatrics—medical residents attend one workshop and advanced practice nursing and master's level social work trainees attend two;
- A 1-day workshop about the team and ethics that combines lectures and a more hands on clinical dialogue;
- A 16-session didactic seminar series, every other week for 3 hours, over two semesters. The content of this series is listed in Table 8.1.
- Interaction with simulated patients and families at Mount Sinai's Morchand Center, where GITT trainees receive feedback from faculty after interviewing patients and families and working as a team in assessing the patient and developing a plan of care.

Most didactic curricula are formally structured. Nonetheless, integration with the clinical curriculum necessitates some flexibility. This allows the didactic component to best meet the needs of the trainees from different disciplines, who may have preceptorships of different length and focus.

TABLE 8.1 The Didactic Seminar Series at Mount Sinai

Orientation to teamwork and gerontology
Introduction to teams and teamwork (I)
Introduction to teams and teamwork (II)
Normal aging and age-related disease
Geriatric assessment and care planning in a managed care environment
Aging diversity
Depression, delirium, and dementia
Formal and informal care systems
Managed care
Quality of life
The extended team
Interface of law, finance, and the health care team
Dying and death
Assessment and care planning revisited
Team building
Case presentations

This chapter will present the basic goals and objectives for GITT didactic curricula. Appendix A provides examples of didactic and clinical curricula from three other GITT sites.

ORGANIZATION OF THE CURRICULUM

GITT Educational Goals

The overall purpose of the didactic curriculum is to ensure that trainees have a shared knowledge base in geriatrics and gerontology and to demonstrate how an interdisciplinary health care team organizes itself to deliver high quality care in different health care settings. Each of the three major themes is framed as a goal.

Geriatrics and Gerontology

Here the goal is to teach core knowledge in geriatrics, including the implications of an aging society, the different processes of aging, the most common diseases and conditions associated with aging, geriatric assessment, and the development and implementation of a care plan.

Interdisciplinary Teamwork

The goal is to improve knowledge about the interdisciplinary team, including understanding the different forms and functions of teams and the roles and responsibilities of the different disciplines, to demonstrate which factors result in a successfully functioning team, and to inculcate the practical skills necessary to work effectively as interdisciplinary team members.

Health Care Systems

The aim is to teach how health care structures and reimbursement systems influence care delivery and to demonstrate the benefits and drawbacks of managed care systems for the older patient and the interdisciplinary team.

Trainee Learning Objectives

The GITT didactic curriculum is designed to help trainees achieve objectives required for team care of older patients and families. After completing the GITT didactic experience, trainees are expected to define a variety of aspects of the interdisciplinary team, demonstrate familiarity with basic gerontologic content, and describe teamwork in a managed care setting. GITT trainees are assessed on the basis of these learning objectives. Table 8.2 lists the objectives of the didactic program at Mount Sinai in detail.

TEACHING METHODOLOGIES

To support the varied components and experiences of the didactic curriculum as well as the diverse disciplines involved in GITT, a variety of teaching methodologies can support the core learning objectives. Because these methodologies serve to bridge the didactic experience with the clinical practicum, case-based interactive training has proved to be especially effective.

Lectures

These are the mainstay of traditional professional school curricula and often carry weight as legitimate means of teaching. Although lacking interactions that are necessary to team training, lectures such as Grand Rounds are useful means of conveying large amounts of information to trainees, especially when they are all of one discipline.

Weekly or Biweekly Seminars

These use a group discussion format to integrate the knowledge and skills gained in the academic curriculum and the practice setting. This group dynamic format is intended to promote critical thinking and role model team behavior through case-based exercises and team teaching. Seminars are also excellent venues for discussions and analyses of readings and journal articles; the presence of multiple disciplines often brings fresh insights to the literature.

Full-Day Workshops

These can provide more comprehensive opportunities to focus on team care in specific settings. At Mount Sinai, for example, we use this format to demonstrate the growing importance of the interdisciplinary team within a managed care environment. Occurring approximately once per month, the workshops include both GITT trainees and those not participating in the intensive GITT experience.

Team-Building Exercises

These are exercises designed to build team skills. They require that trainees work together to perform specific tasks and need not involve patient care issues at all. Examples

TABLE 8.2 Trainee Learning Objectives

Geriatrics/gerontology

Assessment
- Identify the biopsychosocial environmental factors that are integral to a geriatric assessment.
- Administer assessment and care planning skills in an interdisciplinary setting.
- Explain the concept of functional assessment.
- Demonstrate familiarity with the most frequently used functional assessment tools and scales.
- Identify appropriate assessment tools and appropriate treatment and care strategies for these conditions.
- Define skills required for ongoing geriatric assessment of chronic conditions.

Aging
- Understand the heterogeneous nature of the aging population and aging as a culture.

Geriatric syndromes
- Identify older persons with special needs and with special health care needs, such as elder abuse, substance abuse, and developmental disabilities.
- Define and distinguish between depression, delirium, and dementia.
- Evaluate the complexity of chronic health conditions in an older frail patient.

Informal care systems
- Identify the critical role of the informal care system—family, friends, and neighbors—in the care of older persons.
- Demonstrate skills in conducting family meetings with the team and/or individual team members.
- Manage conflict between family/patient/team in care planning and management.

Ethics
- Define quality of life in relation to older patients.
- Support the value of self-determination and autonomy in maintaining independence and self-esteem for both the older patient and the individual team members.
- Affirm death and dying issues for the older patient, the family, and the interdisciplinary health care team.
- Discuss palliative care and end-of-life decisions and their impact on health care management and team functioning.
- Illustrate the framework of advanced directives and the role of the health care team in educating the patient and the family.

Interdisciplinary teamwork

Diversity
- Relate diversity content to interdisciplinary teamwork, recognizing the influence of culture on team members.
- Demonstrate cultural competency in interactions with team members, patients, their families, and communities.

Interdisciplinary care planning
- Describe concepts of a geriatric interdisciplinary team approach and differentiate it from other care models.
- Identify the members of the team and describe their competencies and range of expertise.
- Compare and contrast the education, unique knowledge and skills, and competencies that different disciplines contribute to a geriatrics interdisciplinary team.
- Define the role and function of the interdisciplinary health care team.
- Describe the function of the disciplines that provide consultation to the interdisciplinary health care team.

(cont.)

TABLE 8.2 Trainee Learning Objectives (*Continued*)

Interdisciplinary teamwork *(continued)*

Interdisciplinary care planning *(continued)*
- Identify conditions under which it is appropriate to include each of these consultative disciplines in the care of older persons.

Team dynamics
- Perceive the effective of ageist beliefs on the work of the interdisciplinary team.
- Appreciate the stereotyping that may occur regarding the core disciplines on the team.
- Discuss the collaborative skills of the team that benefit patient care.
- Affirm the value of the interdisciplinary team in geriatric care.
- Identify the dynamics and stages in the development of an interdisciplinary health care team.
- Define barriers to team development and explore solutions to overcome these barriers.
- Discuss teamwork knowledge and skills.
- Assess interdisciplinary team experiences and use in group problem solving around team events.
- Recognize individual styles of communication and how diverse styles contribute to team function.
- Demonstrate a collaborative spirit by showing respect and support for other members' skills in providing patient care.

Health care systems/reimbursement
- Expand the team knowledge to include information regarding law and finance and its impact on the individual, patient, and family.
- Define managed care and the philosophy, terms, and driving forces behind a managed care system.
- Delineate the new and the changed role of the health care professional in this new arena.
- Identify the benefits and disadvantages of different payment systems on care for the older patient and functioning of the interdisciplinary team.

might include using nonverbal communication to solve puzzles, describing how family conflicts are handled, and other ice breakers.

Role Play

This can be part of team-building exercises or can help trainees develop other important skills of geriatric care such as cultural sensitivity and interviewing techniques. Trainees can play themselves, patients, or other team members.

Case Studies

Having trainees develop care plans for case studies is a common and popular tool, as it combines both team building and clinical skills training. The GITT program is developing standardized case studies for both training and evaluation.

Computer-Based Teaching Tools

Computer programs allow trainees to study independently and can provide background material to serve as a leveler when trainees' knowledge of geriatrics may vary widely from school to school and from month to month. These technologies are discussed in greater detail in chapter 7.

Simulated Patient Exercises

An innovation of The Mount Sinai GITT Project is the use of a standardized patient teaching approach, with trained actors simulating the behaviors and clinical manifestations of actual patients. GITT trainees evaluate and develop care plans as a team for a simulated patient. This technique exposes trainees of many disciplines to a uniform, high quality educational experience and ensures experience with specific clinical topics. These interactions are videotaped live and then reviewed by both the trainees and faculty to identify strengths and weaknesses in trainees' clinical and team skills.

Journaling

This method of reflection enables trainees to acknowledge and share impressions, issues, experiences, unanswered questions, and outcomes both privately and with the faculty and group. Journaling provides a structured complement to the didactic curriculum by allowing perceptions, values, and curiosity to emerge within the framework of more formal teaching. Although open entries to the entire GITT experience are welcomed, each seminar session ends with a specific journal question that each trainee must address. These journals are reviewed by the preceptors throughout the semester.

TEAM TEACHING

Team teaching developed in both professional and elementary education with the advent of integrated curricula. Garner (1977) defines team teaching as "a concept which involves instructors from two or more academic disciplines in the planning, preparation, presentation and evaluation of lessons to accomplish common learning objectives for two or more groups of learners" (p. 27).

As an educational strategy, team teaching involves choice, compromise, and consensus. Team members are interdependent and meld their individual philosophies, goals, objectives, skills, and interests together through flexibility, cooperation, and compromise (Tarpey & Chen, 1978). Faculty teaching in teams are better able to address the unique learning needs of trainees, especially in a diversified group, and to create a sense of community and totality within the curriculum. GITT projects all involve at least three disciplines and require the integration of learning objectives for all; team teaching has provided role models for team interaction and facilitated the growth of the team within the trainee groups.

Team teaching is intended to enhance trainee and faculty learning and facilitate interdisciplinary involvement. Teaching collaboratively can serve as a model for teaching trainees useful attitudes, knowledge, and skills (Robinson & Schaible, 1995).

This philosophy of teaching imparts not only knowledge that is rich and diversified but also its own interpersonal dynamic, group process, and organizational structure that in this case embodies the goals of the GITT Program. Team teaching is a valuable and flexible approach to trainee learning, blending strengths of each discipline, allowing a venue for group assessment and evaluation versus individual autonomy in problem solving, and promoting interaction and collaboration of efforts. Table 8.3 describes the approaches that each GITT project has taken.

COORDINATION AND PROBLEM SOLVING

Particularly in the developmental stages, there are a number of administrative, logistic, and communications issues in designing, piloting, and implementing the didactic curriculum. In the Mount Sinai GITT management model, a co-director is responsible for the day-to-day management of the GITT project, assisted by a part-time administrative assistant. The co-director works closely with educational coordinators in each of the specific disciplines, medicine, social work, and advanced practice nursing. These individuals are responsible for serving as the liaisons between the schools and the clinical sites, coordinating schedules and placements, and serving as GITT preceptors and advisors. Monthly management meetings, attended by the educational coordinators and school and clinical site representatives, facilitate communication and identify and resolve problems.

As all the project sites have gained experience in crafting didactic training, several challenges have emerged. These include:

- Determining the appropriate balance between time spent in training and time spent in evaluation;
- Deciding when participation in a module should be elective and when it should be required;
- Successfully integrating didactic and clinical programs, including scheduling, communicating between academic and clinical sites, and determining the appropriate sequencing;
- Ensuring active participation of all the disciplines.

These challenges have been the subject of discussions both within and across GITT sites; we expect that we will need several years of experience as GITT implementation sites before we can devise meaningful solutions.

CONCLUSIONS

The didactic content is a value-added component of GITT. It provides an opportunity to develop and deliver an interdisciplinary curriculum on both aging and interdisciplinary team skills. A strong didactic curriculum ensures that a training program is comprehensive, even when trainees cannot work with a wide variety of patients. A rich variety of methodologies is available to accommodate the needs of any site wishing to implement GITT and to foster exciting opportunities in curriculum innovation and replication for other interdisciplinary educational projects.

TABLE 8.3   GITT Educational Programs by Implementation Sites

Project	Baylor	Great Lakes	Mt. Sinai	On Lok	Rush	UCHSC	U MN	USF
Teaching approach for didactic course								
Team/geriatric didactic content taught with students from each discipline present	Y	Y	Y	N	Y	N	N	Y
Didactic systematically incorporates students' practicum experiences	Y	Y	Y	Y	Y	Y	Mixed	Mixed
Team practicum includes students from each discipline present at each clinical site	Y	Y	Limited	Y	Y	N	Y	Y
Didactic emphasizes lectures	Y	Y	Major	Major	Major	Major	N	Major
Didactic incorporates team exercises/simulations	Major	Major	Major	N	N	N	Some	Y
Didactic incorporates case presentations	Y	Major	Y	Major	Major	Y	Major	Y
Didactic requires readings prior to sessions	Y	Y	Y	N	Y	Y	Y	Y
Computer-assisted learning	Y	Y	N	N	N	N	N	N
Disciplines requiring geriatric training prior to GITT experience	RN, SW	N	RN, MD	RN	N	N	RN	N
Other experience								
Pilot (# students)	70	13 (Staff)	30	N		Y	Y	N
Pilot disciplines	All	All	All		All	No MDs	All	
Faculty development								
Clinical faculty development (hours)	3	16	8	36	2			15
Academic faculty development (hours)	3	16		8	2			12
Required geriatric curriculum								
Behavior management	2	1		2				1
Caregivers/family issues	2	1	2	1	1		1	1
Cognitive impairments	1	1		1	2			1
Community care and resources	2	1		1	2			
Counseling/patient education	1	1		1				1
Death and dying	1	1	2	1	2			1
Demographics	2	1	1				1	
Depression/dementia/delirium	2	1	2	1	2		1	1
Diversity/ethnogeriatrics	2	1	2	1	2	1		1
Ethical issues/autonomy	1	1	1	2	1	1	1	1
Geriatric assessment	1	1	2	1	2		1	
Normal aging	1	1	2				1	1
Sensory changes/compensations	1	1		1			1	1

1 = Required of all disciplines.
2 = Required of some disciplines.

REFERENCES

Garner, A. E. (1977). Is your School of Nursing ready to implement interdisciplinary team teaching? *Journal of Nursing Education, 16*(7), 27–30.

Robinson, B., & Schaible, R. (1995). Collaborative teaching: Reaping the benefits. *College Teaching, 43*(2), 57.

Tarpey, K. S., & Chen, S. P. (1978). Team teaching: Is it for you? *Journal of Nursing Education, 17*(2), 26–29.

CHAPTER 9

Structuring the GITT Clinical Experience

Mary S. Gleason, Judy Farness, Ann Schneider, Nancy L. Wilson, and Vaunette Fay

The challenge of any health education innovation is translating classroom concepts and practicum skills into seamless clinical service. The impetus for the development of team training in geriatrics has been well described in previous chapters. The next step in the transformation is to provide a practicum that blends newly acquired didactic knowledge with actual clinical experience. We will describe the processes involved in structuring a practicum for trainees that, by successfully combining team training with patient care, results in a workable and reproducible learning experience that also enhances health care for older people.

CONTEMPLATING INTERDISCIPLINARY TEAM TRAINING

Exploring the Possibilities

When the Houston Geriatric Interdisciplinary Team Training (HGITT) Project was in its early planning stages, we, like our counterpart sites, used existing professional and personal relationships to begin exploring which hospitals and group practices might be interested in participating as clinical training settings. These existing relationships were especially helpful when we made initial contact with the large multispecialty group practices involved in our project. Because of the growth of Medicare risk programs, we made a special effort to identify and secure clinical training settings with Medicare risk contracts (Butler, 1994).

Coordinated by the Huffington Center on Aging at Baylor College of Medicine (BCM), the HGITT site is a collaborative endeavor of six primary care clinical and seven educational programs at three academic institutions. The academic programs include four within BCM (internal medicine, family medicine, physician assistant, and psychiatry), one at The University of Texas Houston Health Science Center School of Nursing, and two at the University of Houston (social work and pharmacy). The participating clinical settings include two multispecialty group practices with Medicare risk health maintenance organization programs (Kelsey-Seybold Clinic through NYLCare 65 and MacGregor Medical Association through Prudential Healthcare SeniorCare), a geriatric ambulatory care and inpatient service of the BCM Department of Medicine (Geriatric Medicine Associates), a nonprofit Medicare-certified hospice (The Hospice at the Texas Medical Center), the comprehensive geriatric programs of the Houston Veterans Affairs Medical Center (geriatrics and geropsychiatry), and the geriatrics comprehensive county-wide health care system (Harris County Hospital District Geriatric Program).

Initially, the leadership group of the training project requested an exploratory meeting with staff at each potential clinical setting. The educational project coordinators used their professional and personal contacts to request the meetings of large multispecialty group practices. We found that successful meetings require attendance by key representatives from the leadership group initiating the project (such as the principal investigator and coinvestigator); representatives from the academic institutions; and representatives of the medical team and management staff of the clinical training settings, including any candidates for clinical preceptors or clinical setting project coordinator.

The leadership group should prepare the agenda and conduct the meeting. It is reasonable to expect 15 to 20 people to attend the meeting, which is the size of the group that attended our first meeting at a large multispecialty practice. Among the topics that should be discussed at this exploratory meeting are:

- An overview of the training project, including the purpose and length of the project, disciplines involved, funding sources, and project costs (Netting & Williams, 1995);
- Benefits to the clinical setting from participating in the project, including access to a pool of well-trained clinicians as future employees, improved patient care, assistance from the trainees placed in the clinical setting, enhanced marketing opportunities for the setting, and recognition as a result of participating in the project;
- Benefits to the community, such as improved service coordination across organizations and increased knowledge of managed care at the educational institutions;
- Expectations of the clinical setting, including the number of trainees, the amount of time that preceptors will devote to trainee education, cash outlays required (if any), logistic demands such as office or meeting space, and coordination of the project at the setting; and
- The feasibility of the clinical setting staff conducting an interdisciplinary team.

At the conclusion of the meeting, the project leadership should propose a time frame within which the clinical setting staff should make a decision about participation in the project. We found that at least a month was necessary to permit the clinical setting staff to evaluate the merits and feasibility of participation, obtain internal approvals, and select a project setting coordinator.

Determining the Feasibility of Participation

Clinical staff evaluated the advantages and disadvantages of participating in the project (Abramson & Mizrahi, 1996). One large multispecialty group, whose process we will examine as an example, approached its study of feasibility by addressing several questions (Table 9.1). These questions are as applicable to a small multispecialty group practice as they are to a large group practice or an academically oriented group practice. After the project leadership considered and answered all of the questions, the large multispecialty practice decided that the advantages of participation outweighed the difficulties of logistics and coordination. Convincing them to say yes were the critical linkages with experts in the field of geriatrics who were involved in the project and the anticipated opportunities to improve interdisciplinary team skills employed in working with trainees (Abramson & Mizrahi, 1996). The representatives decided that introducing additional trainees into the academically oriented group practice would not compromise the system and, in fact, would enable it so serve more patients after the trainees' initial orientations.

CRITICAL COMPONENTS OF THE INTERDISCIPLINARY TEAM TRAINING APPROACH

Interdisciplinary Teams

Successful GITT necessitates a wide range of clinical experiences with outstanding teams. Each GITT project has a variety of clinical settings for trainee practica. These are summarized in Table 9.2. At each HGITT clinical setting, we identified existing interdisciplinary teams and explained the purpose of each team, methods of team communication, and frequency of meetings. The HGITT project leaders determined that all team meetings were potential training opportunities in which trainees could observe and participate in interdisciplinary team work.

For the HGITT Project, we decided that trainees could either be observers or actual participants. To determine the effectiveness of a team as a teaching mechanism, we conducted a pilot study by introducing trainees from two different disciplines (psychiatry and pharmacy) into large multispecialty group practices during the planning stages of the project. These pilot projects were considered successful interdisciplinary experiences and have been continued in the full project implementation.

Clinical Setting Coordinator

Each clinical setting should select a clinical setting coordinator. We suggest that the clinical setting coordinator have the following qualifications: (a) represent one of the disciplines from which trainees are drawn (medicine, nursing, or social work, for example) and be involved in supervising providers or providing services in the area of the training project (for example, in the HGITT project, all of the clinical setting coordinators are actively involved in services to older adults); (b) be able to work with all levels and with various disciplines at the setting; (c) have sufficient stature within the setting to get the job done; (d) be able to articulate the purpose of the project and the advantages of participation; (e) be able to understand the complexities and political climate of the setting and those of the other organizations participating; (f) have the time to spend on organizational meetings and project implementation (during the planning

TABLE 9.1 Determining the Feasibility of Participation in a Geriatric Team Training Project

Groups determining the feasibility of geriatric team training participation should weigh their answers to the following questions:

- Do the goals of the project complement the goals of the clinical setting?
- What will be the impact of the training program on patient care and patient satisfaction?
- Will patients receive more care, a higher quality of care, or will the level of care suffer with trainees in the system?
- Are there any legal implications of providing on-setting training to trainees?
- How will patients feel about being seen or assisted by trainees?
- Which disciplines can the setting accept for training?
- How many trainees can the setting accept in each discipline?
- Do the potential preceptors have the time and interest to teach trainees?
- How will the introduction of trainees at the clinical setting affect provider productivity and compensation? Where providers' compensation is based on productivity, will the project cover any compensation lost if devoting time to trainees lowers productivity?
- Is the setting using an interdisciplinary approach to the care of older patients already?
- If not, are the potential preceptors willing and able to work in an interdisciplinary setting?
- What skills do the preceptors need to work as members of an interdisciplinary team and to mentor trainees?
- Will the trainees be assigned caseloads or independent projects, or will they only tag along as the preceptors work?
- Will trainees have the chance to observe the work of other disciplines?
- Is there space in the facility for trainees?
- Will the project be continued after the funded period is completed?
- How will activities at the setting be coordinated?
- Must the setting provide any special group training or orientation for trainees?
- In a for-profit group practice, will participation affect the profitability of the practice?
- In an academic group practice, how will the introduction of additional trainees affect the system?
- Can the project be successful in managed care and traditional Medicare fee-for-service practices?

stages of the project several hours a week may be required); and (g) be able to gather needed information and coordinate project activities. The role of the clinical setting coordinator should be defined by the clinical setting project leadership and may include the attributes in Table 9.3.

The clinical setting coordinator may also act as the team learning facilitator. Or, the team learning facilitator may be drawn from one of the educational organizations. For the large multispecialty practices, we determined that the clinical setting coordinator should not act as the team learning facilitator because of other job demands. In the academically oriented practices, the clinical setting coordinators are serving as team learning facilitators. The role of a team learning facilitator is described below.

Clinical Setting Steering Committee

The success of the multiyear project depends on each clinical setting's commitment to its viability. Success and continuity will require that the clinical setting project coordi-

TABLE 9.2 Educational Requirements of GITT Projects by Implementation Sites

Project	Baylor	Great Lakes	Mt. Sinai	On Lok	Rush	UCHSC	UMN	USF
Required practicum training sites								
Adult day care		2	1	1	2	2		
Assisted living			2		2	2		
Home care	2	2	2	1	1	2	2	2
Hospice/palliative care	2	2	2		2	2	2	2
Inpatient	2	1	1		2	2		2
Managed care	2	2	1	1	1	2	1	2
Nursing home	2	2	1		2	2	1	
On Lok/PACE		2	1	1		2		
Primary care—outpatient	1	1	1	1	1	1	1	2
Rehabilitation	2	2	2	1	2	2		
Senior housing	2		2		2			2

1 = Required of all disciplines.
2 = Required of some disciplines.

nators have the involvement and support of key geriatric providers and decision makers as the project matures. We determined that clinical setting steering committees could assist in implementing and directing the training project, and these committees have been established at each clinical setting.

Members of the clinical setting steering committee should include the project's principal investigator and coinvestigator, the clinical setting coordinator, the team learning facilitator, and key physicians involved in managed care and the care of geriatric patients. As needed, the clinical setting preceptors and representatives from various academic disciplines may be invited to participate in steering committee meetings.

The clinical setting steering committee should meet at least quarterly. Its role includes the following: (a) reviewing existing training structure and evaluating its effectiveness for patients and trainees, (b) identifying new interdisciplinary team training opportunities at the setting and developing them, (c) selecting clinical preceptors and determining the number of trainees to be trained, (d) ensuring that the project focus remains on interdisciplinary team training in geriatrics, and (e) reviewing the overall impact of participation in the project on the clinical setting and quality of patient care.

Implementing these administrative guidelines was key to developing on-going support for the program; however, the HGITT leadership realized that another person was needed to support and enhance the day-to-day functioning of the clinical setting by being a liaison with the HGITT academic partners and ensuring that program goals were consistently being met. This agent was the clinical team learning facilitator.

Clinical Team Learning Facilitator

The clinical team learning facilitator is the individual who is responsible for interdisciplinary content and coordination of the team experience at the clinical setting. This professional may be a preceptor who is already in place at this setting or it may be someone new to the setting. The facilitator must be able to link the multiple disciplines,

TABLE 9.3 Roles of the Clinical Setting Coordinator

- Explores the feasibility of participation in the project
- Acts as an interface between the leadership group and the clinical setting
- Provides the leadership group with specific information about the ability of the clinical setting to train trainees
- Negotiates the parameters of the clinical setting's participation with the project leadership
- Generates support within the clinical setting for the project
- Identifies preceptors from various disciplines and obtains approval for the preceptors to participate in the project
- Maintains communication between the clinical setting, project leadership organization, and educational institutions

including preceptors, with their academic counterparts for team training. The facilitator creates two opportunities for trainees: to view and be part of a functioning team, and to assess the effectiveness of patient care provided by the interdisciplinary team. To provide this experience for trainees, the clinical team learning facilitator must be familiar with the clinical setting, know how teams function, and understand geriatric issues.

Often, the clinical team learning facilitator is the cheerleader for team training. Depending on the setting, the approach varies. At some settings, the facilitator focuses on organizational issues to promote team training; at others the facilitator may handle preceptor issues or work to convince others of the advantages of teams and the necessity of team training. Time constraints are often challenging and sustaining this program may be difficult. Overall, the clinical team learning facilitator may spend about 2 to 4 hours per week attending to duties. How this position will continue to be reimbursed is unknown, especially if the facilitator is not integral to the setting.

INITIAL PROBLEMS WITH GITT AND THEIR SOLUTIONS

Some of the problems that arise in an attempt to prepare trainees with experience in a team training setting include the following (University of North Carolina at Chapel Hill, 1993):

- Trainees who are not familiar with their own roles,
- Trainees who are overwhelmed with trying to maintain their role identity while performing their duties in a team of other disciplines,
- Trainee teams or trainee experiences on teams that are short lived,
- Trainees with little training in teams or teamwork or without experience in working on teams,
- Trainees who are often focused very narrowly on goals of their own and their individual discipline,
- Preceptors with all of the above problems.

Preceptors may be new to team training and in the process of learning it themselves (see chapter 5).

FACILITATING LEARNING

Because many different types of clinical settings are used for GITT in our setting, we developed a training manual. We designed this manual to help clinicians, clinical faculty, and academic faculty develop strategies for supporting team learning by health professionals of all disciplines. Specifically, it addresses the overall concepts, goals, and objectives of the project; provides a bibliography of journal articles and other resources for team training; supplies evaluation and self-assessment tools; and ensures uniformity of training programs across different settings. Also important to maintaining a cohesive approach across a multitude of settings and disciplines were orienting participants to the setting of training, identifying goals of the training, and actively examining communication and decision-making processes.

Orienting Trainees to the Setting

Setting the stage to learn GITT requires not only painting a broad background of interdisciplinary teams, but also providing specific details of team meetings at that setting. Integral to understanding a team is, at minimum, an introduction to and understanding of the different disciplines one might encounter on that team. Currently, an understanding of other health care disciplines is not a required part of any health discipline education. Because different disciplines often bring different values, problem-solving methods, and terminology, taking time to emphasize the setting's tolerance for these differences and the collective worth this often brings to patient care is often necessary to set the tone for team meetings (Qualls & Czirr, 1988).

Identifying Goals and Objectives
of Team Training

Although individual trainee goals are important, preceptors must clarify their expectations of trainee responsibilities and roles within the team. A brief overview of the worth of interdisciplinary health care teams, especially in geriatrics, may be necessary to those who have not had this and may serve as a reminder to those who have. If some patient care occurs outside of the team, an explanation of who benefits from team care and when one might transition into the team is useful. Clarifying the variety of teams and how team members come and go, depending on the setting, the problem, and the patient, is often necessary.

Formal meetings represent only a small fraction of the work of interdisciplinary health care teams. For instance, planning for discharge from an acute care setting usually necessitates many encounters with multiple team members (including social work, nursing, medicine, pharmacy, and any specialized therapies the patient requires) to make sure an appropriate plan is in place. Although the general plan may be established in a formal meeting, often the details are worked out in numerous small exchanges. Pointing out how often encounters take place in the course of routine geriatric care—informally as well as formally—often clarifies for the trainee the importance of this training.

Monitoring Communication, Conflict, and Decision Making

Communication between disciplines can lead to misunderstanding, conflict, and even decision making by default. Trainees must know their formal and informal responsibilities, including expectations for attendance at meetings and the nature and format of the information that the team will demand of them. In our setting, we review a calendar of meetings and an outline or handbook of the different communication tools.

Conflict between disciplines is often part of this communication and can be disconcerting to trainees. Reassurance that this is not personal, often normal, and constructive to both team growth and patient outcome is helpful (Drinka, 1994). Sharing examples of constructive conflict and providing training in conflict management skills can alleviate the pressures that the trainees feel. For instance, after doing a complete workup and consulting a surgeon about a patient who had fallen, a medical resident was upset when others suggested that avoiding surgical intervention might be an appropriate option. After discussion with the family, consideration of quality-of-life issues, and full analysis of the implications of surgery in light of this patient's many other medical problems, the team (including the resident) developed a clearer understanding of an appropriate plan of care.

Communication in an interdisciplinary health care team is a complex dynamic among multiple members; the division of labor is usually based on function, not status, and the feeling of shared responsibility for the outcome. A few questions after the first team encounters can help clarify what is happening within any given team and make team function clearer to trainees.

1. What is the team's mission?
2. Who is the leader? Does this leadership change? If so, why? When?
3. What is the climate of this team?
4. How does the team identify and solve problems?
5. Is there a communication pattern?

ROLE MODELING

The teaching value of the clinical setting cannot be overestimated. A smoothly functioning team can motivate trainees, allowing them to witness problem solving, decision making, and conflict resolution. It can be especially empowering to team members who are not physicians if during these team meetings the medical partners are able to let go of their presumed right to lead and permit other partners to assume leadership roles with confidence. For instance, a team meeting that requires the expertise of a discipline other than medicine—such as a rehabilitation problem whose solution requires physical therapists' leadership—might be such an opportunity.

ENSURING FEEDBACK AND EVALUATION

The frequency with which the facilitator meets with the clinic setting staff, the preceptors, and the trainees may be dictated by time constraints, logistics of the facility, or severity of problems that may be occurring. The facilitator's role is evolving differently in each setting. Formal evaluation is necessary, but informal feedback is often just as informative and may allow problems to be resolved earlier and easier. Having trainees in any setting implies more work and is often time intensive. How the clinical team learning facilitator can minimize this impact again varies with the setting, but assisting with evaluation and coordination at the project level will ease the burden on the preceptors and encourage and promote team training.

CLINICAL TEACHING METHODOLOGIES

Teaching clinical skills and behaviors has always been a challenging part of health care trainee education. Challenges become even more pronounced when the focus of education moves to a system model (that is, the role and/or function of teams in solving geriatric problems). What are the teaching methodologies that help translate expert practice into discrete, learnable skills?

Teaching methodologies in clinical settings have traditionally depended on same-discipline learning, transmission of knowledge from expert to novice, and return demonstrations of competency. It is often the responsibility of the trainee to integrate a new competency into the overall approach to a patient. Offering clinical teachers an array of options to incorporate into their own teaching skills library, the HGITT Project has sought to develop a matrix model of teaching methodologies.

Teaching team performance necessitates a different model of expert–novice interaction. The traditional model features discrete, linear efforts in which each clinician, working within a single discipline, develops plans or treatment goals independent of other clinicians. In this model, the patient is the object of, but not a participant in, the care process. The team-based model, on the other hand, emphasizes multidisciplinary communication (often using different language for similar issues), acquisition of more plastic communication skills applicable to both patients and coworkers, and integration of skills or concepts to achieve group goals. This model features interrelated and overlapping roles of clinicians, collegial relationships with trainees, and a care planning process in which the patient becomes an involved participant.

To ensure a successful clinical teaching experience, the clinical team learning facilitator serves as a resource for trainees and preceptors, who may want new teaching strategies. Because different clinical settings require different teaching modalities, the clinical team learning facilitator must first look at the system-wide organization of the particular clinical setting and determine its overall goals. These may include: (a) transmission of geriatric concepts and skills, (b) managing complex cases, (c) developing standards of care, (d) reviewing clinical performance, (e) monitoring continuous quality improvement, (f) developing alternative solutions to problems, (g) developing policies and procedures, and (h) coordinating discharge plans.

The challenge is to match teaching methodology to the team's responsibilities, so that both learning and task performance occur simultaneously and do not detract from the team's daily functioning.

The HGITT Project is developing a resource manual for the clinical team learning facilitators that serves as a reference of teaching resources, cases, and exercises. A panel of expert teachers from multiple disciplines in both academic and clinical settings selected materials for the manual. HGITT Project planners asked participants to submit their own teaching resources, and they undertook a comprehensive review of the literature to ascertain the current practice in clinical teaching. The panel then reviewed the materials and ranked them in several areas, including utility for multiple disciplines, time frame to completion, limitations, clinical relevance, and suggestions for follow-up.

The expert review committee has identified several different teaching styles and methodologies for the varied clinical settings participating in the HGITT Project. They include case studies, chart reviews, computer-assisted technologies, group practicum exercises, observational experiences, performance and feedback, prepared presentations, self-assessment strategies, seminars and conferences, and team-building exercises.

Case studies can be standardized or derived from the clinicians' personal experiences. They are most effective when the number of teaching points is limited to three or fewer and are clearly identified. The exercises are appealing to trainees because of their basis in actual practice and their interactive nature.

Chart reviews are useful strategies, but they require preparation. They are most effective when used in small to medium group settings. This strategy can be used to examine the team's effectiveness in planning discharges or long-term health plans for complex cases. For trainees with limited clinical time at a setting, chart reviews can impart a broader view of how teams have handled patients and problems over time in that setting.

Computer-assisted technologies such as the hypertext system being developed by HGITT allow for self-directed learning. Hypertext is a process that allows special connections or hot links to be embedded in text or graphics displayed on a computer monitor. With these links, the users can progress through the clinical topic at their own pace and toward the material that they wish to access. This technology can be adopted for instruction in both geriatric topics and team content. Chapter 7 describes the range of technologies that settings are using to teach GITT.

Group practicum exercises can encompass projects or presentations that are the product of a team of trainees. Trainee teams require a faculty resource to assist in this process, and that time commitment should be delineated before beginning the project. The benefit of this approach is the real experience of joint planning and problem-solving with a tangible outcome. Trainees respond best to a group practicum exercise that is based on an actual clinical problem rather than a standard or theoretical assignment. Preceptors can use this methodology to teach geriatrics and team skills simultaneously.

Observational experiences are learning situations that preceptors arrange for trainees in which trainees observe different team experiences and then discuss their experiences. It is a method effective for individuals or small groups of trainees. Trainees often fail to understand the purpose of observational experiences unless specific goals are delineated. The preceptor enhances the experience by identifying key points in the team interaction.

Observing performance and giving feedback are a clinical preceptor's most important responsibilities, but these duties are often overlooked in the daily rush of events. This is an opportunity to provide trainees with an objective appraisal of their performance that can improve clinical skills (Ende, 1983). This strategy is most effective when it is well-timed, expected, and focuses on remedial behaviors and specific performances

(Weinhotz & Edwards, 1992). It is also an opportunity to reinforce good clinical performance or improvement.

Requesting *prepared presentations* is a strategy to direct the trainees' reading into areas that may be too complex to address fully during a clinical encounter. This is appropriate for trainee groups of all sizes and involves assignment of a presentation on a topic to the team. This approach prompts trainees to develop a deeper understanding of a specific topic and to become responsible for disseminating this knowledge to the team.

Self-assessment strategies employ standardized assessment tools to measure attitudes, communication styles, and group dynamics. The faculty preceptor must be familiar with interpreting results. These assessments are effective for self-directed individual trainee activity. Group debriefing adds to overall learning objectives, but requires time commitment away from clinical responsibilities.

Seminars and conferences offer group learning experiences that are ideal for medium to large groups of trainees. The content can be tailored to specific needs of trainees and can incorporate role playing, simulation, and observation. It requires the commitment of faculty and trainee time away from clinical responsibilities.

Team-building exercises consist of structured, facilitated group interactions meant to help identify sources of bias and conflict in teams and to develop strategies to enhance functioning, improve communication, and resolve conflict. These exercises can vary from one-time experiences to programs of several weeks' duration. They require clinical faculty preparation and group consent to participate in the activity. They are good for medium to large groups of trainees.

ADAPTING TRAINING TO DIFFERENT TIMETABLES

One of the major challenges of GITT is how to involve trainees of different disciplines in the all-important learning-by-doing experiences. The creation of clinical geriatric training experiences for interdisciplinary teams may involve a range of different disciplines beyond the minimum three disciplines specified by the John A. Hartford Foundation for GITT Projects (medicine, advance practice nursing, and social work). The disciplines represented by a setting's clinical team (usually defined by the clinical mission) and the clinical learning opportunities available for trainees will most likely determine who will be included in team training activities.

The HGITT Project has developed interdisciplinary training experiences for trainees of eight different disciplines from three academic institutions. Each of the six HGITT clinical settings provides training for medical residents, advanced practice nurses, and social work; the other disciplines are trained in only some settings: psychiatry residents at three; physician assistants at four; pharmacy trainees at three; and psychology trainees at two. Other Hartford GITT Projects have created experiences for trainees of additional professions, for example, physical and occupation therapists, chaplains, and dietitians. Regardless of the disciplines involved, there are some clear challenges inherent in structuring the clinical experiences for different groups of health professions trainees. These challenges include matters of logistics (differing academic calendars, programmatic requirements) and conceptual issues (variability in preclinical knowledge and skills of trainees of different disciplines). Interdisciplinary program leaders and faculty must address both to ensure that trainees of different disciplines will be available to participate.

The HGITT Project used a three-step process to determine which trainee disciplines could be trained effectively at a given clinical setting.

1. An HGITT coinvestigator and the clinical setting coordinators identified the current or proposed clinical preceptor for each discipline, and these individuals were interviewed by their respective academic counterparts using a structured guide. This information was summarized to inform overall planning for all project activities. The interviewers solicited information in the following areas from each clinician or potential preceptor: current practice settings (home care, clinic, or other), primary clinical responsibilities, methods and frequency of communication with other disciplines, existing expectations for clinical competency and productivity of trainees' self-development training needs, and perceived barriers to interdisciplinary training.

2. After individual interviews were completed, a large meeting was held at the clinical setting involving an expanded interdisciplinary group of all academic coordinators, preceptors from other clinical settings, and persons crucial to the successful integration of training at that setting. These meetings covered the exchange of information about overall clinical operations and the academic preparation, practicum needs, and logistics of each discipline.

In addition to building communication bridges between academic faculty and clinical preceptors, these meetings produced a menu of options for team learning experiences, identified additional clinical and administrative personnel necessary for project activities, and highlighted resources available to support training.

3. After the general meeting, a series of smaller meetings was scheduled to produce the design of discipline-specific rotations and to delineate how team training would proceed in a particular setting. These meetings are ongoing. Ultimately, each clinical setting must have a defined schedule for trainee involvement in team meetings and learning opportunities. Table 9.4 includes some of the logistic challenges encountered by HGITT and the corresponding strategies used to overcome these challenges.

The total length of a given clinical rotation will determine the ultimate mix of activities that a trainee in a given discipline is able to participate in, which will logically influence the development of competencies. Disciplines whose main objective is exposure to the process may have a more superficial experience, while others will attain a higher level of skill.

Although many disciplines in health and social services recognize the importance of functioning as members of the health care team, no accrediting bodies mandate training in interdisciplinary teams. Both the American Boards of Internal Medicine and Family Practice and the American Nurses Credentialing Center require that trainees have experience caring for the elderly; they do not mandate that this include an interdisciplinary setting, however. Because the majority of health professional educational programs do not have required interdisciplinary educational experiences, developing an interdisciplinary clinical experience is generally based on local arrangements and negotiations across departments and fields.

TABLE 9.4 Common Logistic Challenges in Structuring Team Training for Multiple Disciplines

Challenges	Potential solutions
Clinical rotations are of different lengths (1 month full-time or 8 months part-time).	Design clinical learning around cycles of shorter rotations to reach all disciplines and consider levels of training for trainees with longer rotations.
Trainees begin on different dates, making a single orientation difficult.	Develop self-instructional materials to facilitate background understanding. Involve experienced trainees in helping orient newer trainees of another discipline.
Schedule conflicts hamper the creation of learning teams.	Negotiate commitments to a common meeting time for all trainees as part of rotation requirements for each discipline.

Trainees must have a clear appreciation of the potential practice roles of each discipline that is incorporated into a clinical setting. As Huff and Garrola (1995) note, even though not all health professions trainees will practice in an interdisciplinary team, they will be in practice settings requiring collaboration, consultation, and coordination. Furthermore, most health professionals will be involved in caring for older adults. Therefore, HGITT program leaders and faculty decided to identify the complex array of skills required for health professionals to practice as members of geriatric interdisciplinary teams. They identified specific learning objectives common to all disciplines involved in the project (Table 9.5). Both academic and clinical faculty of each discipline had the opportunity to contribute to the development and refinement of these learning objectives, recognizing that learning objectives would have unequal weights, and that issues of timing and skill were specific to each trainee.

EVALUATING INTERDISCIPLINARY TRAINING

The supervision and evaluation of trainees in the interdisciplinary team training setting occur in two distinct areas. The first area of supervision and evaluation is by the discipline-specific preceptor in the clinical setting and concerns the trainee's comprehension of learning objectives for discipline-specific roles. In the second, the clinical preceptor evaluates the trainee for knowledge of interdisciplinary content and participation in the interdisciplinary team process.

The roles of the discipline-specific preceptors are determined by the individual disciplines and negotiated between the preceptor and the academic institutions. Learning objectives, clinical hours, and evaluation mechanisms for each discipline are set by the academic institution and are evaluated by the preceptor and faculty for that discipline.

Communication between the clinical preceptors and the academic faculty is essential. The academic faculty must clearly outline the goals and learning objectives for the trainee's clinical experience, expectations of the clinical preceptors, and requirements

TABLE 9.5   GITT Learning Objectives

The geriatric team training curriculum is designed around core learning objectives for the essential knowledge, skills, and attitudes required for team care of geriatric patients and families. Upon successful completion of the geriatric team training didactic and clinical experiences, trainees should be able to:

1. Describe concepts of a geriatric interdisciplinary team approach and differentiate that approach from other care models.
2. Identify the different training attitudes and philosophies that distinguish professional subcultures.
3. Identify the unique capabilities of different disciplines required for particular geriatric problems.
4. Articulate the roles of patient, family, and community in caring for the older adult.
5. Recognize the dynamic process of leadership within a team and demonstrate appropriate leadership roles.
6. Recognize cultural, gender, age, ethnic, racial, and socioeconomic barriers that may affect communication and exchange among providers, patients, their families, and communities.
7. Identify how diverse styles of communication contribute to team function.
8. Communicate effectively with other team members, patients, family members, and community representatives.
9. Demonstrate role negotiation skills and effective involvement of other team members in patient care.
10. Determine treatment and management goals with other team members and the patient and describe methods that maximize outcome evaluation in geriatric interdisciplinary team care.
11. Demonstrate an ability to adapt behavior to changing team dynamics and patient care demands.
12. Demonstrate cultural competency in interactions with team members, patients, and their families.
13. Demonstrate skills at resolving problems between team members.
14. Demonstrate a collaborative spirit by showing respect and support for other members' skills in providing patient care.

of the setting (such as patient population, space needs). The clinical preceptors must communicate the skill level expected of the trainees who enter the program, setting expectations (such as the days per week the trainees need to be in clinic, hours at the setting), and evaluation of trainees' clinical performance. The clinical evaluation and input from the clinical preceptor should be utilized to evaluate the curriculum, as well.

At the clinical settings, the trainee's performance is evaluated primarily on evidence of applied knowledge and skill (Headrick, Norman, Gelmon, & Knapp, 1995). The trainees are generally evaluated by their discipline-specific preceptor, and this evaluation usually affects the trainee's grade. If there is an interdisciplinary team at the setting and the trainee is working with the team, the team should have input into the trainee evaluation. If the clinical team learning facilitator is not the clinical preceptor, these two individuals must discuss the trainee's evaluation.

Some of the disciplines will have collaboration and team concepts as a part of the clinical learning objectives, and others will not. If there are learning objectives, there should also be some method to evaluate how the trainee meets these objectives. Trainees of all disciplines are very aware of the evaluation criteria for a clinical experience or rotation, and if interdisciplinary content or practice is not evaluated, the trainee may not feel the need to participate in or value this interdisciplinary content.

Examples of evaluation criteria that can be included on trainee evaluations include:

- Demonstrates knowledge of roles and functions of other disciplines
- Identifies when it is appropriate to make referrals to specific disciplines
- Develops professional relationships with practitioners from various other disciplines
- Promotes professional behavior
- Works collaboratively with the preceptor and other members of the health team.

Chapter 10 describes many of the evaluation tools that are available. Appendix B contains the core measures that the GITT Project will be using to measure change in behaviors and knowledge across all project sites.

CONCLUSIONS

The goal of the HGITT Project is to make the practicum a learning experience for trainees that leads to improved patient care. Our initial experiences in HGITT have reinforced the dynamic nature of clinical teaching, and over time, we hope to further refine and expand our strategies for teaching and modeling team training.

REFERENCES

Abramson, J. S., & Mizrahi, T. (1996). When social workers and physicians collaborate: Positive and negative interdisciplinary experiences. *Social Work, 41,* 270–281.

Butler, R. (1994). *Ten geriatric messages for managed care: How to be responsive to the growing older adult population.* Paper presented at the American Society for Aging meeting for Managed Care Professionals and Executives, Atlanta, GA.

Drinka, T. J. K. (1994). Interdisciplinary geriatric teams: Approaches to conflict as indicators of potential to model teamwork. *Educational Gerontology, 20,* 87–103.

Ende, J. (1983). Feedback in clinical medical education. *Journal of the American Medical Association, 250,* 777–781.

Headrick, L. A., Norman, L., Gelmon, S., & Knapp, A. (1995). *Interdisciplinary professional education in the continuous improvement of health care: The state-of-the-art.* (Final Report to the Health Services Resources Administration, Bureau of Health Professions). Washington, DC: Department of Health and Human Services.

Huff, F., & Garrola, G. (1995). Potential patterns—Conceptual and practical issues in interdisciplinary education. *Journal of Allied Health, 24,* 359–365.

Netting, F. E., & Williams, F. G. (1995). Integrating geriatric case management into primary care physician practices. *Health and Social Work, 20,* 152–155.

Qualls, S. H., & Czirr, R. (1988). Geriatric health teams: Classifying models of professional and team functioning. *Gerontologist, 28,* 372–376.

University of North Carolina at Chapel Hill. (1993). *Education for interdisciplinary rural health care: A program director's resource manual* (Bureau of Health Professions, Contract #240-920030). Chapel Hill, NC: UNC-CH.
Weinholtz, D., & Edwards, J. (1992). *Teaching during rounds: A handbook for attending physicians and residents.* Baltimore, MD: Johns Hopkins University Press.

Evaluating the Effects of Geriatric Interdisciplinary Team Training

Terry Fulmer and Kathryn Hyer

The Geriatric Interdisciplinary Team Training (GITT) Program provides a remarkable opportunity to explore the effects of team training in the context of geriatric care. The Program's mission is training, and it is not a clinical trial. Nonetheless, we can gain important insights into how trainees learn to work on teams by systematically collecting information across the projects. We will be summarizing pretests and posttests administered to GITT trainees to help determine what the essential features of an interdisciplinary team training curriculum might look like. We also hope to learn how students from different disciplines master the goals and objectives that teachers of GITT find essential.

We recognize that each of the individual projects is specially tailored to its site's needs, with different trainee populations, clinical experiences, and interventions. In obtaining information across projects and sharing these data, the Resource Center can help project personnel find ways to improve their curricula and understand the trainees' perceptions of the GITT experience. The core measures activity, as we have come to call it, will also provide each site with benchmarks and will enrich the efforts of the external Program Evaluation, which a team from the University of California at Los Angeles is undertaking.

WHY GITT CORE MEASURES?

Our approach to core measures is consonant with the goals of the overall GITT Program, which are to:

- Improve the responsiveness of academic institutions to the educational and training needs of health care providers;
- Develop well-tested curricula for geriatric team training;
- Create a cadre of well-trained professionals competent in geriatric and interdisciplinary skills;
- Test staff development training models for practicing health professionals.

We believe that the core measures will help the sites and the Hartford Foundation answer the following questions:

- What did students learn about interdisciplinary teams in terms of team leadership, roles on teams, conflict management, and communication skills?
- What did students learn about the care of older people as evidenced by their ability to identify proper care and their understanding of the role of other disciplines in providing care?
- How satisfied were the students with GITT training?
- How interested are GITT graduates in working in geriatrics or in team settings?
- How frequently have trainees used the team skills during the practicum training?

A summary of available instruments that focus on selected aspects of the clinical encounter can be found in Tables 10.1–10.6. These tables have been developed from two summaries prepared by the Resource Center evaluation consultants Teresi and Holmes (Teresi & Holmes, 1996; Teresi, Holmes, Hyer, & Totten, 1996), and have served as the foundation from which the Resource Center then selected, modified, or created the core measures we now use. Searches of MEDLINE, CINHAL, and personal communications provided the information. Although the instruments have different foci, all have relevance to the goals of GITT.

Core measures are meant to provide an ongoing assessment of the projects' progress, and a large common pool of uniform data that will facilitate collaborative analyses and interpretations. In this chapter, we provide a summary of evaluation measures that are available in the literature, measures that guided our conceptualization of the core measures. We then discuss the final core measures created by the Resource Center in collaboration with the project investigators and evaluators for use in the GITT Program (see Appendix B).

Because the GITT Program is foremost a training model, the core measures focus on the trainees, the ultimate unit of analysis. The Hartford Foundation's reason for funding this program is to enable other institutions to learn about and replicate successful training models. To do this, the Foundation is supporting both formative and summative measures. The formative perspective, captured by the Foundation through annual site visits and annual reports, captures programmatic and clinical data that we believe will be very important for disseminating the lessons learned by the sites during project implementation. The formative approach also allows sites to collaborate on implementation strategies, modify their training over the 3 years of implementation, and celebrate their successes within and across projects. The GITT core measures are summative and have been developed to focus primarily on any changes in trainee knowledge, attitudes, and behaviors regarding teams and geriatric care.

THE GITT CORE MEASURE CONSTRUCTS AND INSTRUMENTS

Kirkpatrick conceptualized evaluation at four levels (Kirkpatrick, 1975):

Level 1   Reaction of participants to training
Level 2   Knowledge obtained through training

Level 3   Behavior changes observed by others
Level 4   Organizational or programmatic impact

GITT core measures focus on feelings about and perceptions of the program and knowledge obtained as a result of participating in the GITT. Appendix B contains the instruments derived and developed for the cross-project core measures in the GITT program. We developed these measures through group consensus, looking for a tool that would capture essential information, yet be practical in terms of the time it would take to collect the data. The four components of the GITT core measures take approximately 60 to 75 minutes to collect. They are given at the beginning of the training experience and again at the end of the training in a pre and post approach. The components are: (a) demographics, (b) students' knowledge, attitudes, and behaviors regarding interdisciplinary teams, (c) case studies for knowledge of geriatric care, and (d) videotapes for knowledge of team dynamics.

Although we have chosen the core measures to assess students' knowledge, attitudes, and behaviors regarding interdisciplinary teams, we sought to assess knowledge, attitudes, and behaviors concerning the care of geriatric clients as well. In an effort to capture the latter, the planning sites expressed great interest in developing case studies based on patient vignettes of fairly typical geriatric cases. This has been done through the intensive efforts of a Case Study Working Group comprised of volunteer members from GITT (Terry Fulmer, Kathy Hyer, Robert Kane, Nancy Whitelaw, and Nancy Wilson). The team dynamics knowledge is measured through the responses to the questions related to the videotapes. At this writing, these measures are new to the program, and data are not yet available for comment.

The demographics collected in the core measures include an identification number, student status, work experience, any formal training in geriatrics (and the nature of the training experience), any previous team training, types of previous employment, educational degrees, gender, and ethnicity.

The pretest includes: (a) a trainee prequestionnaire, comprised of 46 items, with sections addressing opinions about teams, self-assessment regarding team behavior, attitudes about teams, and career goals regarding geriatric teaming; (b) clinical case studies with five test questions related to appropriate geriatric care and team involvement; and (c) a 3 to 4 minute videotape of a team in progress with five questions that address team dynamics. The posttest includes 53 items, with the same pretest questions along with seven evaluation items of the GITT experience, a post case study, and a post videotape. All are pencil and paper measures. The case and video at posttest are different from the pretest, but the questions remain the same.

Effective teaming depends not only on the intellectual expertise of the team members, but also on the way individuals behave in teams. This is most often referred to in the literature as team skills or team dynamics. The literature on group dynamics (Clark, 1994; Drinka & Ray, 1991; Heinemann, Schmitt, & Farrell, 1991; Toner & Meyer, 1988) suggests that there are certain basic concepts: (a) common goal perception, (b) democratic leadership and decision making, (c) resource availability, and (d) free flow of communication. The GITT Trainee Questionnaire addresses some these domains; qualitative case studies and videotaped teaming vignettes address others.

TABLE 10.1 Course, Trainee, and Instructor Evaluations

Tool	Source	Comments
Course and Instructor Evaluation Form	University of Houston, Graduate School of Social Work, undated	This final student evaluation is comprised of eight items. Six are rated on a five-point continuum from poor to outstanding, and two are rated from very little to very much. Respondents rate the course on four items, such as, "I would rate the overall quality of this course as . . ."; and the instructor on four additional items, such as, "I would recommend this course instructor to a fellow student" and "Considering lectures, readings, class discussions, student presentations, and term papers, how much content of this course pertained to women, women's issues or the changing role of women in our society?"
Geriatric Assessment Core Class Participant/ Enrollee Evaluation	Columbia/New York Geriatric Education Center (GEC), 1995	Participants rate performance using a five-point continuum from strongly agree to strongly disagree, applied to 10 items, such as, "The content was relevant to the core class objectives," and "The speaker was knowledgeable, organized, and effective in the presentation." Three open-ended items elicit opinions regarding strengths, weaknesses, and ways in which the course did or did not meet the respondent's objectives.
Geriatric Experience Assessment–Student	University of North Carolina, Division of Physical Therapy, 1994	This tool contains eight items. The first five reflect the worth and impact of the experience, such as, "The time devoted to this experience was well spent and worthwhile." Statements are scored on a five-point continuum from strongly disagree to strongly agree. The three remaining (open-ended) questions are "What was the most valuable aspect?" "What about this experience will help you offer better physical therapy to geriatric clients?" and "What would you recommend changing and how?"
Harlem Valley Psychiatric Center Treatment Team Seminar & Evaluation Form	Toner and Meyer, 1988	This form is a 38-item evaluation of team seminars by participants. The scoring is on a five-point continuum from strongly agree to strongly disagree. Typical questions include: "I had no trouble understanding the presentations

TABLE 10.1 *(Continued)*

Tool	Source	Comments
		during the seminar," "I felt that we had adequate time to integrate the material," and "The concepts I have learned during the seminar have helped me to understand the Uniform Case Record."
Harvard Upper New England GEC (HUNEGEC) Intake Questionnaire	HUNEGEC, not dated	Trainees respond to 13 questions: six items on trainee background and training experience, three items on geriatric training at the trainees' institution, and four open-ended questions on goals for training and future goals in geriatrics. Typical open-ended items are "On return to your academic institution, what obstacles do you anticipate in trying to implement goals in geriatrics?" and "Please describe specific goals you have in each of following areas . . ."
HUNEGEC 1-Year Follow-Up Questionnaire	HUNEGEC, not dated	This is an eight-item questionnaire measuring changes in the home institution and in the trainee as a result of the GEC experience. Three questions ask about geriatric courses and programs at the trainee's institution and about the disciplines and academic levels of the courses. Five open-ended questions request details about the changes, such as, "Since your experiences at the HUNEGEC, have any additional faculty members or professionals at your institution become involved in geriatric activities?" and "Did your experience contribute to your new level of involvement in geriatrics?"
HUNEGEC Posttraining Questionnaire	HUNEGEC, not dated	This is a 10-item questionnaire: one item requests an estimate of the hours spent at specific geriatric services, a second measures satisfaction with time spent using a three-point scale (too little, about right, too much); the remaining eight questions are open-ended. Examples include: "Which of the goals you had for your training were most fully met?" "Please describe your experience in training and include problems experienced and suggestions for program improvement." and "Did your attitudes toward the field of geriatrics change as a result of your experience?"

(cont.)

TABLE 10.1 Course, Trainee, and Instructor Evaluations *(Continued)*

Tool	Source	Comments
Midsemester Course Evaluation	University of Houston, Graduate School of Social Work, not dated	The evaluation contains six items. Two items are ratings of the course and instructor on a seven-point continuum from totally unacceptable to outstanding, with questions such as "How would you rate this course thus far?" Three multiple choice items measuring the appropriateness of the level, pace, and instructor demeanor are included, such as, "The instructional pace is too fast, the pace is just right, the pace is too slow." One open-ended item elicits suggestions and comments.
Residency Objective Structured Clinical Exam (OSCE)–Student Evaluation Questionnaire	Baylor College of Medicine, Department of Family Medicine, © 1995	This is a 31-item resident evaluation of work load, quality of support services, interactions with and performance of attending physicians on a service. Seven items ask residents to estimate the number of patients they have seen with various conditions. Fourteen items such as "Evaluate your performance on the following stations" are rated on a five-point continuum from poor to excellent. Nine items are resident ratings of their experiences on a five-point continuum, such as, "Please rate how comfortable you felt overall while you were taking the OSCE," from very uncomfortable to very comfortable. One open-ended question asks for additional comments on the experience.
Student Evaluation of Course	University of Texas-Houston Health Science Center, School of Nursing, Center for Nursing Research, May, 1993	This is an 11-item measure, with nine items scored on a four-point continuum from needs improvement to excellent and two open-ended questions. Typical questions are "The course requirements in the syllabus were clearly stated," "The course encouraged problem solving and creative thinking." Items evaluate the course requirements, objectives, texts, and assignments; two open-ended questions measure the strengths of the course and elicit suggestions for course improvement.
Geriatric Fellowship: Self-Assessment	University of North Carolina, undated	Four open-ended items on faculty-fellow interaction and the relevance of the experience, and seven pages of items split into skill areas (clinical, teaching, research, administration) are rated on a

TABLE 10.1 *(Continued)*

Tool	Source	Comments
		three-point scale (limited, moderate, and considerable skill). No psychometric information is available.
Field Experience Evaluation	Area L Area Health Education Center Interdisciplinary Student Training Program, undated	This measure contains six open-ended questions related to evaluation of student contributions to the team, ability to provide resources for patients, benefits of team participation, most useful activity during rotation, elements that were confusing or unhelpful, and suggestions for improvement. No psychometric information is available.

TABLE 10.2 **Individual and Team Functioning**

Tool	Source	Comments
Strength Deployment Inventory	Porter (1976) © 1989 Personal Strengths Publishing, Inc. (There is a charge for the test.)	Based on the work of Elias Porter (1976, 1983, 1987) including the Relationship Awareness Theory (RAT), the Strength Deployment Inventory (SDI) assesses the motivational value system of the respondents under two kinds of conditions: when everything is going well, and when faced with conflict and opposition. RAT holds that there are three basic sets of motivations (Altruistic-Nurturing [A-N], Assertive-Directing [A-D], and Analytic-Autonomizing [A-A]) from which seven motivational value systems are derived. The measure consists of 20 items, which take a total of 10 minutes to complete and 20–30 minutes to interpret. For 10 of the items, respondents assume things are going well and for the remaining 10 items they assume they are in conflict. Items consist of incomplete sentences followed by three different endings. Respondents are asked to allocate a total of 10 points among these three possible sentence endings based on how frequently each sentence ending is self-descriptive. Typical questions include: (a) "Most of the time I am apt to be . . ." "a feeling person who is quick to respond to the feelings of others," "an energetic person who is quick to see the opportunities and advantages," "a practical person

TABLE 10.2   Individual and Team Functioning *(Continued)*

Tool	Source	Comments
		who is careful not to rush into things before I am ready," (b) "In getting along with difficult people, I usually . . ." "change what I am doing and try to make it more acceptable to the person," "find the holes in that person's argument and press the strong points in mine," "appeal to the person's sense of respect for logic and fair play." Test-retest reliabilities for each scale were: A-N, $r = .78$; A-D, $r = .78$; and A-A, $r = .76$. Each item ending was analyzed to determine the extent to which it discriminated between high scores on a scale and low scores on a scale using the chi-square method; results indicated a high degree of ability to discriminate.
Styles of Teamwork Inventory	Hall, O'Leary, and Williams (1964), Hall and Williams (1971). © 1994 Teleometrics International (There is a charge for test.)	A revised version of the Teamwork Appraisal Survey, the Styles of Teamwork Inventory is an 80-item measure of how individuals function on work teams. It is based on the team behaviors model (Hall, O'Leary, & Williams, 1964) that provides a two-dimensional analysis of individual behavior in a team setting, according to which individuals in teams have a concern for the accomplishment of the work at hand and a concern for the relationships that exist with other team members. The model identifies five distinct styles of behavior. The measure is designed to elicit preferences for behaviors and feelings in four areas: individual attitudes toward team situations, leadership preference, conflict resolution, and intergroup relations. Items are scored on a 10-point continuum ranging from completely characteristic to completely uncharacteristic and are designed to elicit preferences and weighting of behaviors that are used to infer a preferred approach to working in task groups. The test-retest reliabilities for the five style subscores range from .69 to .81 with a median coefficient of .77. Chronbach's alpha is .76 for the total measure. The test takes about 30

TABLE 10.2 *(Continued)*

Tool	Source	Comments
		minutes to complete, 20 minutes to score, and 30 minutes to interpret to the group. Teleometrics recommends spending another 30 minutes to explain the theory behind the test. It is recommended that this be done in one setting, which may suggest that this test is not practical for GITT.
Intensive Care Unit Physician Questionnaire	Shortell, Rousseau, Gillies, Devers, and Simons (1991). Copyrighted but there is no charge. (Permission to use in our research has been obtained.)	The authors claim that although the measure was developed for use in intensive care units (ICU), it has applicability for other hospital settings. It takes 20 minutes to complete. It consists of 67 items divided into five sections. Relationships and Communications within the ICU (physician/physician relationships, nurse/physician relationships, general relationships, and communications), Teamwork and Leadership (nursing leadership, physician, general), Managing disagreements between physicians and nurses, Authority, and Satisfaction. All items are rated on a five-point Likert scale, most from strongly agree to strongly disagree, and some are rated from not at all likely to almost certain. The authors indicate that other services or units can be substituted for ICU without loss of reliability. For example, a typical item measuring physician to physician relationships is "It is easy for me to talk openly with physicians on this ICU (other unit, specialty, etc)." Although the questionnaire is discipline- and setting-specific, there are some sections that appear more general and seem to examine team function. It is impossible to know how well adaptations would perform psychometrically. Cronbach's alphas for the scales range from .61 to .88, with all but three scales about the .70 level. The full psychometric characteristics on construct development, reliability, and validity of the ICU Nurse–Physician Questionnaire are summarized by the authors in Shortell, Rousseau, Gillies, Devers, and Simons (1991).

(cont.)

TABLE 10.2 Individual and Team Functioning *(Continued)*

Tool	Source	Comments
Conflict Management Survey: A self-assessment of your management of the dynamics of conflict	Hall (1975), Hall and Williams (1971). Revised measure © 1995 Teleometrics International Hall, 1995. (There is a charge for the test.)	This survey is based on the team behaviors model (Hall, O'Leary, & Williams, 1964; Hall & Williams, 1971), representing a two-dimensional analysis of an individual's behavior in conflict. Hall asserts that individuals determine conflict from two perspectives along a 2 x 2 matrix from low to high: concern for personal goals and concern for the relationship. The model identifies five models of conflict behavior. The authors assert that by displaying 120 different patterns of conflict management, the tool permits members to learn alternative methods of resolving conflict. Total administration is at least 1 hour; 15 minutes to complete, 15 minutes to score, and 30 minutes to interpret to the group. Teleometrics also recommends another 30 minutes to explain the theory behind the test. The administration time and the cost may preclude this from serious consideration. Factor analytic results reflect .93 average commonality across the five styles. Spearman–Brown reliability coefficients for the five conflict management modes are: Collaborative = .87; Compromise = .73; Accommodative = .70; Forcing = .83; and Avoidant = .75. Reliability (Cronbach's alpha) ranges from .70 to .87.
Conflict Management Appraisal: An assessment of an associate's reactions to, and management of, conflict	Hall (1975). Revised test © 1994 Teleometrics International. (There is a charge for test.)	This measure is used in conjunction with the Conflict Management Survey measure. Forty questions are divided into two 20-item sections: Your Manager's Practices and Your Practices With Your Manager. Two process scales, Exposure and Feedback, are created. The measure takes about 20 minutes to complete, 20 minutes to score, and 30 minutes to interpret. Teleometrics also recommends another 30 minutes to explain the theory behind the test. The internal consistency estimated using Cronbach's alpha is .78 for Exposure and .80 for Feedback.
The Rahim Organizational	ROCI-I: Rahim and Bonoma (1979) and	The 21-item ROCI-I takes 6 minutes to complete. It provides scores on three

TABLE 10.2 *(Continued)*

Tool	Source	Comments
Conflict Inventories (ROCI)	Rahim (1983b). ROCI-II: Rahim, (1983a). © Consulting Psychologists Press, Inc. (There is a charge for the test.)	components of conflict management: Intrapersonal Conflict (seven items, alpha = .84), Intragroup Conflict (eight items, alpha = .79), and Intergroup Conflict (six items, alpha = .79). For each item, subjects respond to a five-point Likert continuum from strongly agree to strongly disagree. Typical questions include, "There is a good match between my needs and the needs of the organization" and "In our group, we do lots of bickering over who should do what job." The 28-item ROCI-II takes 8 minutes to complete. It has five dimensions that represent different styles of handling interpersonal conflict along a 2 x 2 matrix: Concern for Self and Concern for Others. High concern for self and others is Integrating (seven items, alpha = .77). High concern for others and low concern for self is Obligating (six items, alpha = .72). Low concern for others and high concern for self is Dominating (five items, alpha = .72). Low concern for others and low concern for self is Avoiding (six items, alpha = .75). Compromising (four items, alpha = .72) is moderate in both concerns. For each item, subjects respond to a five-point Likert continuum from strongly agree to strongly disagree. Higher scores indicate greater use of conflict style. Questions in ROCI-II include, "I avoid an encounter with my peers," "I use my influence to get my ideas accepted," and "I win some and I lose some."
Field Experience Self-Assessment– Initial and Final Evaluation	Area L Area Health Education Center Interdisciplinary Student Training Program, undated	Ten statements of activities/knowledge are each rated on a five-point continuum (1 = low to 5 = high). Questions include, "I feel comfortable in interviewing patients and families" and "I feel that I can participate on an interdisciplinary team to form a treatment plan." An open-ended item on the initial evaluation form asks how past academic and clinical experiences would benefit involvement on a team. The final item inquires about the value of the experience.

(cont.)

TABLE 10.2   Individual and Team Functioning *(Continued)*

Tool	Source	Comments
Small Group Process: Reflection and Analysis	R. Hunter, UNC-Chapel Hill, undated.	This instrument measures 11 domains with questions to guide reflection or discussion following the observation of a team meeting. Typical prompts under Leadership include, "Who are the group's leaders?" and "Is the leadership style autocratic or democratic?"

TABLE 10.3   Trainee Knowledge

Tool	Source	Comments
Alcohol Problems in Later Life and Depression and Suicide in Later Life	Pratt, Wilson, Benthin, and Schmall (1992)	Two quizzes assess the knowledge of community-dwelling adults and social service providers about mental health issues. The Alcohol Problems Quiz contains 10 items, and the Depression Quiz contains 12 items rated as true, false, or I don't know. Pilot testing with participants of three hour-long community education sessions showed that most of the incorrect answers were I don't know responses. The internal consistency, using the KR-20, was .83 for the Alcohol Problems Quiz and .85 for the Depression Quiz. No research has yet examined the relationship between knowledge measured by the quizzes and actual behavior (predictive validity). The authors state that these quizzes were not targeted to people with significant knowledge of mental health and that the items may be too easy for individuals with experience in mental health or inappropriate as an evaluation of an in-depth or intensive training experience. The measures may not be useful for this effort because the items are too easy and too specific, focusing on alcohol and depression rather than on more generic topics. Moreover, the scales are underdeveloped psychometrically, with little published validity data.
Basic Test of Geriatric Medicine	McMillan and Robinson (1991)	The authors developed a 66-item multiple choice test from a published set of objectives related to medical students' knowledge of concepts regarding the care of the elderly. The Content Validity Index (CVI) for the original

TABLE 10.3   *(Continued)*

Tool	Source	Comments
		118 item set yielded CVIs of greater than .66 for 85% of the items. For the 66 items in the final version, the reliability estimate using the KR-20 is .67, and the mean scores for two groups of students (one that had a short course in geriatrics and one that did not) are significantly different. A brief description of the test development process is provided in *Academic Medicine* 1991; 66:560; however, the test questions have not been published. Dr. Robinson, from the University of South Florida, believes the test is dated and does not recommend its use.
Geriatric Intern Rotation Test and Post-Test	Lindberg and Sullivan (1996)	A 35-item Knowledge Test and a 24-item Attitudes Questionnaire were given to residents at the beginning and again at the end of a 4-week inpatient geriatrics rotation. Information is not provided on the time required for the tests. The Knowledge Test contains 20 multiple choice and 15 true-false items developed by a panel of geriatricians, based on the goals and content of the rotation. Examples of knowledge questions are "Which of the following is the most reliable screening test to detect hearing impairment in an older person?" and "Weight loss or failure to regain weight after an acute illness is a poor predictor of increased morbidity and mortality." The alpha for the true/false items is reported as 0.83. A modified version of the Maxwell and Sullivan questionnaire (Maxwell & Sullivan, 1980, described below) was used as the attitude test, but the modifications are not described. Items such as "Elderly patients need too much attention and social support" are scored on a five-point continuum from 1 = strongly agree to 5 = strongly disagree. Alphas for Part B (five items on time concerns) and Part C (seven items on response to care) are reported as .70 and .65, respectively.
Resident Questionnaire (Evaluation Working Group of the John A.	Unpublished, not copyrighted.	This Resident Questionnaire was developed by medical residency programs that are participating in a

(cont.)

TABLE 10.3   Trainee Knowledge *(Continued)*

Tool	Source	Comments
Hartford Foundation Geriatrics in Primary Care Initiative [1996])		Foundation-funded program to increase the geriatric content in primary care medical residencies. The purpose of the questionnaire is to collect uniform information across seven sites participating in the initiative on the knowledge, attitudes, and behaviors of medical residents. The eight-page questionnaire requires 20 minutes to complete and contains six sections. The first section collects identifying and demographic information and asks three questions on future career plans (one item asks for identification of the type of career the respondent desires from a list of choices; and two items ask the respondent to rate on a five-point continuum the extent to which the resident plans to emphasize geriatrics and the likelihood of seeking additional training in geriatrics). The second section lists 19 activities related to medical treatment (such as, Functional assessment and History assessment and physical exam). The respondent is asked to rate each on a 5-point continuum (1 = low and 5 = high) for the following four items: Importance in your care of geriatric patients, your confidence in performing with geriatric patients, your likelihood of performing with geriatric patients, and your confidence in teaching to fellow house staff and students. The third section focuses on the perceived impact of the training experience. Using the same scale, residents are asked to rate the usefulness of their experience and their confidence in caring for patients in each of the settings in which they trained. Respondents are asked then to rate the degree of positive impact the experience will have on their practice of medicine (1 = very small; 5 = very large) and the amount of training in geriatrics in their program (1 = not enough; 5 = too much). The fourth section consists of 17 items developed to measure attitudes toward both elderly patients and the elderly in general (four items on personal experience

TABLE 10.3 *(Continued)*

Tool	Source	Comments
		with medical care for the elderly, eight items on medical care for the elderly population in general, and five items on the characteristics of elderly people). Respondents are asked to indicate on a five-point continuum whether they strongly disagree (1), disagree (2), are neutral (3), agree (4), or strongly agree (5) with each statement. The fifth section contains five items about the respondent's satisfaction with the training: the first two items request a rating of the level of satisfaction with the program's training in geriatrics (1 = not at all; 5 = highly satisfied) and the quality of geriatrics teaching (1 = poor; 5 = excellent). The remaining three items are open ended, asking what the respondent would tell an incoming resident, what was the most significant experience in the program, and for suggestions as to how the program could be improved. The sixth section contains 23 multiple choice knowledge questions derived from the American Geriatrics Society syllabus (19 focus on diagnosis and course of treatment for individual patients and four are questions on health services use and functional status of the older population in general. Psychometric data on sections four (attitudes) and six (geriatric knowledge) are available in advance of a paper soon to be published. These data are based on responses of 121 residents, fellows, and faculty used to pilot test the complete questionnaire. The correlation of the attitude test with the Maxwell-Sullivan Too Much Time to Care and No Benefit of Treatment subscales is .59. The internal consistency reliability as estimated by Cronbach's alpha was .77. Item correlations with the total score were all statistically significant. For section six (geriatric knowledge) the alpha was .66. For both of these sections, the discriminant validity of the tests was estimated by comparing the differences in scores across levels

TABLE 10.3   Trainee Knowledge *(Continued)*

Tool	Source	Comments
		of training and by level of career interest in geriatrics using pairwise t tests.
Test of Clinical Geriatrics	Jackson, Wiederholt, and Katzman (1990)	Developed as part of the evaluation of a mini-residency offered at the University of California, San Diego, a test of clinical geriatrics was given to 71 health professionals from nursing (35%), medicine (27%), social work (20%), and psychology (13%) as part of the evaluation of a 2-week mini-residency. Participants completed pretests and posttests to assess knowledge of geriatrics; their scores significantly improved following the mini-residency.
The Service Knowledge Quiz	Hill, Tuttle, Johnson, and Morrow-Howell (1993)	Respondents are given 10 minutes to answer 20 true–false items designed to assess knowledge of national programs and services generally available to the elderly. The true–false format was selected so this would be comparable with the Facts on Aging Quiz. A sample of 312 respondents generated a coefficient alpha of .36. Test–retest reliability over a 6-week period was .65 among 39 graduate nursing students. Typical questions include, "If I need a nursing home over a long period of time, my Medicare coverage will pay for it"; "About 35% of older adults live in nursing homes at the present time"; and, "Older adults use counseling services more often than younger adults." A significant positive correlation between self-reported years of formal education and score was found; further analysis confirmed that graduate nurses and older adult caregivers scored significantly better than did either undergraduate nursing students or older adults who were not caregivers. The authors conclude that the quiz has good stability over time and that the low internal consistency is to be expected because the quiz measures a heterogeneous body of knowledge.
Biology of Aging Exercise	National Institute on Aging, not copyrighted	Ten multiple choice items, each with four possible answers focus on a general knowledge of the aging process.

TABLE 10.3 *(Continued)*

Tool	Source	Comments
		Examples of questions are "Human functional capacity diminishes with age, beginning at about age: a. 20, b. 30, c. 40, d. 50." and, "With the process of aging, the incidence of autoimmune diseases . . . a. increases, b. decreases, c. decreases rapidly, and d. stays the same." No additional information about reliability is available at this time.
Facts on Aging Quiz	Palmore (1988)	Palmore has authored three versions of the Facts on Aging Quiz. The first (FAQ1, 1977) and second (FAQ2, 1981) each contain 25 true-false items. Items in both quizzes cover the demographics of aging, perceptions of aging individuals, resource use, functional capacity, and the biology of aging. The Mental Health Quiz (FQMHQ) contains 25 true-false items addressing the prevalence, causes, characteristics, and treatment of mental illness in the elderly. Items reflect characteristics of the elderly as well as their roles and their use of resources. The FAQ1 has been revised by the author based on the suggestions of researchers both in the United States and in other countries. (Studies include: Klemmack, 1978; Intrieri, Kelly, Brown, & Castilla, 1993; Palmore, 1988; Shahidi & Devlin, 1993). Palmore summarizes their collective experience noting that scores increase with the test taker's level of education, and that in 23 studies where the FAQ was used to measure changes in knowledge, all but four reported a significant increase in knowledge accompanying educational input. A multiple choice version of the FAQ2 has been created (Harris & Changas, 1994). A sample question from the FAQ2 is "The majority of old people live alone." The multiple choice version is: "The majority of old people live: a. alone, b. in institutions, c. with their spouses, d. with their children." Mean scores on this version were lower than on the original FAQ2, suggesting that the multiple choice format

(cont.)

TABLE 10.3   Trainee Knowledge *(Continued)*

Tool	Source	Comments
		is more difficult. Biserial correlations were low, but higher than for the true–false versions. The internal consistencies of the test items are unacceptably low for both versions (.07 for the true–false and .36 for the multiple choice).
What's Your Aging IQ?	National Institute on Aging, not copyrighted	Twenty true–false items including demographics ("Baby boomers are the fastest growing segment of the population"), health ("Heart disease is a much bigger problem for older men than for older women"), function ("You can be too old to exercise"), and general perceptions related to the elderly. No additional information on reliability is available at this time.

TABLE 10.4   Team Effectiveness

Tool	Source	Comments
Team Effectiveness Survey	Hall, O'Leary, and Williams (1964), Hall (1975), Hall and Williams (1971). © 1994, Teleometrics International. (There is a charge for test.)	The Team Effectiveness Survey is a 20-item behavior description rated on a 10-point continuum from extremely uncharacteristic (1) to extremely characteristic (10). Examples of questions include, "Person X is open and candid in dealing with the entire team," or "Person X gives support to members who are on the spot and struggling to express themselves . . ." Adapted from a model of interpersonal relations *(Johari Window),* the technique assesses how individuals present and process information. Team members receive a score that characterizes their team behavior and their interpersonal styles graphically within a four-part table to reflect the interaction of two sources of information—self and others. The assessment can be a rating of as many team members as the team chooses. The time for test administration varies. Teleometrics estimates that the instrument requires (per person evaluated): 15 minutes to complete, 15–20 minutes to score, and at least 30 minutes to understand. There are no psychometric data to report. Given the

TABLE 10.4 *(Continued)*

Tool	Source	Comments
		length of time to take and score, this may be an impractical test.
Team Progress Diagnostic	Hall, O'Leary, and Williams (1964), Hall (1975), Hall and Williams (1971). © 1989, Teleometrics International. (There is a charge for test.)	An earlier version of the Team Effectiveness Survey. This thirty-two item matrix describes team member behavior. Behaviors are classified into modes (problem solving; fight; flight). Self-assessment occurs by processing team members' views of an individual's behavior. Teleometrics estimates that the instrument takes (per person evaluated) 15 minutes to complete, 15–20 minutes to score, and at least 30 minutes to understand. There are no psychometric data to report. Given the length of time to take and score, this may be an impractical test.

TABLE 10.5 **Attitudes**

Tool	Source	Comments
Aging Semantic Differential	Rosencranz and McNevin (1969)	The instrument consists of 32 pairs of polar adjectives, such as Productive-Unproductive and Tolerant-Intolerant; the respondent is asked to mark on a seven-point continuum where an elderly person falls on the scale between the two adjectives. The stated goal is to measure attitudinal dimensions; based on a factor analysis, the items are divided into three subscales: Instrumental-Ineffective Dimension (9 items), Autonomous-Dependent Dimension (9 items), and Personal Acceptability-Unacceptability Dimension (14 items). Authors suggest that this approach has an advantage over approaches that require responses to specific statements as these may not differentiate between misconceptions and more objective attitudes. Studies that have used this measure include Adelman, Fields, & Jutagir, 1992; Eyison, 1992; Fields, Jutagir, Adelman, Tideiksarr, & Olson, 1992; Intrieri, Kelly, Brown, & Castilla, 1993; Reuben, Fullerton, Tschann, & Croughan-Minihane, 1995; Shahidi & Devlin, 1993. A revision of this

(cont.)

TABLE 10.5 Attitudes *(Continued)*

Tool	Source	Comments
		instrument is included in Knox, Gekowski, & Kelly (1995), and a confirmatory factor analysis was published by Intrieri, von Eye, & Kelly, 1995. A modified version of the scale (Woolliscroft, Calhoun, Maxim, & Wolf, 1984) was able to detect positive change in attitudes of first year medical students after exposure to groups of well elderly; however, no control group was included.
Attitudes Toward Old People	Kogan (1961)	The Kogan attitudes measure contains 34 items; there are 17 sets of items with two versions of each, one phrased positively, one negatively, such as: "Most old people make one feel ill at ease" and "Most old people are very relaxing to be with." Respondents are asked to score each item on a six-point Likert continuum from strongly disagree to strongly agree. In testing with college undergraduates, the author found that people were more likely to disagree with negative statements about old people than to agree with positive statements. The authors conducted several tests to identify correlations between this scale and existing measures of authoritarianism, anomie, antiminority attitudes, and personality dimensions. Adelman & Albert (1987) in a review of several attitudinal measures, regard the scale as one of the better validated, if outdated instruments measuring attitudes toward older people; however, no reliability estimates were provided in the original article. Studies that have used this scale include Nieman, Vernon, & Horner (1992) and Perrotta, Perkins, & Schimpfhauser (1981).
Tuckman–Lorge Questionnaire	Tuckman and Lorge (1953)	Developed to measure stereotypical attitudes toward the elderly, this instrument consists of 137 statements about them. Respondents are instructed to circle yes if they generally agree with the statement and no if they disagree. The items are general statements covering several categories, such as, affect ("They are grouchy"), normal

TABLE 10.5   *(Continued)*

Tool	Source	Comments
		activities ("They like to just sit and dream"), and health ("They suffer from constipation"). Several are dated ("They object to women smoking in public"). An analysis by Axelrod & Eisdorfer (1961) resulted in a modification of the questionnaire after finding that only 70% of the original statements had construct validity. In a review of studies of medical students' attitudes toward the elderly, Adelman and Albert (1987) state that the revised version is preferred.
Attitudes to Elderly People	Deary, Smith, Mitchell, and Maclennan (1993)	Based on their perceptions that more general scales on attitudes toward the elderly might not capture the impact of a geriatrics educational intervention, the authors developed this instrument specifically for use in medical settings. After pilot testing, 33 items in the original form were reduced to 15 statements that required a yes or no response. Varimax rotation (see Child, 1990) resulted in identification of two factors: Negative Attitudes and Medical Intervention. The first factor (nine items) contained items such as, "I find it difficult to treat the elderly as normal people" and "I feel impatient and uneasy with the elderly." The second factor (six items) contains items such as, "Renal dialysis should be used for elderly people with renal failure" and "Powerful narcotics should only be given to a cancer patient if he has severe persistent pain, and they should be withdrawn as soon as possible." The authors suggest that the emphasis on inquiry about patience, empathy with elderly, and treatment, rather than general attitudes may allow better measurement of change. As reflected in the content of this last item, there is overlap between knowledge and attitude; moreover, the question is double-barreled in that more than one statement is being rated. No reliability statistics are presented. Post hoc analyses following analysis of variance showed more positive attitudes of clinical phase (fourth

(cont.)

TABLE 10.5 Attitudes *(Continued)*

Tool	Source	Comments
		or fifth year) medical students following a 4-week course in geriatric medicine. However, no control group was studied, and precourse and postcourse scores did not appear to be matched.
Attitudes Toward the Geriatric Patient	Maxwell and Sullivan (1980)	This instrument was developed to measure attitudes of family practice residents towards caring for elderly patients. However, items are generically worded so that the measure could be used with other disciplines. The measure is comprised of 28 statements; respondents are asked to indicate their agreement or disagreement on a five-point Likert continuum from strongly agree to strongly disagree. Items were assigned on an a priori basis to five categories: General Attitudes (six items), Cost Effectiveness (four), Time and energy (six), Therapeutic Potential (six), and Educational Preparation (six). Initial testing with first-, second-, and third-year medical residents found significant differences among the three cohorts in all categories except cost effectiveness when comparing residents from different years. (It is noted that the directions of the difference varied across comparisons; for example, for General Attitudes and Time and Energy, attitudes were worse for second year students than first year students. Third year students had significantly more positive attitudes than second year students. However, the analyses are flawed because students were not followed longitudinally. Differences may represent cohort effects.) The internal consistency was assessed using the Kuder-Richardson intracategory coefficient; the coefficients were .63 for General Attitudes, .50 for Cost Effectiveness, .61 for Time and Energy, .62 for Therapeutic Potential, .62 for Educational Preparation, and .78 for the total measure.

TABLE 10.6 Team Member Behavior and Perceptions

Tool	Source	Comments
Collaborative Practice Scales	© Weiss and Davis (1985)	The scale consists of nine items for nurses and 10 for physicians. Both are scored on a six-point Likert-type scale ranging from never to always. All items relate to the characteristics of interactions with other professions. Typical questions for nurses are "I ask MDs about their expectations regarding the degree of my involvement in health care decisions" and "I suggest to MDs patient care approaches that I think would be useful." Physician questions include "I acknowledge to nurses those aspects of health care where they have more expertise than I do." Cronbach's alpha coefficients were .85 for physicians and .83 for nurses.
The Interprofessional Perception Scale	© Ducanis and Golin (1979)	The scale is comprised of 15 true-false items addressing the respondent's own and other professions. Each item requires three responses: Level 1, How would you answer; Level 2, How would they answer; Level 3, How would they say that you answered? Typical questions ask "Persons in this profession . . . seldom ask others' professional judgments" or "have a higher status than other professions." Reliability as measured by percent of exact agreement within profession had a mean of .80 for level 1 and .79 and .74 for levels 2 and 3, respectively.
Disciplinary Perception Scale (DPS)	© Drinka and Ray (1991)	Twenty-nine upper-level trainees from multiple disciplines completed a modified version of Ducanis & Golin's Interprofessional Perception Scale. The DPS uses a five-point Likert scale ranging between yes and no with yes = 1 and no = 5. Trainees were asked to complete the 12-item DPS for medicine, nursing, social work, and physical therapy professions. Questions include "Perception of persons in discipline . . . are competent? . . . fully utilize the capabilities of other professions? . . . trust the professional judgment of those in my profession." No psychometric data for the revised version are included in the article.

(cont.)

TABLE 10.6   Team Member Behavior and Perceptions *(Continued)*

Tool	Source	Comments
Interdisciplinary Education Perception Scale	© Luecht, Madsen, Taugher, and Petterson (1990)	This is an 18-item questionnaire with items scored using a six-point scale ranging from strongly agree to strongly disagree. Typical questions include, "Individuals in my profession are well-trained," "Individuals in my profession trust each other's professional judgment," and "Individuals in my profession have good relations with people in other professions." Validated on 143 students and administrators in allied health disciplines (occupational therapy, medical records, speech pathology, and recreational therapy). Analysis yielded an overall alpha of .87.
Interdisciplinary Team Weekly Inventory	Clark (1994)	This is a 17-item inventory of feelings and attitudes toward teams; the items are used as prompts for journal review. Using a 1 through 5 continuum, respondents indicate how comfortable and confident they feel in response to such questions as: "This week, as a professional: 1 = I am confident in my role to 5 = I am confused about my role and 1 = I identify with my own professional discipline and 5 = I identify with the team as a group." Another example is: "This week I believe that teams: 1 = are ineffective in developing solutions to problems to 5 = are effective in developing solutions to problems." No instrument psychometrics are reported.
Modified Family Assessment Device for Teams	Waite and Harker (1993). Sepulveda Veterans Administration Interdisciplinary Team Training Program, California. (not copyrighted).	This instrument is a 54-item adaptation of the McMaster Family Assessment Device (Epstein, Baldwin, & Bishop, 1983; Miller, Epstein, Bishop, & Keitner, 1985). It uses a 4-point Likert-type scale from strongly agree to strongly disagree. The measure creates scores for problem solving, communication, roles, affective response, affective involvement, behavior control, and general function. Typical questions include, "We often don't say what we mean," "Anything goes on our team," and "We try to think of different ways to solve problems." There are no psychometric data available.

TABLE 10.6 *(Continued)*

Tool	Source	Comments
Team Building Measures	© Dyer (1995)	Three scales are included: The Team-maturity scale, a 22-item questionnaire with a five-point Likert-type scale that is used as a diagnostic tool to measure perception of team maturity. Respondents are asked: "How are decisions made in your unit? 1 = The boss tells us what the decisions are, 3 = We discuss issues, but the boss makes all final decisions, 5 = We all make appropriate decisions by consensus," and "Is your unit leader capable of building your group into an effective team? 1 = Not capable at all, 3 = Somewhat capable, 5 = Completely capable." Higher scores indicate a respectively higher level of team maturity. The Team-building Checklist, a problem-identification checklist with 14 items scored on a five-point continuum from low evidence = 1 to high evidence = 5. The checklist asks, "To what extent is there evidence of the following problems in your work unit? conflicts or hostility; apathy; ineffective staff meetings." Higher scores imply more team-building efforts. The Team-development scale, a 10-item questionnaire scored on a five-point Likert-type scale that helps to identify areas that may need team development. Typical questions include, "How well does the team work at its tasks? 1 = coasts, loafs, makes no progress, 5 = works well, achieves definite progress," or "How are differences or conflicts handled in our team? 1 = Differences are denied or avoided at all costs, 5 = Differences are recognized and the team usually is working them through satisfactorily." These are primarily training tools and no psychometric data are reported on any measure.
The Team Effectiveness Measures	Schmitt, Farrell, and Heinemann (1991) (Copyrighted, no charge for researchers who use subscales	The Team Effectiveness Measures were developed and tested among four types of Veterans Administration geriatric teams—Geriatric Evaluation and Management, Nursing Home Care,

(cont.)

TABLE 10.6 Team Member Behavior and Perceptions *(Continued)*

Tool	Source	Comments
	developed by Schmitt, Farrell, & Heinemann but some of the 14 subscales are copyrighted to others and include charges.)	Hospital-based Home Care, and Adult Day Health Care Teams—in 34 VA Medical Centers across the country. The entire questionnaire takes an average of 1 hour to complete. There are 122 items with 14 subscales that measure 10 team components. Schmitt, Heinemann, & Farrell (1994) developed and copyrighted four of the 14 subscales. Attitudes Toward Health Care Interdisciplinary Teams consists of three subscales: quality of care by teams, costs/benefits of teams, and MD centeredness. The responses for the subscales are scored along a six-point continuum from 1 = strongly disagree to 6 = strongly agree. Questions from the quality of care by teams (11 items) include "Hospital patients who receive team care are better prepared for discharge than other patients." The alpha is .80. Typical questions on the five items on costs and benefits of team care (alpha = .64) include, "Working in teams unnecessarily complicates things" and "In most instances, the time required for team meetings could be better spent in other ways." The five items about the degree the team should be physician-centered state, "Physicians are natural team leaders" and "Physicians have the right to alter patient care plans developed by the team." Cronbach's alpha = .68. The Anomie scale is a 20-item single factor scale measuring member uncertainty about team goals, responsibilities, roles, and group norms. Typical questions include, "My team's basic mission is clear to me" and "My job makes me feel like a juggler with too many balls in the air." Chronbach's alpha is .88. The following team components used by Schmitt, Heinemann, & Farrell are adaptations with copyright permission of other researchers' measures. Team Cohesion consists of two Moos Group Environmental subscales (Moos, 1994) (Cohesion and Leader Support) and

TABLE 10.6 *(Continued)*

Tool	Source	Comments
		Team Communication consists of two of Moos' subscales (Anger and Aggression and Expressiveness). Each Moos Group Environmental subscale consists of nine items; response format is true = 0, and false = 1. Moos reports reliabilities for the subscales of .86, .74, .83, .70, respectively. In Schmitt, Heinemann, & Farrell (1994) the reliabilities were .87, .84, .79, and .65. Moos Group Environmental Scales are copyrighted and may be adapted with permission. Three subscales have been adapted and modified (with copyright permission) from the ICU Nurse/ Physician Questionnaire by Shortell, Rousseau, Gillies, Devers, and Simons (1991). All items are scored along a six-point continuum: 1 = strongly disagree to 6 = strongly agree. These scales are designated Team communication, a 10-item subscale with questions like, "It is easy to ask advice from team members"; Quality of external relations, a five-item subscale with questions such as, "Other hospital units and programs have a low opinion of us"; and an eight-item subscale of Team effectiveness; "Our team is very good at responding to crisis situations." Chronbach's alphas for the respective scales are .87, .70, and .88. Three subscales from the Maslach & Jackson Burnout Inventory (Maslach & Jackson, 1986) were also adapted and used with permission to measure stress and burnout. All items are scored from 0 (never) to 6 (everyday). The scales are an eight-item Personal Accomplishment subscale, a nine-item Emotional Exhaustion measure, and a five-item Depersonalization measure. The internal reliabilities reported by Maslach and Jackson are .71, .90, and .79, respectively. In the study Schmitt, Heinemann, & Farrell reported reliabilities of .75, .90, and .74. It may be possible to use some of these subscales for team measures. Psychometric characteristics have been presented only at

TABLE 10.6   Team Member Behavior and Perceptions *(Continued)*

Tool	Source	Comments
		professional meetings, and published in proceedings (Farrell, Heinemann, & Schmitt, 1992; Heinemann, Schmitt, & Farrell, 1991; Schmitt, Heinemann, & Farrell, 1994). However, a full manuscript on the development of the Attitudes Towards Interdisciplinary Health Care Teams scale/subscales has been submitted for publication, and a full manuscript on the Anomie scale is in final preparation.
Team Skills Questionnaire	University of Colorado Health Sciences Center, undated	This 42-item questionnaire contains items measuring the use of team skills, rated on a six-point continuum. Domains include Collaboration (eight items); Participation (five items); Communication (four items on listening; five items on speaking); and Formal Decision-making (seven items on goalsetting; six items on problem-solving; and seven items on conflict resolution.) We would recommend changing the end-points to measure frequency of actual use of the skills. There are no validation data for this instrument.

THE FOUNDATION REPORTS AS FORMATIVE DATA

It is important to understand the clinical aspects and impact of the GITT experience. Formative data are captured through site progress reports to the Foundation and from ongoing discussions with projects' staffs. The charts and appendices submitted by each site as part of the implementation program proposals constitute an important component of these formative data. These data are updated regularly. One potential product of these formative data is the how-to manual under development by the Resource Center that will describe the steps necessary to create academic and clinical partnerships and provide recommendations for implementing GITT in a variety of clinical settings.

THE CURRICULA AS THE DRIVER OF CHANGE

Chapters 8 and 9 explored curricular issues in geriatric team training. Obviously, the curricula, both didactic and clinical, drive the effect of GITT on the trainees. The eight projects have each developed model curricula, and our understanding of those curricula will help us understand changes in trainee core measures. As a first step in providing a basis for the characterization of didactic and practicum GITT experience, we have developed a glossary of terms (Appendix B). The goal of the glossary is to develop a consistent lexicon that will facilitate recognition of both the commonalities and the differences across the project curricula. A GITT curriculum workgroup has already expanded and refined this glossary, which is expected to be revised considerably over time. We understand that developing a glossary promotes the evolution of same thinking, which can impede creative strategies and concept development. On the other hand, in the absence of a standard nomenclature, different projects may use the same word to mean different things. We have accepted the first limitation to achieve consistency in our communication. All sites receive summary characterizations of the implementation programs that enhance the understanding of how terms are being used.

STUDENT CHARACTERISTICS

Each of the GITT trainees comes with a unique set of experiences, which, of course, influence the effect of training. The Resource Center captures key aspects of the trainee demographic profiles for the project sites and sends a uniform set of data back to each site. Each site receives from the Resource Center a data log and computer disk prepared using Microsoft Access, which site personnel use for their own purposes in understanding their trainees. Further, they obtain a pooled set of trainee profiles from the other sites. Although they cannot identify individuals or sites, they can review how their trainee profiles differ from or mirror Program trainees. The demographic information we have included are gender, age, discipline, semester of professional school training, background in geriatrics and team training, and work experience in geriatrics and teams. The goal is to link student demographic information to the clinical setting and track changes in students' attitudes, knowledge, and behavior over time. We have developed a mechanism for assigning student identification numbers, which ensures student confidentiality at the Resource Center level.

CONCLUSIONS

Measuring the effect of a team training project on the knowledge and attitudes of student trainees across a variety of disciplines is, to say the least, complicated. The GITT Program provides an opportune moment for an intensive, national effort to do so. This chapter describes the GITT core measures effort, which we believe will help determine what these projects may or may not have in common, and the different ways the students learn as the overall program matures. The GITT Program is in a position to capture information about the way students are affected by geriatric team training and to explore those effects within the context of the unique curricula at each of the projects. It is our way of tackling the question, "Why teams?"

REFERENCES

Adelman, R. D., & Albert, R. C. (1987). Medical student attitudes toward the elderly: A critical review of the literature. *Gerontology & Geriatrics Education, 7,* 141–154.

Adelman, R. D., Fields, S. D., & Jutagir, R. (1992). Geriatric education. Part II: The effect of a well elderly program on medical student attitudes toward geriatric patients. *Journal of the American Geriatrics Society, 40,* 970–973.

Axelrod, S., & Eisdorfer, C. (1961). Attitudes toward old people: An empirical analysis of the stimulus-group validity of the Tuchman Lorge Questionnaire. *Journal of Gerontology, 16,* 75–80.

Child, D. (1990). *The essentials of factor analysis* (2nd ed.). London: Cassell.

Clark, P. G. (1994). Learning on interdisciplinary gerontological teams: Instructional concepts and methods. *Educational Gerontology, 20,* 349–364.

Deary, I., Smith, R., Mitchell, C., & Maclennan, W. (1993). Geriatric medicine: Does teaching alter medical students' attitudes to elderly people? *Medical Education, 27,* 399–405.

Drinka, T., & Ray, R. O. (1991). Perceptions of upper-level trainees in an interdisciplinary geriatrics practicum: Implications for curriculum development. *Gerontology & Geriatrics Education, 12,* 47–59.

Ducanis, A. J., & Golin, A. K. (1979). *The interdisciplinary health care team* (pp. 3–40). Germantown, MD: Aspen.

Dyer, W. G. (1995). *Team building: Current issues and new alternatives* (3rd ed.). Reading, MA: Addison-Wesley.

Epstein, N. B., Baldwin, L. M., & Bishop, D. S. (1983). McMaster Family Assessment Device. *Journal of Marital and Family Therapy, 9,* 171–180.

Eyison, J. (1992). A comparative study of the attitude of dental students towards the elderly. *European Journal of Prosthodontics & Restorative Dentistry, 1*(2), 87–90.

Farrell, M. P., Heinemann, G. D., & Schmitt, M. H. (1992). A measure of anomie in health care teams. In J. R. Snyder (Ed.). *Interdisciplinary health care teams: Proceedings of the Fourteenth Annual Conference.* Chicago, IL: School of Allied Health Sciences Indiana University School of Medicine, Indiana University Medical Center.

Fields S. D., Jutagir, R., Adelman, R. D., Tideiksarr, R., & Olson, E. (1992). Geriatric education. Part I: Efficacy of a mandatory clinical rotation for fourth year medical students. *Journal of the American Geriatrics Society, 40,* 964–969.

Hall, J. (1975). Interpersonal style and the communications dilemma: II. Utility of the Johari awareness model for genotypic diagnosis. *Human Relations, 28,* 715–736.

Hall, J., O'Leary, V., & Williams, M. (1964, Winter). The decision-making grid: A model of decision making styles. *California Management Review,* pp. 43–54.

Hall, J., & Williams, M. S. (1971). Personality and group encounter style: A multivariate analysis of traits and preferences. *Journal of Personality and Social Psychology, 18*(2), 163–172.

Harris, D. K., & Changas, P. S. (1994). Revision of Palmore's second Facts on Aging Quiz from a true-false to a multiple-choice format. *Educational Gerontology, 20,* 741–754.

Heinemann, G. D., Schmitt, M. H., & Farrell, M. P. (1991). Developments of the attitudes toward health care teams scale: Phase two*. In J. R. Snyder (Ed.), *Interdisciplinary health care teams: Proceedings of the Thirteenth Annual Conference.* Baltimore, MD: School of Allied Health Sciences, Indiana University School of Medicine, Indiana University Medical Center.

Hill, R. D., Tuttle, S. M., Johnson, M., & Morrow-Howell, N. (1993). Assessing knowledge of services for older adults: The service knowledge quiz. *Gerontology & Geriatrics Education, 13*(4), 53–64.

Intrieri, R. C., Kelly, J. A., Brown, M. M., & Castilla, C. (1993). Improving medical students' attitudes toward and skills with the elderly. *Gerontologist, 33,* 373–378.

Intrieri, R. C., von Eye, A., & Kelly, J. A. (1995). The aging semantic differential: A confirmatory factor analysis. *Gerontologist, 35,* 612–621.

Jackson, J. E., Wiederholt, W., & Katzman, R. (1990). Teaching the multidisciplinary team approach in a geriatrics miniresidency. *Academic Medicine, 65,* 417–419.

Kirkpatrick, D. L. (1975). Techniques for evaluating training programs. In D. L. Kirkpatrick (ed.), *Evaluating training programs.* Alexandria, VA: ASTD Press.

Klemmack, D. (1978). Comment: An examination of Palmore's Facts on Aging Quiz. *Gerontologist, 18,* 403–406.

Knox, V. J., Gekoski, W. L., & Kelly, L. E. (1995). The age group evaluation and description (AGED) inventory: A new instrument for assessing stereotypes of and attitudes toward age groups. *International Journal of Aging & Human Development, 40,* 31–55.

Kogan, N. (1961). Attitudes toward old people: The development of a scale and an examination of correlates. *Journal of Abnormal and Social Psychology, 62,* 44–54.

Lindberg, M. C., & Sullivan, G. M. (1996). *Effects of an inpatient geriatrics rotation on internal medicine residents' knowledge and attitudes.* Unpublished manuscript, University of Connecticut, Geriatric Medicine.

Luecht, R. M., Madsen, M. K., Taugher, M. P., & Petterson, B. J. (1990, Spring). Assessing professional perceptions: Design and validation of an interdisciplinary education perception scale. *Journal of Allied Health,* pp. 181–191.

Maslach, C., & Jackson, S. E. (1986). *Maslach Burnout Inventory* (2nd ed.). Palo Alto, CA: Consulting Psychologists Press.

Maxwell, A. J., & Sullivan, N. (1980). Attitudes toward the geriatric patient among family practice residents. *Journal of the American Geriatrics Society, 28,* 341–345.

McMillan, S. C., & Robinson, B. (1991). Development of a basic test of geriatric medicine. *Academic Medicine, 66,* 560.

Miller, I. W., Epstein, N. B., Bishop, D. S., & Keitner, G. I. (1985). The McMaster Family Assessment Device: Reliability and validity. *Journal of Marital and Family Therapy, 11,* 345–356.

Moos, R. H. (1994). *Group environment scale manual: Development, application, research.* Palo Alto, CA: Consulting Psychologists Press.

Nieman, L. Z., Vernon, M. S., & Horner, R. D. (1992). Designing and evaluating an episodic, problem-based geriatric curriculum. *Family Medicine, 24,* 378–381.

Palmore, E. B. (1988). *The Facts on Aging Quiz: A handbook of uses and results.* New York: Springer Publishing Company.

Perrotta, P., Perkins, D., & Schimpfhauser, F. E. (1981). Medical student attitudes toward geriatric medicine and patients. *Journal of Medical Education, 56,* 478–483.

Porter, E. (1976). On the development of relationship awareness theory: A personal note. *Group & Organization Studies, 1,* 302–309.

Porter, E. (1983). *Relationship Awareness Theory,* Manchester, UK: Training Officer Marlebone Press.

Porter, E. (1987). The truth, the half-truth, and something less than the truth: A modern look at four style behavior models. *American Society of Training and Development.*

Pratt, C. C., Wilson, W., Benthin, A., & Schmall, V. (1992). Alcohol problems and depression in later life: Development of two knowledge quizzes. *Gerontologist, 32,* 175–183.

Rahim, A., & Bonoma, T. V. (1979). Managing organizational conflict: A model for diagnosis and intervention. *Psychological Reports, 44,* 1323–1344.

Rahim, M. A. (1983a). A measure of styles of handling interpersonal conflict. *Academy of Management Journal, 26,* 368–476.

Rahim, M. A. (1983b). Measurement of organizational conflict. *Journal of General Psychology, 109,* 189–199.

Reuben, D. B., Fullerton, J. T., Tschann, J. M., & Croughan-Minihane, M. (1995). Attitudes of beginning medical students toward older persons: A five-campus study. *Journal of the American Geriatrics Society, 43,* 1430–1436.

Rosencranz, H. A., & McNevin, T. E. (1969). A factor analysis of attitudes toward the aged. *Gerontologist, 9,* 55–59.

Schmitt, M. H., Heinemann, G. D., & Farrell, M. P. (1994). Discipline differences in attitudes toward interdisciplinary teams, perceptions of the process of teamwork, and stress levels in geriatric health care teams. In J. R. Snyder (Ed.). *Interdisciplinary health care teams: Proceedings of the Sixteenth Annual Conference.* Chicago, IL: School of Allied Health Sciences, Indiana University School of Medicine, Indiana University Medical Center.

Schmitt, M. H., Farrell, M. P., & Heinemann, G. D. (1994). *The quality of geriatric team functioning.* (National Institute of Aging, RO1-AGO8957).

Shahidi, S., & Devlin J. (1993). Medical students' attitudes to and knowledge of the aged. *Medical Education, 27,* 286–288.

Shortell, S. M., Rousseau, D. M., Gillies, R. R., Devers, K. J., & Simons, T. L. (1991). The organizational assessment in intensive care units (ICUs): Construct development, reliability, and validity of the ICU nurse-physician questionnaire. *Medical Care, 29,* 709–727.

Teresi, J., & Holmes, D. (1996). *GITT common core and optional measures: Conceptual model and background literature.* Unpublished data.

Teresi, J., Holmes, D., Hyer, K., & Totten A. (1996). *Review of GITT student measures.* GITT Resource Center, June 17, 1996.

Toner, J., & Meyer, E. (1988). Multidisciplinary treatment team training in the management of dementia: A stress management program for geriatric staff and family caregivers. In R. Mayeux, B. Gurland, V. Barret, A. Kutscher, L. Cote, & Z. Putter (Eds.), *Alzheimer's disease and related disorders, psychosocial issues for the patient, family, staff, and community* (pp. 81–102). Springfield, IL: Charles C. Thomas.

Tuckman, J., & Lorge, I. (1953). Attitudes toward old people. *Journal of Social Psychology, 37,* 249–260.

Waite, M., & Harker, J. O. (1993). *Modified Family Assessment Device for Teams* (Adapted with permission of the developers). Sepulveda, CA: Sepulveda Veterans Affairs Hospital.

Weiss, S. J., & Davis, H. P. (1985). Validity and reliability of the collaborative practice scales. *Nursing Research, 34,* 299–305.

Woolliscroft, J. O., Calhoun, J. G., Maxim, B. R., & Wolf, F. M. (1984). Medical education in facilities for the elderly. *Journal of the American Medical Association, 252,* 3382–3385.

PART 4

Organizing Team Training in Different Sites and Settings

CHAPTER 11

Geriatric Team Training in Managed Care Organizations

Janet C. Frank and Richard Della Penna

> *Managed care is better than unmanaged care.*
> —Ernest Sayward, MD; first medical and research director
> of Kaiser Permanente's Northwest Region

Many elderly today receive their health care from a variety of medical organizations that want to manage care. We are interested in geriatric training in these new environments because older people may be put in double jeopardy by placing themselves in the hands of well-meaning professional staff who are trained in neither geriatrics nor the principles of managed care. Older persons, especially the most frail, have complex and multiple health problems that intersect with the psychosocial dimensions of their lives. We believe that we can address these problems most effectively through well-functioning teams of health and social professionals who work in concert to solve or manage multifaceted problems. We will explore the potential for team care in this new environment and describe some model programs that will provide much needed answers.

The words "managed care" have come to represent simultaneously the best and the worst aspects of today's health care delivery system. Opinions vary on whether it is a *bete noire* or the hope for a health care system whose costs are out of control. Arguments usually hinge on whether the current rush to managed care has had a positive or a negative effect on the individuals or institutions presenting their viewpoints. Is managed care good or bad? The answer—the concept is good, but in practice it may be either, depending on the health plan and providers under discussion.

Regardless of one's viewpoint, it is important to recognize that the current dynamics of change in health care financing and delivery have evolved over many years. Its recent rapid growth has come about because of the shortcomings in the way health care has been traditionally structured, delivered, and financed. The problems of run-away inflation in medical costs, fragmentation in care, gaps in coverage, wasteful competitive duplication of high technology, and financial incentives that foster excess care all helped set the stage for change.

With change being the only certainty in health care delivery today, academic medical centers and other professional graduate training programs must respond by providing training that is relevant to the systems in which their graduates will provide care. Such new content demands will combine the current scientific and clinical care standards with new information on the organizational and business function aspects of health care. In the managed care world of health care, trainees' vocabularies will include such terms as population-based medicine, management of resources, cost effectiveness, and team care. Training programs that include either coursework or clinical training in managed care organizations are quite rare, with the majority of new professionals entering their practice fields, often in managed care environments, without one single course or clinical experience in a managed care organization (Council on Graduate Medical Education [COGME], 1995).

Academic medical centers and professional graduate programs have been struggling for the past two decades with limited success to infuse geriatrics content into health and social service professional training programs (Health Resources Services Administration [HRSA], 1995). The majority of today's health and social service professionals continue to graduate and begin their care careers without the benefit of one single course that addresses the special needs of the elderly. The collision course of unmet training needs in both geriatrics and managed care began in 1973, with the passage of the HMO Act, allowing Medicare beneficiaries the option of selecting to receive their care through health maintenance organizations (HMOs).

This chapter will focus on the dual demands of preparing geriatric and gerontologic health and social service professionals to function most effectively in a changing health care environment, dominated by managed care. The major issues this chapter will address include:

- The evolution of managed health care
- An analysis of the current major models of managed care
- The importance of educating future practitioners about managed care for older adults
- Training programs in and about managed care organizations
- Competency requirements for professional caregivers in managed care
- The role of teams in managed care
- The challenge of providing Geriatric Interdisciplinary Team Training (GITT) in various managed care environments

EVOLUTION OF MANAGED CARE

What Is Managed Care?

Managed care is no longer a simple concept or single system. It was developed as an alternative to the traditionally dominant fee-for-service delivery system. In general, managed care describes a structure of health care delivery and financing that employs various techniques to control and manage the delivery of health services and their cost. Prepayment, cost control, shared financial risk among providers, and some limitation of consumer choice are common attributes of managed care organizations (MCOs). The distinguishing organizational characteristics of a given managed care program derive largely from the contractual arrangements between health plans and physicians. These arrangements influence the processes of care and incentives, which, in turn, affect the potential for integrating health care delivery, training health care professionals, and developing programs that are not traditionally part of a benefit structure. Figure 11.1 shows the percentages of different MCO models today.

History of Managed Care

Prepaid health care is not a new concept. Its roots go back at least two centuries when, in 1798, the Fifth Congress of the United States established the Marine Hospital Service, an organized network with salaried physicians to care for sick and disabled seamen through deductions from their wages (Schwartz, 1965).

Beginning in 1929, several developments significantly altered the organization and delivery of medical care. In disparate parts of the country, a prepaid hospital care plan, a consumer medical cooperative, and a prepaid comprehensive health services plan employee contract were quietly established, the harbingers of future managed care.

In the 1930s, industrialist Henry J. Kaiser entered into a prepaid arrangement with Dr. Sydney Garfield and his group of physicians. This group was the first of the Permanente Medical Groups, and their arrangement was to become the largest of the early managed care programs. The Kaiser Plan initially provided medical care for work-related injuries of Kaiser employees. Capitation was added for general medical care and eventually, medical care for workers' families was incorporated into the program. In 1932, the Committee on the Cost of Medical Care, a former president of the American Medical Association, and a group of health care leaders and consumers issued a report favoring the joining of prepayment plans with group practice (Kay, 1979).

At the end of World War II, the Kaiser Plan was opened to the general public. Unions and large employers became major supporters of the Kaiser Plan, which has grown exponentially and currently provides care for over 7 million people across the country (Kay, 1979). Group Health of Puget Sound and the Health Insurance Plan of New York followed in 1947, and Group Health of Minneapolis was established in 1957 (Kay, 1979).

Organized medicine was not receptive to the report or the development of alternatives to fee-for-service reimbursement. The American Medical Association's position at that time was strongly against prepaid physician groups, instead supporting indemnity insurance with its fee-for-service reimbursement coverage. County medical societies barred physicians who participated in prepaid programs from membership.

Medicare and the Health Maintenance Organization

The growth in private health insurance in the United States after World War II was rapid, with 139 million of the 194 million total U.S. population covered by some type of health insurance by 1965. The employer typically sponsored health insurance as a benefit for its employees. This excluded large groups of the elderly and the poor. President Johnson signed legislation that established Medicare and Medicaid in 1965 to provide health insurance protection to these two groups. Fee-for-service reimbursement for physicians and cost-plus reimbursement for hospitals were program components added to mollify

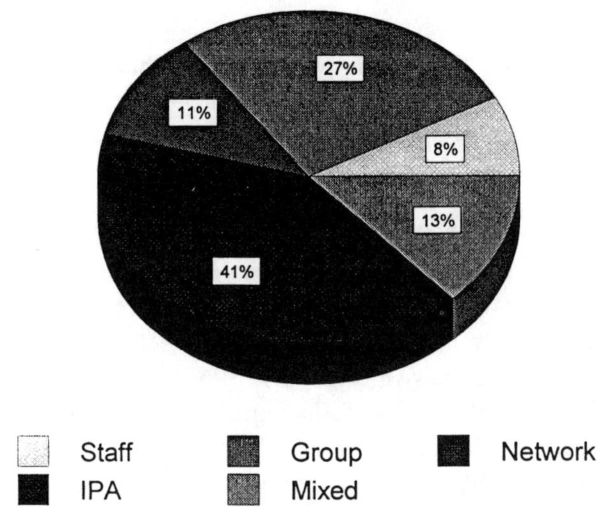

FIGURE 11.1   HMO enrollment by model type. Data from Wagner (1995).

the American Medical Association. Medicare altered the financing of care for the elderly but did not change the fundamental way health care was delivered.

The designers of Medicare did not anticipate the rapid evolution of expensive technology and the demand for services. Spectacular cost escalation began as hospitals became the dominant site of care. Academic health centers increased the sophistication of hospital care with their contributions to patient care, health professional education, and research. Medicare provided significant funding for care and training and strengthened these institutions.

Within 5 years of the establishment of Medicare, the Nixon administration became concerned about the rapid inflation of health care costs. The leaders of the Department of Health, Education, and Welfare invited Paul Ellwood, M.D., to assist in developing a strategy to control costs. Their efforts resulted in the passage of the Health Maintenance Organization Act in 1973. HMOs, the first name applied to a type of MCO, were designed to cover all health needs—preventive and curative—of a person for a set predetermined price. As the name implies, this new type of organization would maintain a person's health. Prevention of more costly adverse health events was a hallmark of HMO care because any money not spent on care would be retained by the organization. One feature of the Act permitted Medicare beneficiaries to choose between traditional fee-for-service payment or HMOs. The expectation was that market forces would halt the cost escalation by fostering competition on quality and cost. The Act also provided start-up grants and nullified state laws that limited the development of HMOs. Most importantly, it required employers with more than 25 employees who offered indemnity coverage to also offer the choice of two federally qualified HMOs, if available. Capitated Medicare-risk contracting directly with MCOs followed in 1982, with the most rapid growth occurring from 1993 to 1995 (see Figure 11.2). By 1995, about 10% of Medicare beneficiaries nationwide were receiving their care in MCOs. In some areas of the country, such as Southern California, over 40% of the elderly have enrolled in MCOs.

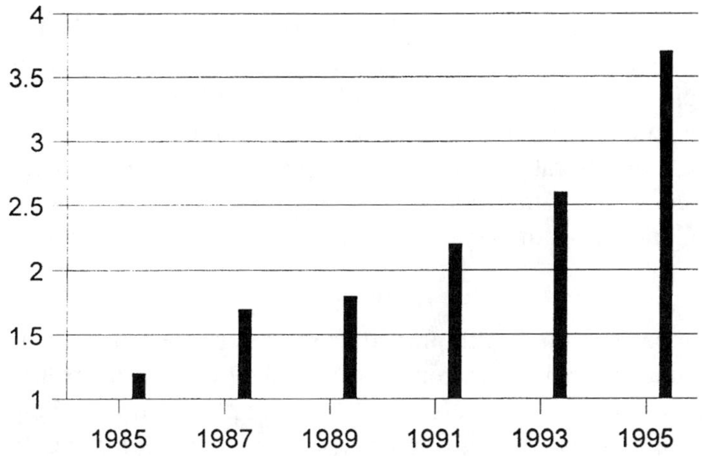

FIGURE 11.2   Growth of Medicare managed care. The figure depicts the growth in yearly enroll-ment of Medicare managed care. Source: Bovner (1996).

MANAGED CARE MODELS

Managed care organizations may be nonprofit or for-profit, with some companies listed on the American Stock Exchange (Shouldice, 1991). MCOs have a contractual rela-tionship with enrollees to provide a defined set of comprehensive preventive and treatment services for a fixed annual fee. Enrollment is voluntary, and out-of-pocket copayments are minimal. The expectation is that individual care will be well integrat-ed, efficient, and managed by plan primary care physicians working with appropriate specialists. The organization assumes the risk of financial loss or benefits from any profit associated with the care of its members. Because enrollment is voluntary, cost, access, and quality of care and service become the ways organizations distinguish themselves and succeed competitively. The addition of specific measures or outcomes for report cards is a more recent method for plans to distinguish themselves and attract new members.

MCOs have three major components: (a) the health plan that enrolls members and provides overall management and organization, such as sales, marketing, and overall regulatory compliance; (b) providers including physicians, hospitals, home health agen-cies, and skilled nursing care facilities; and (c) subscribers, members, or enrollees. In the early days of HMOs and managed care, there were fewer ways in which these three components were organized and related. Model classification derives primarily from the relationship between the health plan and its physicians. It is important to remem-ber that most MCOs are no longer pure but often have elements of several models (Wagner, 1995).

Staff Model

Physicians in the staff model are direct employees of the health plan. They are salaried but usually also have financial incentives based on performance and productivity. In the strict staff model, members must obtain their care from these physicians. Specialty care is provided by physician staff or contracted out to community physicians. The practice settings are typically large, centralized medical office buildings. Social workers, non-physician providers, and ancillary features such as maintenance of a common medical record, radiology, or laboratory services are typically available on site. The staff model MCO usually contracts with hospitals and other facilities for nonphysician services. Group Health Cooperative of Puget Sound is an example of a staff model.

Advantages

The staff model permits the health plan to exert greater control over the staff. This can be seen as advantage when improvements in clinical care result from appropriate utilization and quality improvement efforts. The health plan also is in the position of scrutinizing the qualifications when hiring new physicians. Ongoing peer review is easier, and continuing professional education can be provided more efficiently. Centralization allows ready access to other health professionals and support services for both members and providers.

Disadvantages

The health plan-physician relationship can be a disadvantage when physicians feel they are constrained by what is perceived as inappropriate heath plan intrusion into the area of clinical judgment. Centralization acts as a disadvantage for current or potential members who do not have ready access to an office facility. This is especially true for many elderly and disabled patients. Development of the staff model requires the investment of time and capital. This is a disadvantage when a health plan seeks to expand quickly into new markets. Staff models are also unattractive to many people because they must abandon their current physician when they join the managed care organization.

Group Model

The group model is similar to the staff model, except that the health plan does not employ physicians directly but instead contracts with a multispecialty group practice. These are the only physicians members may see. The group is the employer of the physician and the physician may actually hold an ownership position in the group. The group receives a capitation for all physician services. Physicians share staff, offices, and equipment. In some arrangements, such as Kaiser Permanente, the physician group agrees to see only members of the managed care plan. In some group models, the health plan contracts exclusively with a group practice, but the physicians also see non-HMO patients. The Geisinger Clinic is an example of this type.

Advantages

The positive attributes of the staff model are applicable to the group practice arrangement. Additionally, physicians are independent of the direct control of the health plan, which permits them to practice medicine without the concern that the health plan employer will penalize them for what they see as appropriate clinical decision making.

Disadvantages

Because the physician group is at some financial risk for performance, physicians may still feel constrained against providing appropriate services when they are expensive. The group model also shares some of the staff model's disadvantages, especially centralization. Centralization and the requirement for members to see only group physicians may be seen as an undesirable limitation of choice.

Network

In network models, the managed care organization contracts with several multispecialty physician groups. The practices may resemble the larger groups typical of a group model, or they may be smaller primary care-based practices that receive a capitation fee and then may directly reimburse specialists they enlist to provide services to members for whom they are responsible. These types of groups of physicians typically contract with several MCOs.

Advantages

Network MCOs allow for wider geographic physician access and greater member choice because more than one group may be available in reasonable proximity.

Disadvantages

The major disadvantage of this model is that there is potential for inappropriate variation in practice patterns among the different medical groups.

Independent Physician Association

In this model, the managed care organization contracts with an association of physicians who are joined together in a separate legal entity. The Independent Physician Association (IPA) becomes a virtual group and contracts with one or more MCOs. The IPA assumes the risks associated with capitation. Physicians continue to practice in their private offices, and patient records and ancillary services are not centralized.

Advantages

The major advantage of this model is its potential for a wide geographic physician presence. This is convenient for members and confers a marketing advantage to the health plan. Member physician choice is greater. Rapid expansion is easier for the network managed care organization.

Disadvantages

Physicians remain relatively independent, and they are deprived of the benefits and satisfaction of group practice. Peer review is more difficult, and inappropriate variation in practice patterns may result. The lack of a critical mass of providers in one location makes coordinated care more difficult. Physicians are also much closer to adverse financial risk than with other models, and this may have a negative impact on their practice.

Direct Contract

The health plan in this model contracts directly with individual physicians who typically have limited risk. Reimbursement is via capitation or on a reduced fee-for-service basis.

Advantages

The biggest advantages to this model are the increased choice of physician and wide geographic presence.

Disadvantages

The disadvantages are similar to IPA models, but with less financial risk to physicians. Physicians with high resource consumption practice patterns may not have their contracts renewed.

Additional Model Variations

Point of service (POS) is an enhancement that many MCOs are adding. This allows members who elect this option to use providers who do not have a contractual relationship with the MCOs. This expanded choice comes at the price of a higher premium and higher out-of-pocket expenses.

A provider hospital organization (PHO) is comprised of physicians and a hospital who have joined forces to form a separate entity whose board is comprised equally of physician and hospital representatives. PHOs usually seek relationships with MCOs and provide their services on a fee-for-service basis or by capitation.

Enhanced Models of Managed Care

Social HMOs, or SHMOs, are health maintenance organizations that provide an array of social support services to Medicare beneficiaries in addition to the usual core medical and hospital services. Financed under a waiver from the Health Care Financing Administration (HCFA), a SHMO receives a higher capitation for members who become nursing home certifiable, but remain in the community. Long-term community-based services are available to qualifying members. Case managers coordinate the available services, which include personal assistance, homemaker services, respite nursing home stays, and transportation for medical care. SHMOs seek to enroll healthy older people so that the risk for the cost of services can be evenly shared. The program has been expanded from the four original sites, and the cost effectiveness of the program is being evaluated.

The Program for All-Inclusive Care for the Elderly (PACE) model is a very comprehensive form of managed care for older people who are already nursing home certifiable. There are currently 10 demonstration sites that are attempting to replicate the experience of San Francisco's On Lok program. Most PACE members are dually eligible for Medicare and Medicaid, and the PACE receives a combined capitation that provides comprehensive services. In addition to the core Medicare services, PACE sites also provide adult day care, a full array of home nursing and social services, transportation, nutrition services, personal care attendants, and homemakers. The goal is to keep the enrollee in the community, but if this is not possible, the PACE site must cover the costs of institutional care as well.

Both the SHMO and PACE models are demonstrations, and their enrollment is very small. The effectiveness of these programs is being evaluated, and the qualifications of the medical staff caring for SHMO members is receiving more attention. One question under study is whether the addition of geriatricians and geriatric nurse practitioners will make a difference.

There are obvious advantages to the additional services available to the SHMO and PACE models. Frail elderly receive services beyond the standard Medicare benefit package and receive attention to problems that are outside the usual medical model. These models both rely on a team approach to care and combine physicians, nurse practitioners, social workers, and others into a care team. Chapter 12 describes the PACE Model On Lok in greater detail.

TRAINING FUTURE PRACTITIONERS IN MANAGED CARE PROGRAMS FOR OLDER ADULTS

There are two basic reasons why we need to provide appropriate training for health and social service professionals in managed care programs for older adults.

1. Older adults, especially frail elderly, constitute a group that will grow exponentially in the next 30 years as the baby boomers age. This group presents multiple challenges due to the myriad of chronic health problems interwoven with social, economic, and psychologic needs. Care professionals in any care setting need better preparation to provide high quality services to older persons.
2. Health care is being provided more frequently within managed care health systems today, and there is no indication that there will be any reversal of this trend (see Figure 11.2).

Greenlick (1995) adeptly summarizes the multiple changes in health care that an older US citizen has experienced in Table 11.1. These changes include the mechanisms and forms of payment, the location of care, the focus of the care, and how care is evaluated. Although Greenlick identifies the year 2005, the characteristics are fairly close to those we are experiencing today. Both older persons and academic institutions must cope with these sweeping transformations in health care, the latter by redesigning curriculum and clinical training to fit the current—and future—systems of care.

Models to Provide Training in MCOs

There are three types of models to provide the necessary training for future practitioners to care for older adults enrolled in MCOs. These include programs sponsored by MCOs, programs within academic MCOs, and student/trainee placements by academic health centers into MCOs.

MCO-Sponsored Training Programs

MCOs sponsor a number of exemplary training programs. Distinct from academic medical centers, organizations such as Kaiser Permanente offer their own nurse practitioner

TABLE 11.1   Changes in the Structure of the US Health Care System in One Lifetime

	1935	1985	2005
Payment mechanism	Out-of-pocket	Private insurance and out-of-pocket	Socially organized payment system
Form of physician payment	Fee-for-service	Mixed	Capitation and salary
Dominant site of care	Physician's office	Hospital	Diffuse network
Function of medical staff	Care	Curing disease	Disease prevention care and management
Measured by	How nice?	How technical?	How cost-effective?

Note. From "Educating Physicians for the 21st Century," by M. R. Greenlick, 1995, *Academic Medicine, 70,* pp. 179–185. Copyright 1995 by *Academic Medicine.* Reprinted by permission.

programs and medical (internal and family medicine) residencies and fellowships. These are accredited programs with organized curricula, clinical training schedules, and internal application and acceptance policies. To date, no MCO offers a special geriatrically focused training program.

In addition to the 1- and 2-year training programs above, postgraduate continuing education programs are offered by many MCOs. The Henry Ford Health System has organized The Managed Care College and sponsors a number of continuing medical education (CME) programs annually. Kaiser Permanente offers regional and inter-regional conferences on geriatrics topics annually. These CME programs are often attended by MCO professional staff, who are provided education release time, and community practitioners who pay a fee to attend.

Newly hired physicians and other professional staff require retraining by the MCO because so few new graduates have had any relevant training or experience in managed care. Nothing is more telling of the inadequacies of current academic training than the fact that MCOs report that up to 1 year of retraining is necessary for the majority of new professionals to orient them to the managed care world (COGME, 1995).

Academic MCO Programs

Academic medical centers are interested in reorganizing to include a managed care component for a number of reasons. One is to provide in-house settings for managed care training. However, this may not be the primary reason. Changes in the health care system have profoundly altered the way providers and hospitals are reimbursed and have eroded both the financial support and patient base of academic health centers. Research, patient care, and teaching make up the core mission of these centers, and managed care has presented daunting challenges to keeping this mission intact. Academic medical centers rely on clinical care incomes, and they must be competitive in their patient care practice to protect clinical revenues (Carey & Engelhard, 1996).

The culture of traditional academic medicine is at odds with the principles inherent in managed care. The decision-making style of universities is decentralized, usually through a hierarchy of departments, whereas the MCO is centralized. This has implications for the ability to respond to change or initiate new activities. Academic medical centers have placed a high priority on specialty training, whereas the MCO relies on primary care. Traditionally, the primary location of training has been the hospital, with an emphasis on use of high technology; MCOs emphasize ambulatory care and low-technology interventions.

Even with these challenges, a number of academic medical centers have embarked on redesigning their training programs to include content in managed care through training partnerships with MCOs. Case Western Reserve University has joined the Henry Ford Health System, New York Medical College is working with Kaiser Permanente, and The University of Delaware has combined efforts with Jefferson Medical, to name a few exemplary programs. Harvard University, George Washington University, and University of California, Los Angeles (UCLA) have each designed programs that include new content and clinical placements utilizing a segment of their practice groups or affiliated community MCOs (COGME, 1995).

Student/Trainee Placements at MCOs

Student placements, preceptorships, and residency rotations are by far the predominant type of training currently received by health and social service students at academic institutions. Much of the information available on this topic addresses medical student placements, but nursing, social work, pharmacy, public health, and allied health graduate students have similar opportunities.

In 1995 about 14% of medical schools required all students to have a clinical training experience in an MCO. Just under half of all students in medical schools actually have an MCO clinical placement (COGME, 1995). A 1-month rotation was the most prevalent type of clinical experience. The placement, or any portion of time spent in the MCO, may or may not have included experience in geriatric care services.

Students in a variety of health professions have opportunities for MCO experience; six Southern California Kaiser medical centers had training affiliations with six nursing programs, four pharmacy programs, three public health, and six social work programs. During one academic year, 66 nursing graduate students, 47 pharmacy students, 6 public health and 16 social work students received clinical training, ranging from 4 weeks to 9 months, as dictated by their program's requirements (Frank & Della Penna, 1996).

What is the clinical training experience in MCOs? Despite considerable variation between programs, Veloski, Barzansky, Nash, Bastacky, & Stevens (1996) have identified some common limitations of clinical training placements. The majority of placements occur in group or staff model MCOs. This is logical because these models generally have large memberships, large staffs available to precept, and centralized facilities. However, the network type models, with great geographic dispersion, are the fastest growing type of MCO. In addition, many health professions schools place students in MCOs, not because of the managed care environment, but because of the large and diverse patient population available; this leaves the unique features of MCOs, such as cost containment, unaddressed. This content could be included in the clinical training, but would require additional preceptor staff time and presumably decrease the efficiency of the MCO.

Funding Graduate Medical Education

Graduate medical education (GME) funding, initially provided to teaching hospitals to offset the higher costs of patient care associated with teaching activities, is provided through Medicare. It has supported the academic medical center's priorities (or may have aided in creating them) by having as its funding base the number of residents in hospital-based or hospital-owned care settings (COGME, 1995). In 1995, over 75% of the some $6.374 billion GME dollars went to training specialty (nonprimary care) medical residents (COGME, 1995).

Until the summer of 1997, GME reimbursement was included in the capitation rates of Medicare risk contracts to MCOs, whether or not they provided training. This practice, along with other issues associated with GME funding policies, was the topic of serious debates in health policy circles (AAMC, 1997a, 1997b). As part of the budget accord reached in the summer of 1997, Congress removed this disincentive. At the same time, however, Congress reduced support for teaching hospitals (AAMC, 1997c). Other policy changes that remain under discussion include (a) a decrease in medical specialty training, with a concomitant increase in training primary care providers; (b) an increase in training in ambulatory care sites; and (c) moving the GME funding out of the Medicare program because a minuscule portion actually relates to geriatric training.

CURRICULUM CONTENT FOR GERIATRIC TRAINING IN MCOS

Core Content Areas

The Council on Graduate Medical Education (COGME) has identified a series of content areas that they consider core training areas to prepare professionals for work in MCOs (1995). The recommended major content areas include:

- Health systems finance, economics, organization, and delivery
- Practice of population-based medicine that is evidence based and epidemiologically sound
- Development of effective patient-provider relationships
- Understanding systems-based care and organizational change
- Ethics
- Promotion of teamwork

All of these core areas are also appropriate for geriatric care training for many disciplines who will work in MCOs. In 1995 the Bureau of Health Professions in the Health Resources and Services Administration convened a group of experts to identify how to better prepare the health care workforce to care for an aging population. The report that resulted from this forum identified a number of similar areas to those listed above. In particular, geriatrics training in MCOs was identified as a clear need, and both MCO and discipline representatives identified a need for geriatric interdisciplinary team training (HRSA, 1995).

Geriatric Interdisciplinary Team Training was subsequently developed as a major national training initiative by the John A. Hartford Foundation of New York. All of the implementation sites have included one or more MCOs in their clinical partnerships (see Table 11.2).

Advantages and Disadvantages of Managed Care Models for GITT

Team effectiveness hinges on proper clinical reality-based preparation and training. Some managed care models lend themselves more readily than others to this task. In choosing MCOs as training sites, academic institutions will maximize the partnership's success and the student's experience by selecting:

- A managed care organization whose mission includes education and training and is willing to partner with academic institutions
- A managed care organization that uses teams effectively and sees the advantage of being able to hire appropriately trained team members
- Appropriate facilities where teams with core professionals are based and where training and team interaction can take place with minimal disruption of the organization's and staff work flow
- Preceptors from the organization's staff who have the appropriate qualifications and skills to participate in the training

Table 11.3 identifies the characteristics of various MCO models and rates how likely these features will be available in them for GITT. The larger, centralized MCO models are more likely to have the mission of education and the staff and facilities for student training. The more decentralized models are often networks of physicians' offices or small clinics; in these, student training, in teams or singly, may intrude into those professionals' patient care. When there is a limited number of professional staff on hand, adding preceptor functions could be extremely burdensome. The most innovative models of MCOs, such as the SHMO or PACE, have team care as an integral part of their

TABLE 11.2   Managed Care Clinical Training at GITT Sites

GITT site	Managed care program model
Ford/CWRU	Nonprofit HMO and Managed Care College (PACE)
Houston GITT	POS and Group Model Health Maintenance Organization (HMO)
Mt. Sinai	PACE
On Lok	PACE
Rush	Staff Model HMO, IPA and POS
University of Colorado	Staff Model HMO, IPA, Group Model HMO, and PACE
University of Minnesota	Staff Model HMO and POS
University of South Florida	Staff Model HMO, IPA and Mixed Model HMO

PACE, Program for All-inclusive Care of the Elderly.
POS, Point of service plan.
IPA, Independent practice association.

TABLE 11.3   Criteria Available for GITT by MCO Model

Managed care model	Centralized training site	Core professionals	Preceptor availability	Care integration	Future employment
Staff	++++	+++	+++	+++	+++
Group	++++	+++	++	+++	+++
Network	+	+	+	+	−
IPA	−	−	−	−	−
Direct service	−	−	−	−	−
SHMO	+++++	+++++	+++++	+++++	+++++
PACE	+++++	+++++	+++++	+++++	+++++

+, Available.
−, Not available.
IPA, Independent practice association.
PACE, Program for All-inclusive Care of the Elderly.
SHMO, Social health maintenance organization.

organizational philosophy and are extremely well-positioned to provide GITT. Although relatively smaller in patient census, these programs attract the frail, older person who is most suited to a team approach to care.

SUMMARY

Health care reform dominated by a managed care environment was initiated to reverse the escalating costs of medical care. MCOs, in one form or another, have grown rapidly, and they currently supply the majority of health care in America. Academic training programs did not proactively respond to the changing health care environment or the demographic imperative of an aging society.

Multiple challenges face academic training programs. How can academic institutions most effectively incorporate needed new content into already crowded and highly competitive curriculum? How can clinical training be provided in MCOs, within or outside the academic institution, without canceling out the cost efficiencies that are the pillars of the managed care environment? How can academic faculty be trained to support and model MCO values when these values may be the antithesis of those they hold? As we are midstream in the health reform current, we have more questions than answers.

We do know that the growing number of elderly Americans require a radical shift in the way care and services are currently provided. We must pay special attention to the frail elderly who develop dependencies that threaten their ability to remain in the community. These people will require not just appropriate medical services, but also social and personal services that are currently not available to them through Medicare. Team care appears to be a promising way to assess and manage the various aspects of the care needs of frail and very ill elderly. Population-based care for disease states, such as advanced congestive heart failure or chronic obstructive lung disease, go beyond the individual provider and involve a team of providers. MCOs are developing an increasing number of team approaches to this area. Unfortunately, health professionals are put on teams with little preparation for the task during their training.

There is growing support for formal training in GITT. Well-integrated managed care provides an opportunity for the organization and delivery of this team care and for the preparation of health professionals in training, the future members of interdisciplinary teams. Nonetheless, we must continue to measure the value of team care in terms of quality and cost in the competitive market of managed care. The GITT Program will provide information on the methods, content, and acceptability of training students in a variety of MCO settings.

REFERENCES

American Association of Medical Colleges. (1997a). *Statement on teaching hospitals and Medicare disproportionate share hospital payments,* 105th Cong. 1st Sess. XX (1997), (testimony of David D'Eramo).

American Association of Medical Colleges. (1997b). *Statement on future financing of graduate medical education,* 105th Cong., 1st Sess. 35 (1997), (testimony of Ralph W. Muller).

American Association of Medical Colleges. (1997c, August 4). Budget agreement reached. *Short Topical and Timely News from AAMC* (AAMC STAT Listserv).

Carey, R., & Engelhard, C. (1996). Academic medicine meets managed care: A high-impact collision. *Academic Medicine, 71,* 839–845.

Council On Graduate Medical Education. (1995). *Sixth report to Congress: Managed health care: Implications for the physician workforce and medical education.* Washington, DC: U.S. Department of Health and Human Services.

Frank, J., & Della Penna, R. (1996). *Kaiser Permanente and UCLA.* GITT planning grant report to the John A. Hartford Foundation.

Freeborn, D. K., & Pope, C. R. (1994). *Promise and performance in managed care: The prepaid group practice model.* Baltimore, MD: Johns Hopkins University Press.

Greenlick, M. (1995). Educating physicians for the twenty-first century. *Academic Medicine, 70,* 179–185.

Health Resources and Services Administration. (1995). *A national agenda for geriatric education: White papers* (Vol. 1). Washington, DC: Department of Health and Human Services.

Kay, R. M. (1979). *Historical review of the Southern California Permanente Medical Group.* Los Angeles: R. M. Kay and the Southern California Medical Group.

Rovner, J. (1996). Clearing the smoke from Medicare and Medicaid. *Business & Health Magazine, 14,* (Suppl. C).

Schwartz, J. (1965, Sept.–Oct.). Early history of prepaid medical care plans. *Bulletin of the History of Medicine,* pp. 470–475.

Shouldice, R. (1991). *Introduction to managed care.* Arlington, VA: Information Resources Press.

Veloski, J., Barzansky, B., Nash, D., Bastacky, S., & Stevens D. (1996). Medical student education in managed care settings. *Journal of the American Medical Association, 276,* 667–671.

Wagner, E. (1995). Types of managed care organizations. In P. Kongstevedt (Ed.), *Essentials of managed health care.* (p. 24–34). Gaithersburg, MD: Aspen.

CHAPTER 12

Turning the Clinical Agency into a Setting for Team Training

Kate O'Malley, Susan Kornblatt, and Carol Van Steenberg

The Geriatric Interdisciplinary Team Training (GITT) Program brings together academic and clinical partners to prepare trainees for high quality interdisciplinary care of the elderly. One major challenge in this venture is enabling the clinical setting to balance its responsibilities to care for elderly clients and provide an excellent learning experience for trainees.

In this chapter we address some of the issues involved in turning the clinical agency into a setting for team training. First, we will discuss the importance of clinical training and the requirements for successful GITT. Next, we will explore the implications of these requirements for an operating agency, pointing out some of the costs and benefits of becoming a clinical training partner. Then, drawing on the experience and insights of the academic-clinical partnerships formed throughout the United States to implement GITT, we will suggest some strategies to manage the communication and staff training concerns as clinical agencies transform themselves into interdisciplinary training settings while continuing their caregiving mission. Finally, we will use a case study of our own organization, On Lok Senior Health Services in San Francisco. We will explain how we are developing the capacity to transfer the richness of our experience in providing care to the frail elderly through an interdisciplinary team to trainees whose experience and interest in our setting may vary widely.

THE IMPORTANCE OF CLINICAL TRAINING

Clinical placements are essential to the development of professional skills in health and social service settings. In the clinical setting, the trainee comes into contact with the real world of providing services, working directly with clients or patients. The most effective clinical training occurs with the guidance of a skilled preceptor, who offers feedback and encouragement as theory is applied under controlled circumstances.

In the best case scenario, the theory matches the practice, the clinical setting provides a stimulating and appropriate experience, the preceptor has skills worth emulating, and the trainee is open and enthusiastic. With repeated experiences, the trainee masters professional skills and learns professional behavior and values. At the same time, newly energized agency staff gain fresh perspectives from trainees and sharpen their own clinical skills as they focus on transmitting them to trainees. By supervising students, staff can evaluate and improve their own performance (Gates & Curtis, 1995).

THE CLINICAL SETTING IN GITT

Requirements, Benefits, and Challenges

Effective GITT curriculum planning occurs only when clinical settings and academic institutions work together. Most academic partners implementing GITT plan to involve multiple clinical settings as placements for GITT trainees. These agencies vary in their organizational sponsors, missions, staffing patterns, and degrees of sophistication in providing care. With these variables, implementing a consistent curriculum and providing a uniform training experience become very complicated.

In GITT, the clinical setting must offer two training opportunities—the practice of clinical skills along with the equally important acquisition and practice of team skills. Preceptors with clinical training skills must also understand and model effective team-member skills, making the implicit activities of teamwork become explicit and obvious to trainees. Preceptors cannot assume sole responsibility for modeling effective teamwork, however, as trainees will interact with many staff in the clinical setting. Thus, GITT offers an incentive for all clinical staff to sharpen their skills and performance.

GITT also offers the agency the opportunity to affiliate more closely with academic institutions in their community and to serve as a catalyst for interinstitutional knowledge transfer and collaboration. The agency, through its relationships with multiple departments of several universities, may facilitate new bonds among its partners, benefiting all concerned. Affiliation with academic institutions may both offer personal and organizational prestige and recognition and bring the community agency new opportunities for learning, program development, public policy advocacy, and funding. Similarly, universities may recognize the academic value of service, coupled with educational and research-related goals.

However, the clinical setting also faces many challenges as it takes on the interdisciplinary team training responsibility. There are tensions between service providers and universities; practitioners in the service field often share suspicion of academics (Clark, Spence, & Sheehan, 1988). How can partners acknowledge these misgivings and address them constructively?

Given the GITT Program expectations that the clinical setting be a learning laboratory on teamwork, any unaddressed or lingering team dynamics problems in the agency will face extra scrutiny. Will the clinical setting be able to withstand such scrutiny? Are the agency's clinical staff able to serve as the role models in team development? If skills and attitudes need some development, how can the clinical agency be supported in that effort? Whose job is it to assess the effectiveness of the agency team and provide feedback to the agency leadership? How is team effectiveness assessed?

Organizational support at the highest level of the agency is essential to develop a training environment appropriate for GITT and address the demands of participation on the agency as a whole. Participation in GITT is stressful for staff; the agency's leadership must take action to manage that stress.

Agencies without training experience prior to GITT involvement must develop preceptor skills both in clinical work and team training and must make time for professional staff to engage in training. Those in managed care settings may face specific productivity guidelines. Time away from clinical work can have an impact on the profitability of the clinical setting, at least in the short run.

Central leadership and effective communication reduce the stress of additional GITT-related work in the agency. The clinical setting must identify who on staff is responsible for training and for precepting. A centralized process for trainee intake, tracking, orientation, and other logistic support should be in place. (Many agencies have been involved in disciplinary training for years without developing an integrated approach to training.) Communications among all parties must be clear and open, and staff must be prepared to sort through myriad details about scheduling, space, data collection, and other logistic issues.

Agency leaders must continuously assess the impact of implementing the training program on the organization to improve training efforts and minimize organizational stresses. For example, conflict may arise between precepting and nonprecepting staff over issues such as an imbalance in work load, the status associated with the precepting activity and role, and the staff or career development opportunities available to preceptors.

STRATEGIES FOR PREPARING CLINICAL SETTINGS FOR GITT PARTICIPATION

During 1996, the planning year prior to the implementation of the GITT Project, academic and clinical partners began to address curriculum development and clinical setting preparation issues in anticipation of starting the training in 1997. In April 1997, sites awarded implementation grants met in Tampa, Florida to share their experiences to date. In several workgroups, academic faculty, clinical faculty, and administrators across sites shared their approaches to preparing clinical settings for GITT.

Based on their collective planning experience and initial implementation activities, the GITT workgroups developed the following recommendations.

1. Clinical agency leadership should demonstrate its support and involvement in GITT by articulating the agency's commitment publicly, participating during the planning phase, and allocating staff time for participation.
2. The GITT Project should establish central leadership at the clinical setting for training coordination to promote problem solving, facilitate clarification of issues, and provide the authority necessary to move ahead.

3. Written descriptions of the local GITT Project should clearly communicate the goals, players, process, timelines, and requirements from the clinical preceptors and the agency.

4. The clinical agency's leaders should meet with agency managers and staff periodically to discuss concerns, clarify the process and expectations of GITT, solve problems, and establish the site's commitment to training.

5. The academic partners and the clinical settings should develop a communication strategy, clearly defining roles, naming individuals responsible in key areas (e.g., scheduling, data collection, trainee orientation), and establishing a regular meeting schedule of clinical agency staff and academic partners.

6. The clinical agency must provide a structured orientation for all staff (preceptors and nonpreceptors) at the beginning of GITT implementation and periodically thereafter, increasing the staff's awareness of the expectations for team and clinical training experiences.

7. The academic partners should provide staff training on topics relevant to GITT to encourage buy-in from staff who will benefit personally from the training and to improve the quality of the practica experience for the GITT trainees.

8. Clinical preceptors should work with academic faculty to develop the GITT training curriculum and articulate preceptor expectations, thereby establishing mutual agreement and buy-in. This curriculum should include sufficient details for each discipline in training to give staff a clear road map of day-to-day activities with trainees, and it should be available for interested staff to review.

9. The GITT Project Director should meet with preceptors on a one-to-one basis to elicit concerns about skills and roles; this will allow identification of areas for further training and enable the preceptors to feel that their contributions are important and valued.

10. Staff should be involved in developing and presenting training sessions for GITT trainees, other staff, and others affiliated with GITT. This activity helps staff develop training skills and reinforces the value of their knowledge and contribution to GITT, even if they are not directly involved in precepting activities.

11. Whenever feasible, long-term trainees should help orient new trainees to the clinical setting, thus decreasing staff involvement in mundane and repetitive activities.

12. Preplacement interviews of trainees can help coordinators make the best match between trainee interest and the setting's characteristics and capabilities (language, culture, etc.).

13. Clinical setting coordinators should arrange work space, mailboxes, and access to telephones and computers in advance to minimize last-minute scrambling as trainees arrive and to help them feel more welcome in the agency.

14. Scheduling trainees whose clinical placement times vary widely between disciplines and levels of experience within disciplines is a universal challenge to clinical settings. Identifying one staff person to support this effort and coordinate scheduling, notification of arrival, and departure dates is critical.

The workgroups also identified a range of problems that could emerge during implementation and proposed some approaches for addressing these problems. Because the GITT Projects depend on effective clinical preceptors, inadequate supply of these preceptors would be a serious threat to success. Reasons for inadequate staffing include insufficient number of clinical preceptors to manage the numbers of trainees participating in GITT, rapid preceptor turnover, and absence of key disciplines at some clinical settings with no plan to expand the team.

Possible strategies for coping with these preceptor difficulties include the creative use of copreceptors, the acceptance of training responsibility as a team function, and supplementation through outside resources. As copreceptors, agency staff members could work with trainees in tandem with their official preceptor to develop team member skills. In this way, discipline-specific preceptor requirements (such as MSW supervision of MSW trainee) could be met, while nonpreceptor staff take responsibility for some of the training activities (for example, the MSW trainees might accompany the staff occupational therapist for a home safety assessment). To minimize the potential impact of preceptor turnover, clinical settings should make efforts to regard trainees as the business of the team rather than the responsibility of a single preceptor. Then, even if an individual leaves midway in the trainee's placement, the trainee who has a strong relationship with other staff should be able complete the placement in a meaningful way. Borrowing staff from other locations or using academic faculty in a part-time staff role can help fill in discipline-specific gaps. Trainees can also travel to other clinical settings to have a full team experience at least some of the time. Part of their learning could include an analysis of the impact of a missing discipline on the full functioning of the team.

Turnover of the clinical agency's leadership requires the academic partners to establish new relationships. GITT might not hold as much interest for a new leader busy learning the job, and GITT might flag if the agency fails to replace its leader quickly. A GITT Project that is firmly integrated into the fabric of the organization should be able to withstand some leadership loss, but probably not for long. On the other hand, if procedures are firmly in place, and the complex logistics of scheduling have been institutionalized in some way, leadership turnover will pose less of a threat to GITT.

No-shows, that is, short-stay trainees who renege on their clinical commitments, are another source of tension. Agency staff feel slighted and are inclined to invest less energy in future encounters. In this event, strategies for managing agency and staff stress are particularly important, especially by devising ways to free staff from routine orientation efforts.

Another source of tension in the agency is the conflict over time for training versus time for caring (especially likely in a managed care environment). GITT must prove its value by helping raise the standard of care for the patients, in part because the staff who serve as mentors for students will hone their own clinical skills in the process of teaching (Gates & Curtis, 1995). GITT Projects thus could make the case that the investment of time in the short run provides a major gain in the long run—better care and improved customer satisfaction. The complexities of managed care, including multiple payers, protocols, limited referral patterns, and productivity requirements, provide a curriculum challenge in matching the didactic training with the clinical setting. GITT Projects could build the case for using teams in managed care settings for targeted groups (frail older patients for example) and strengthen the setting's ability to manage care effectively for these groups (see chapter 11).

CASE STUDY—ON LOK'S EXPERIENCE IN LAUNCHING GITT

On Lok is the only GITT grantee that is an operating clinical agency rather than an academic institution. Because of our mission and our experience as a service provider, we probably have focused thus far more intensively on issues related to the preparation of the clinical setting for GITT than have the other GITT sites. We enjoy an advantage not available to most of the other GITT grantees, namely the central management of all six of the clinical settings where our GITT trainees will be placed. Five of our clinical settings are the day health centers and primary care clinics operated directly by On Lok SeniorHealth Services (OLSHS); our sixth clinical setting is operated by the Goldman Institute on Aging, which has a subcontract with On Lok to deliver the On Lok SeniorHealth service package. In contrast, most of the other GITT Projects involve several or many clinical settings that have no operational relationships. Although starting up the GITT Project has posed numerous challenges for us that we anticipate will be shared by all the other GITT sites, clinical setting preparation probably has been more straightforward.

On Lok's Mission and Health Care Model

The mission of OLSHS is "to provide quality and affordable services for the well-being of the frail elderly." In San Francisco, OLSHS delivers a complete continuum of health and long-term care services: primary care, adult day health care, home care, specialty care, and inpatient services (both hospitalization and nursing home care).

Beginning in the early 1970s, On Lok responded to a community need in San Francisco's Chinatown-North Beach area by creating a consumer-oriented health care model for the older person who requires long-term care but does not want to go into a nursing home. The On Lok model is a fully integrated managed care system for the frail elderly. It meets complex medical and social needs by putting in one place all medical, restorative, social, and supportive care. On Lok's model has been shown in the last few years to work effectively in all sorts of communities and is being replicated across the United States through the Program of All-Inclusive Care for the Elderly (PACE).

Most of On Lok's 550 enrollees attend an adult day health center for many of their services; a primary care clinic is adjacent. On Lok's centers and clinics are located in North Beach, the Polk Gulch area, and the Mission/Noe Valley area. Through a subcontract between On Lok and the Goldman Institute on Aging (IOA), On Lok SeniorHealth by IOA/University of California, San Francisco serves frail older clients in the Richmond, Western Addition, and Sunset sections of San Francisco.

In addition to creating a care delivery system that includes the full range of health care professionals and facilities, On Lok has developed an integrated reimbursement system. Medicare and Medicaid both provide per capita payments to On Lok Senior Health Services each month, based on its census of entitled enrollees. These funds are pooled and used without regard to traditional restrictions, eliminating unproductive paperwork and barriers to optimal care.

The Participant and the Team in On Lok

The average age of On Lok participants is 82 years. They have an average of seven medical diagnoses each. Almost all participants (89%) are eligible for Medicare and Medicaid, with 5% eligible for Medicare alone, and 6% eligible for Medicaid alone. Individuals ineligible for Medicaid make private capitation payments.

In the On Lok model, an interdisciplinary team of primary care physician, nurse, social worker, rehabilitation therapist, home health workers, and others uses a systematic method for assessing need that recognizes the complex interrelationships among social, emotional, and physical factors. They formulate, coordinate, and control the implementation of a treatment plan that addresses the whole person (not just disease manifestations) and incorporates all care settings. The team monitors the impact of treatment and the progress of the individual over time and adjusts the care plan as indicated by the individual's ever-changing needs. This same interdisciplinary team gives care, usually in a day health center or at home, for the balance of the participant's life. On Lok also contracts with hospitals and nursing homes for inpatient care, and these services are managed by the team.

For the fixed monthly rate, On Lok provides as much care as is needed, as long as necessary, regardless of how costly this becomes. On Lok has no out and no place to shift costs. Cost control must be achieved by keeping the participant as healthy as possible. On Lok's comprehensive, integrated model of care depends on team effectiveness.

On Lok's clinical staff use a state-of-the-art electronic medical record system. Although the system is still under development, it enhances interdisciplinary problem identification and resolution. Individual providers can input, retrieve, and manage information on their patients; see clinical changes in patients over time; and appreciate aggregate changes in specific patient populations.

The interdisciplinary team approach to care planning and delivery has been key to On Lok's positive results in quality, client satisfaction, and cost-effectiveness. On Lok and the other mature PACE settings have experienced a consistently lower level of hospital utilization among the program's frail enrollees than occurs in the general 65 and over population. For 1995, PACE enrollees (at On Lok and the eight senior replication sites) averaged 2,399 hospital days/1,000 persons per annum and 4.9 days/admission; the average for On Lok's participants was 1,200 days/1,000 persons per annum and 4.15 days/admission. These rates compare favorably with the general Medicare population, which includes the well elderly, where the utilization averaged 2,448 days/1,000 persons per annum in 1994 and length of stay of 7.6 days/admission (U.S. Department of Health and Human Services, 1995).

GITT at On Lok

On Lok's GITT Project, in clinical cooperation with the Goldman IOA, builds on previous relationships with academia and service staff. On Lok formed the GITT Steering Committee, made up of representatives from On Lok, the IOA, and their academic partners, to serve as the primary vehicle for academic-community agency planning, curriculum development, and partnership. The GITT Steering Committee's 25 members began with the premise that learning how to use On Lok's well-developed interdisciplinary health care teams effectively in primary and continuing education processes would make a valuable educational contribution (Drinka, 1991).

Academic partners that had an interest in placing trainees at On Lok or the IOA were invited to join the GITT Steering Committee. On Lok and IOA staff were invited to join the GITT Steering Committee based on their organizational responsibilities or their interest in supervising trainees. Table 12.1 lists the academic partners and staff participants on the GITT Steering Committee.

The purposes of the GITT Steering Committee are to (a) identify and articulate On Lok models of GITT, (b) agree on key interdisciplinary learning objectives and activities for GITT trainees, (c) identify barriers to implementation of GITT, (d) participate in development and implementation of evaluation measures, (e) develop preclinical and clinical orientation materials regarding GITT, (f) review and participate in the development of GITT cross-setting data collection instruments, (g) agree and articulate interdisciplinary preceptor responsibilities and competencies, and (h) develop and use preceptor skills' measures. These purposes, together with the Committee's extensive provider-academic membership, enable the Steering Committee to function as a strong force in guiding the development of the clinical training setting.

The On Lok GITT Steering Committee met approximately six times during the GITT planning year. The GITT Project Director developed agendas, facilitated meetings, directed and worked with all subcommittees, produced minutes of meetings, and identified future GITT planning needs. Because all levels of agency staff, from Executive Director to clinical staff, have worked with academic faculty on the Steering Committee as a team consistently, it has been possible to build strong consensus around key planning issues.

The GITT Steering Committee was very productive during the planning year. Academic faculty, formerly peripherally aware of On Lok's clinical services, became much more familiar with On Lok's delivery system, staff, and educational curriculum. Service staff and academic faculty developed new working relationships. They developed written curricula for five models of team training with input and agreement from clinical staff and academic faculty, identified interdisciplinary responsibilities of preceptors, and facilitated consensus among service staff and academic faculty regarding these responsibilities. Service staff and academic faculty also became familiar with the GITT Program cross-site data collection instruments and the importance of consistently participating in the use of them. By the end of the planning year, each GITT Steering Committee member had become part of the GITT team.

On Lok has used part of its award to defray some of the costs of the universities with which we hoped to develop working relationships. We realized that the planning process would be time consuming not only to our agency staff but also to the faculty employed by our academic partners. Financial support for faculty to become involved in the development of clinical curriculum added motivation for their consistent participation. We are continuing to provide modest support to our academic partners during the implementation of GITT to enhance on-going curriculum review, evaluation, and revision.

Through its experience with GITT thus far, On Lok has learned that a number of factors are critical to making the changes required to implement GITT. These include:

TABLE 12.1   On Lok GITT Steering Committee Participants

Academic partners	Staff participants
UCSF, Department of Medicine	GITT Project Director
UCSF, Department of Medicine/Mount Zion Hospital	Executive Director
	Director of On Lok SeniorHealth Services
UCSF, Department of Family Medicine/San Francisco General Hospital	Medical Director
	Five On Lok Center Managers
St. Mary's Medical Center, San Francisco	Medical staff
UCSF, Department of Physiological Nursing, Gerontological Nurse Practitioner Program	Nurse Practitioner
	Social Work Specialist
UC, Berkeley School of Social Work UCSF/ San Francisco State University, Joint Program in Physical Therapy	Physical Therapy Specialist
	Occupational Therapy Specialist
	Director of Home Care
San Francisco State University, School of Social Work	IOA Director of Education
	IOA Medical Director
Samuel Merritt College, Departments of Physical Therapy and Occupational Therapy, Oakland, CA.	IOA On Lok SeniorHealth Director

- Commitment of agency leadership to training in general and to the GITT in particular
- Consolidation of responsibility for GITT coordination in one position
- Ongoing collaboration by clinical staff and academic faculty to structure and refine expectations for preceptors
- Communication and support to reduce agency and staff stress
- Training of clinical staff, both preceptors and collateral staff, to fulfill new roles and responsibilities created by GITT.

Leadership

On Lok's GITT Project has had the support of On Lok's Executive Director/Chief Executive Officer from the beginning. The Executive Director's background includes several years as an academic faculty member prior to joining On Lok and a personal commitment to clinical training and to staff development. The Director of Senior Health Services, who is responsible for overseeing daily clinical operations, also embraces the commitment to training. On-going support, training, and professional development of clinical staff contribute to an unusually low turnover of staff in the five On Lok SeniorHealth centers. That low turnover bodes well for GITT, of course, as it ensures continuity in preceptors and organizational learning.

Coordination

At On Lok, GITT operates under the leadership of the GITT Project Director (PD), who reports directly to the Executive Director. The PD provides agency-wide coordination for clinical training and maintains working relationships with clinical preceptors and with academic faculty. The PD oversees all clinical training for medical residents and other clinical trainees at On Lok; is responsible for all aspects of GITT program development, implementation, and evaluation; and works closely with key clinical faculty in each specialty area where clinical internships are offered (medicine, nurse practitioner, social work, physical therapy, and occupational therapy). Coordination functions include developing protocols for intake and exit of all trainees, working with clinical faculty to ensure that discipline-specific as well as interdisciplinary learning objectives are addressed for all trainees, preparing written interdisciplinary curricula, overseeing the planning and implementation of clinical faculty development efforts, designing and overseeing evaluation efforts, and taking responsibility for all facets of GITT Project implementation.

Communication

To clarify the role of clinical staff in teaching, On Lok's clinical staff have worked with academic faculty through the GITT Steering Committee to reach consensus about realistic responsibilities. The GITT PD has facilitated small group and one-to-one meetings to ensure common understanding among academic faculty, On Lok and IOA administrators, and the clinical staff involved with clinical precepting. On Lok is making sure that training responsibilities are in staff job descriptions where appropriate. This way staff know when they are hired what some of their teaching responsibilities ultimately will be.

Staff and Preceptor Training

Recognizing that staff need knowledge, skills, and ongoing support to implement GITT while maintaining their productivity, On Lok has designed a faculty development program that involves both general On Lok staff and preceptors. Elements include didactic geriatric interdisciplinary case conferences, and courses, lectures, grand rounds, and other conferences at the academic sites.

Preceptor training at On Lok focuses on improving teaching skills—technical competence, organizing workload, ethical professional behavior, and interpersonal communication techniques as an interdisciplinary team member. The relationship between preceptor development and the successful transformation of the clinical agency into a team training setting is critical.

As the role of community settings in the education of residents and students enlarges, these kinds of development programs become increasingly important. Community practitioners so developed are a significant, effective, and potentially abundant resource in the education of students and residents. The key to realizing the educational potential in community settings lies in the skill of the preceptor, both as clinician and as educator. Ideally, the community preceptor is an excellent clinician with enthusiasm and ability for imparting skills to others (DeWitt, Goldberg & Roberts, 1993).

On Lok is using the following strategies to support preceptor development.

1. Completion of a preceptor development needs assessment. The Preceptor Self-Assessment, which is based on the GITT Steering Committee's work to clarify preceptor roles and responsibilities and expected competencies, includes a pretest and posttest to measure preceptor skills. The GITT PD uses this instrument with all preceptors to develop Individual Learning Plans for them, with personal learning objectives, activities, and timelines for completion. The posttraining Preceptor Self-Assessment highlights skills that have been enhanced and identifies skills for future development.

2. Preceptor observations. Our preceptors observe effective preceptors at other clinical settings to learn how to structure clinical experiences for trainees. Because structuring learning experiences for trainees can be time consuming, preceptors can benefit from seeing how creative scheduling is done at other community settings. Observing a completely different setting takes preceptors out of their regular routine and gives them the opportunity to learn new or different ways to provide a wider cross section of experiences for trainees.

3. Brief interdisciplinary lectures. Preceptors develop and present brief lectures to trainees. Clinical precepting and brief presentations are the two main methods for teaching residents and students, and we place special emphasis on developing faculty skills in these areas (DeWitt, Goldberg & Roberts, 1993). Making presentations may be a new experience for some clinical preceptors, although they may have many years' experience as excellent clinicians. Providing support for staff as they develop presentation skills is an appropriate use of GITT resources.

4. Staff exchanges. On Lok and IOA preceptors participate in staff exchanges across our clinical settings. Staff take the day off from their regular clinical responsibilities and become trainees in another discipline. For example, a nurse practitioner may spend the day with a social worker to see what it is like to be a social work intern. We expect this experience will give preceptors a unique opportunity in interdisciplinary teaching and learning.

5. Managing agency and staff stress. To minimize stress on staff, On Lok's GITT staff and Steering Committee are providing orientation materials to trainees prior to placement, educating academic faculty about the complexity of the On Lok program, developing an interactive CD-ROM to orient trainees to On Lok and interdisciplinary team care, and providing introductory training on computer access to On Lok's unique computerized medical record system.

SUMMARY

Turning the clinical agency into a team training setting presents a multifaceted challenge; strategies for successful metamorphosis include: (a) a solid commitment from the clinical agency leadership; (b) central leadership for interdisciplinary training, written curricula, project descriptions, and job descriptions for all preceptors; (c) constant communication and coordination with academic partners; and (d) effective and on-going preceptor training. With these factors taken into consideration, the clinical agency can turn into a team training setting to the benefit of all.

REFERENCES

Clark, P. G., Spence, D. L., & Sheehan, J. L. (1988). Challenges and barriers to interdisciplinary gerontological team training in the academic setting. *Gerontology & Geriatrics Education, 7*, 93–110.

DeWitt, T. G., Goldberg, R. L., & Roberts, K. B. (1993). Developing community faculty: Principles, practice and evaluation. *American Journal of Diseases of Children, 147*, 49–53.

Drinka, T. J. K. (1991). Development and maintenance of an interdisciplinary health care team: a case study. *Gerontology & Geriatrics Education, 12,* 111–125.

Gates, G. E., & Curtis, M. (1995). Characteristics of effective preceptors: A review of allied health literature. *Journal of the American Dietetic Association, 95,* 225–227.

U.S. Department of Health and Human Services (1995). *HCFA statistics.* (HCFA Publication Number 03373, p. 32). Washington, DC: U.S. Government Printing Office.

CHAPTER 13

Integrated Health Care Systems: GITT As a Core Capability

David A. Lindeman, Lois Halstead, Stan Lapidos, Denis A. Evans, and Patricia Rush

Over the past decade the United States has experienced a major restructuring of health care delivery. Through the early 1980s health care system reconfiguration consisted primarily of the horizontal integration of hospitals. In recent years, health care delivery has made a shift toward vertical integration of delivery systems, as hospitals have acquired other hospitals, physician practices, home health agencies, and information systems. Although vertically integrated systems have not yet unequivocally demonstrated their ability to lower costs while providing higher quality care and improved patient satisfaction, the pressure to develop broader health care systems is building inexorably.

Just as health care delivery in the United States is in the process of undergoing a change, the population that is served by these evolving service systems is also changing markedly. The general patient population is becoming older and more in need of care for chronic conditions. This transformation has led to increased use of services such as home health care, ambulatory care, and assisted living. Concurrently, the elderly are entering managed care environments at an accelerated pace (see chapter 11).

The growth of the older population, the rapid expansion of the old-old, and the shift from acute to chronic care needs, combined with the advent of new forms of financing and delivery of care are posing dramatic challenges for integrated health care systems. Although health care systems continue to evolve, it is somewhat ironic that health professions education has changed little. For the most part, providers for senior care and integrated health systems are still being trained through traditional methods at schools of medicine, nursing, social work, pharmacy, and allied health professions, often without significant input regarding the changing health care delivery system. Nor do these students have much opportunity to work closely with professionals from other disciplines.

This chapter addresses provision of Geriatric Interdisciplinary Team Training (GITT) to professionals by looking at trends in integrated health care systems and the experiences of one such organization, The Rush System for Health (RSH). Through the Rush GITT Project, RSH has attempted to introduce innovative geriatric training to improve both the content and effectiveness of geriatric education and the delivery of health care to geriatric patients. We anticipate that the Rush GITT Project will become an instrumental force within the RSH in modifying both education of health care trainees and provision of health care to the elderly.

BACKGROUND

Integrated Health Care Systems

Recent estimates indicate that there are at least 320 health care systems throughout the United States (Bellandi, 1996). In the 1970s and 1980s, horizontal integration of hospitals characterized the transformation of health care delivery in the United States, with hospitals merging at an unprecedented rate (Starkweather & Carman, 1987). By the mid-1980s the organizational dynamics of health care systems had changed. As control of health care costs took precedence, and patient characteristics and utilization patterns changed, many health care executives and policy makers saw the benefits of developing vertically integrated systems to control the entire array of health care services, providers, and costs (Campbell, 1995; Conrad & Dowling, 1990; Robinson, 1994). These health care systems expanded outward from the hospital and purchased physician practices, home health care agencies, nursing homes, and an array of ambulatory care and other programs (Shortell, Gillies, Anderson, Erickson, & Mitchell, 1993; Shortell, Gillies, & Devers, 1995; Zelman, 1996). Although the number of freestanding hospitals has continued to decline to only 5,200 nationwide, health care systems are showing a steady increase in numbers and scope of services. No one has yet demonstrated that these systems provide higher quality patient satisfaction while lowering costs (Conrad & Shortell, 1996; Goldsmith, 1996; Shortell et al., 1995). Because of change in culture and the length of time these systems take to become fully operational, we are not likely to have proof of their effectiveness for many years (Zelman, 1996).

Several observers suggest that these systems are well positioned to respond to the healthcare challenges of the 21st century and will be key players in the redesign of health care for years to come (Altman & Reinhart, 1996; Conrad & Shortell, 1996; Griffith, 1996). However, with the health care system evolving so rapidly, we cannot predict the specific configuration of future integrated health care delivery systems.

In the early 1990s, it was projected that there would only be three or four major integrated financing and delivery systems serving patients in each major health care market, each integrated horizontally and vertically to offer economies of scale, scope, and cost effectiveness across their respective systems (Cochrane, 1997). The development of vertically integrated systems has not progressed in quite so linear a manner. Although some health care systems continue to integrate vertically, others that have integrated are to some extent disaggregating, including Harvard/Pilgrim, Kaiser Permanente, and FHP (Nash & Parks, 1997). Cost control is the underlying factor driving the organizational dynamics of these health care systems.

An additional development that is particularly relevant to integrated health care systems and the way they serve the elderly is the burgeoning number of managed care programs, especially health maintenance organizations. The expansion of managed care is occurring for Medicare recipients just as it is for the population as a whole (see chapter 11).

The new millennium may find the majority of seniors receiving their health care through managed care, and much of that care will be provided by integrated health care systems.

Geriatric Training and Health Care Systems

Health professions students receive training in care of the elderly generally through the traditional system of academic medical centers, professional schools of graduate education, and specialized programs such as Department of Veterans Affairs Geriatric Research, Education and Clinical Centers, Administration on Aging Long-Term Care Gerontology Centers, and Bureau of Health Professions Geriatric Education Centers, among others (Zeiss & Steffen, 1996). Although geriatric education has had greater visibility in advanced training programs, faculty shortages, insufficient curricular emphasis on geriatrics, and a dearth of clinical training settings have limited health professions training in geriatrics (Health Resources Service Administration, 1995). In light of the insufficient availability of discipline-specific geriatric curricula, it is not unexpected that interdisciplinary geriatric education has been even more limited in its availability and impact, primarily due to the epistemology of the interdisciplinary approach, curricular considerations, and limitations in academic and administrative resources (Clark, 1991; Clark, Spence, & Sheehan, 1987; Qualls & Czirr, 1988).

Health care systems are dependent on highly qualified, well-trained professionals; yet the forces that have shaped the reformation of these systems have also tended to restrict interaction with educators and academic centers, and especially with the geriatric education system (Farrell, Schmitt, & Heinemann, 1988; Weisbrod, 1976). These new systems of care place highest priority on the control of health care delivery, both in terms of efficiencies and costs, with minimal attention to the issues of training and its potential impact on processes and outcomes (Kaluzny, 1985; Shortell, et al., 1995). Only when the leaders of these integrated health care systems recognize how central geriatric training is to their basic goals and objectives will geriatric education receive the attention it deserves.

Strategies of Integrated Health Systems

To best relate training in general and GITT specifically to the evolving health care delivery systems, it is important to consider how integrated health systems are felt to succeed. Cochrane (1997) suggests that integrated health care organizations will be successful if they achieve the goals of (a) superior customer service, (b) the coordination of care and management of the continuum, (c) the integration of management systems, (d) the integration of clinical processes, (e) economic alignment of all elements, and (f) a unified culture. Although underlying this framework are fundamental economic incentives and the need for changes in the infrastructure of health care systems, it is telling that the author concludes that clinical integration and process redesign are "keys to making any integrated healthcare system work in the end," and healthcare systems "will need to completely reengineer the way they do business" (Cochrane, 1997).

Just as it will be critical for health care systems to develop new information systems to help manage care, it will be the training and the retraining of the health care provider that will ultimately lead to better integration of clinical processes and help coordinate care. Shortell and Hull (1996) frame these priorities slightly differently: (a) improve measures of cost, quality, and outcomes of care; (b) improve risk management; (c) speed up the pace of downsizing acute inpatient bed capacity; (d) accelerate the formation of physician group practices; (e) increase the number of primary care physicians and related primary care providers; (f) determine how to best structure medical education and residency programs; and (g) meet the health needs of the poor and those with inadequate financial coverage for care more effectively.

From another perspective, systems will be successful through investment in core capabilities of functional integration, physician-system integration, and clinical integration (Gillies, Shortell, & Young, 1996). As Gillies et al. suggest, clinical integration is "the most important core capability because it is where the ultimate value is added to the consumer." This will require the control of clinical variation in practices, procedures, and outcomes. Successful systems will have to move from developing protocols and pathways within individual operating units and coordinating across units and settings for a given episode of illness, to the community, where community health protocols and pathways will prevent disease and improve the health of populations. Geriatric education, and more specifically, GITT, are central to a system's ability to improve this core competency.

THE RUSH SYSTEM FOR HEALTH

With the establishment of Rush University in 1972, Rush-Presbyterian-St. Luke's Medical Center (RPSLMC) laid the foundation for an integrated healthcare system that would serve the residents of greater metropolitan Chicago. Today, the RSH is a comprehensive, cooperative health delivery system that includes 10 hospitals and an array of services capable of delivering health care to more than 2 million people in northern Illinois and Indiana. RSH is vertically integrated, with an academic health center, a teaching hospital, community hospitals, managed care offices, and home and community-based programs that serve communities of diverse socioeconomic and cultural backgrounds. Staffed by over 4,700 physicians and 18,000 employees, the health care providers in RSH were responsible for over 102,000 admissions; 929,000 outpatient visits; 260,000 home care visits; and 211,000 emergency room visits in 1996. RSH has 3,263 acute care beds, 669 long-term care beds, and 180 rehabilitation beds.

RPSLMC is the academic health center that supports RSH. Located in the near west side of Chicago, it is among the largest medical centers in the metropolitan Chicago area. It includes Presbyterian-St. Luke's Hospital and the Johnston R. Bowman Health Center for the Elderly for rehabilitation and skilled nursing care. In addition to offering tertiary medical care to patients throughout the Midwest, it is the home of Rush University, with colleges in medicine, nursing, and health sciences. Its seven Rush Institutes provide multidisciplinary and interdisciplinary approaches to disease and conduct research that is used to improve diagnosis and treatment of patients throughout RSH.

RSH includes a continuum of outpatient and community-based services, including primary medical care, health promotion, preventive care, and behavioral health services.

Known regionally for its geriatric services, it provides a comprehensive array of geriatric care, including skilled nursing, subacute and long-term care, adult day care programs, and retirement communities. Rehabilitation services, including in-home physical, occupational, and psychological therapy; home health services; and hospice services round out the continuum of care under RSH.

The goals of RSH are to (a) offer a full range of patient services, from primary to tertiary; (b) provide community-based health care, backed by the strength of a system; (c) educate physicians, nurses, and other healthcare professionals to ensure quality care for the future; (d) engage in research devoted to patient care; and (e) support the professional development of physicians and foster the private practice of medicine. RSH was founded on the belief that member organizations can learn from one another and build on their individual strengths to benefit patients served by the whole system.

Geriatric Training in the Rush System for Health

Until recently, geriatric training in RSH has generally been offered through a traditional framework: discipline by discipline, care setting by care setting. The amount of geriatric training has varied, depending on discipline requirements, faculty preferences, and individual student interests. Although many trainees have received a thorough grounding in geriatrics through their training at Rush University, there have been no comprehensive geriatric curricula for most graduate trainees, except for the few geriatric-oriented programs, such as the master's program for geriatric nurse practitioners.

Trainees at Rush University have benefited significantly from a specific strength of the Rush University educational philosophy, however. The University employs a very successful teacher-practitioner model of training throughout all disciplines and programs, a model that has been nationally recognized since the early 1970s. This approach to training future healthcare providers uses faculty who are practicing clinicians. Rush University has employed the general teacher-practitioner model of education in health and social services delivery in all its geriatric and gerontological educational programs, resulting in strong clinical skills and significant hands-on experience for all geriatric and gerontological trainees.

THE RUSH GERIATRIC INTERDISCIPLINARY TEAM TRAINING PROJECT

The Rush GITT Project is a collaborative initiative on the part of Rush-Presbyterian-St. Luke's Medical Center and Loyola University of Chicago School of Social Work. It has targeted nurses, medical residents, social workers, and trainees from many other disciplines to learn the methods and advantages of interdisciplinary geriatric service delivery.

The academic disciplines being trained in the Rush GITT include nursing; medicine; social work; occupational, physical, and speech therapy; audiology; clinical nutrition; pharmacy; ethics; religion; and health systems management. Departments or programs within these disciplines include Gerontological Nursing, Family Nursing, Geriatric Medicine, Family Medicine, Physical Medicine and Rehabilitation, Psychiatry, Social

Work, Occupational Therapy, Physical Therapy, Audiology, Speech/Language Pathology, Clinical Nutrition, Pharmacy, Health Systems Management, Spiritual Care, and Ethics.

Taking full advantage of RSH's extensive clinical operation, six clinical settings within it will serve as the clinical training environment. These include Rush Home Care Network, a home health care agency; Rush Prudential Health Plans, a managed care organization with a network of staff model primary care offices; Rush Alzheimer's Disease Center, an assessment and treatment program serving dementia patients; Neighborhood Family Practice of Pilsen, a family practice clinic serving a largely low income Hispanic community; Johnston R. Bowman Health Center, an acute care, rehabilitative, and skilled nursing facility; and Illinois Masonic Medical Center, a community hospital. We have placed special emphasis on minority and ethnic communities, taking full advantage of the ethnic diversity of Chicago and the integrated system of care available throughout RSH.

We have developed three core modules or team training practica to provide team experience through both didactic and practice activities. These modules—Community, Continuity of Care, and Frail and Impaired Older Adults—correspond to the major challenges health professionals will face in a changing health care system and combine a 10-week didactic curriculum with corresponding clinical practicum appropriate for each module. We have implemented the practica in a modular format and tailored them to meet the needs of individual programs and, for more senior trainees, individual practitioners. The practica's educational approach incorporates problem-based learning to develop clinicians who have excellent clinical reasoning competencies and are skilled at creative problem solving. The modules emphasize (a) the promotion of wellness and disease prevention in the elderly, rather than the treatment of disease; (b) the teaching of values and attitudes, not just skills and techniques; (c) the importance of patients and families in reasoning and decision making; (d) the role of social supports relative to aging populations and their families; (e) the roles of health care economics and information systems in decision making; and (f) the need to achieve a balance of professional autonomy and shared expertise.

The didactic content is structured around 10 weekly curriculum sessions emphasizing four major content areas: working in teams, working with patients and families, understanding ethical issues in patient care, and understanding health and economic systems. Rush and Loyola faculty as well as preceptors from participating clinical settings teach the didactic sessions. Supplementing the didactic program, trainees meet 1 hour per week to discuss a practice case that requires input from multiple disciplines.

Teams of trainees representing a minimum of three disciplines, but often consisting of individuals from five or six different disciplines, are assigned to a clinical setting for their practice experience. Teams vary in size by setting but include a physician resident, social worker, advance practice nurse, and other allied health science professionals as appropriate. Trainees are precepted by an individual from their own discipline who is drawn from Rush or Loyola faculty or staff from participating clinical settings.

Implementation Strategy

To introduce this new educational framework consisting of multiple disciplines, three different content modules, four core competencies, and six different clinical training settings, the Rush GITT staff selected an incremental implementation strategy. That is, rather than attempting to introduce an entire new program at once, orient all clinical settings, select and train all faculty, recruit and coordinate dozens of trainees, and, most importantly, introduce new collaborative working relationships between academics and colleagues in clinical settings, we determined that a more gradual approach would be warranted for program start-up. We introduced one GITT content module at a time, using one clinical setting, and educating a carefully selected cohort of trainees using a core group of faculty. This strategy has been highly successful, resulting in an efficient and relatively problem-free start-up for the project. Each of the remaining two modules was brought on line in turn, as were a total of four training sites as of fall 1997. This procedure allowed us to make adjustments as needed to respond to the needs of trainees, preceptors, or faculty and promote the most efficacious program. In the initial implementation phase, staff involved in the introduction of each new module and clinical setting have benefited from the experiences of all other module and clinical setting start-ups.

RUSH GITT: INITIAL IMPLEMENTATION EXPERIENCES

Although RSH can generally be viewed as representative of integrated health systems, in many areas it has very specific or unique features. Several of these features have had a direct impact on the implementation of the Rush GITT Project. Of greatest significance is the fact that RSH is integrally tied to an academic medical center, which in the case of the GITT has provided many excellent opportunities for developing training and clinical options not available to projects where the academic partners are not an integral part of the health care delivery system. Other elements, such as the teacher-practitioner model, are not often present in other health care training programs, and are even less common in integrated health care systems. Although these different and sometimes unique characteristics of the Rush approach to GITT are important, some specific items have played an important role in the success of this program and challenged its implementation in the start-up year.

Factors That Have Facilitated GITT Implementation
Congruence with the Goals of the Rush System for Health

The Rush GITT Project clearly would have had a much lower likelihood of success were it not compatible with the mission and long-range goals of RSH. The philosophy of the GITT staff from the outset has been to identify the confluence of interest between the larger RSH and the training opportunities that the GITT initiative has made available. The Rush GITT Project and its method for training teams in the care of older persons have been proposed as the primary training model for all health professionals throughout RSH. Thus, a general initiative for improving and expanding interdisciplinary geriatric training has been adopted specifically to improve and expand interdisciplinary geriatric training throughout the RSH. Since the inception of the Rush GITT, all departments training professionals in care of the elderly have been monitoring the progress of the GITT Project and determining how to introduce their trainees into it.

Similarly, while providing more comprehensive care for the aged in the short term, the immediate modifications that the Rush clinical system arranged to implement the Rush GITT Project are also contributing to long-term changes in the Rush health care delivery system. The initial pilot teams developed and refined as part of the GITT Project will assist in establishment of interdisciplinary teams within other clinical settings in RSH. These include teams that provide care in the home, in outpatient clinics, and in the growing managed care population served by the Rush System. Ultimately, this confluence of agendas between the GITT initiative and RSH can be summarized as a common interest in improving quality and outcomes of care for patients, by among others, expanding health promotion and disease prevention activities; expanding home and community-based care; and reducing inappropriate admissions, length of stay, and readmissions throughout RSH.

As the focus on training for RSH begins to change to meet the changes in the health care environment, it is clear that the GITT initiative represents the direction that training at Rush will be taking. At the highest levels, Rush policymakers are committed to developing a program that will eventually be a template to be used throughout RSH.

Administrative Support

The implementation of a team training program could not succeed solely on the basis of a good fit between the goals and mission of GITT with those of RSH. In fact, the ease with which the Rush GITT Project was able to commence has as much to do with the extensive administrative support, from the leadership of participating disciplines and clinical settings all the way to the senior administration of the health care system. The chief executive officer of RSH not only pledged support to underwrite faculty, staff, and physical plant costs required for start-up, including substantial in-kind resources, but also made a commitment to the long-term integration of interdisciplinary education throughout training programs systemwide. The administration-sponsored systemwide Long-Term Care Planning Task Force adopted the Rush GITT Project as the vehicle for providing geriatric training, reinforcing the support generated for the program at the highest system levels.

Academic Partners

Although Rush University has historically had extensive cooperation among the faculty of its professional schools, the GITT initiative has created an even more harmonious environment for collaboration. Through this project, the Colleges of Medicine, Nursing, and Health Sciences have found a unique opportunity to address the challenges of providing state-of-the-art advanced training in geriatrics in a collaborative fashion. Staff have met over an extended period of time to design, modify, implement, and evaluate a program that provides concurrent training for trainees from multiple disciplines.

The dean of each participating school demonstrated commitment to the GITT Project by contributing senior staff time to work on the initiative, in some cases at the level of associate dean, along with faculty, space, and financial support. Finally, chairs of the many participating departments have demonstrated universal support by providing access or referral to large numbers of potential trainees and the commitment of faculty time for the development and implementation of GITT. As the implementation phase has progressed, each college has added more staff time, enrolled more trainees, and played a greater role in developing the Project curriculum. In the long term, this greater level of buy-in will lead to an even stronger commitment on the part of these academic partners to the ultimate success of the program.

By design, the GITT Project has developed successful partnerships with other academic entities beyond the three schools within Rush University. Loyola University of Chicago School of Social Work, while serving as a key source of trainees and faculty for the team training program, has been instrumental in the implementation of the program. The GITT Program has also resulted in several unexpected benefits for the academic programs, such as enhanced partnerships with other institutions, including the Chicago College of Pharmacy at Midwestern University. The inclusion of pharmacy trainees has substantially improved the training environment for all participating disciplines and provided a unique opportunity for pharmacy trainees to work very closely with other members of the clinical community.

It is important not to overlook the many pragmatic issues that have facilitated the implementation of the Rush GITT from the perspective of the academic partners. First and foremost is the fact that the GITT Project has provided a timely solution to an increasingly persistent problem facing most of the academic partners: a lack of placement opportunities for students. The Department of Internal Medicine, for example, needed to identify 80 geriatric placements for its residents to satisfy new national internal medicine residency requirements. Not only does the GITT Project offer a large number of placements, but it provides them on an organized, systematic basis. The GITT Project has also provided trainees with the opportunity to work with new settings that had not been available previously, opening a rich array of training venues to trainees.

Clinical Partners

RSH has provided a complete continuum of geriatric clinical settings from which the Rush GITT Project could choose. All potential clinical training settings are under one administrative umbrella, facilitating the process. As GITT has been introduced, a new phenomenon has occurred—the academic partners have begun to see the clinical partners and the specific clinical settings as their customers.

By introducing an array of trainees from many disciplines into the clinical training settings, GITT has changed the clinical partners' perspectives about professional training in general and interdisciplinary team training specifically. They perceive GITT trainees as adding value to the clinical setting. This is crucial development for clinical settings that must demonstrate their effectiveness and importance to the larger health care system. The GITT Project is felt to be a cost effective way of improving care for elderly patients while providing students with state-of-the-art training; it is also perceived as a means of improving consumer satisfaction, through both greater attention to family issues and increased availability of highly trained staff. Staff at clinical training settings have acknowledged their appreciation for being in a learning environment and benefiting from exposure to state-of-the-art knowledge and faculty with national reputations. It is clear that the Project has led to improved collegial interaction, both between clinical and academic partners and within clinical settings. Clinical setting administrators and preceptors alike have acknowledged that the rewards of participating in a research and development environment have been instrumental in initiating and maintaining interest in GITT. Finally, while the GITT Project is still in its initial stages, representatives from RSH recognize that the initiative is educating future clinicians and preparing a pool of professionals who will be candidates for employment within the health care system—a long-term benefit.

System Change

As previously identified, a measure of success will be how RSH and the Rush GITT Project achieve their common goal: system change. To date, the teacher-practitioners in the academic settings and the preceptors in the clinical settings have accepted that this initiative offers benefits and have subsequently begun expanding collaborative activities and changing the way geriatric education and clinical care have traditionally interfaced. Middle management in several units within RSH have started the process of adapting to the new training program, gradually changing the way services are provided. The Rush GITT Project is even demonstrating its ability to provide continuity in training, as clinical setting staff have changed during the course of the implementation period.

In an exciting development, the GITT Project has already been influential in the restructuring of one of the GITT academic partners. The College of Health Sciences is in the process of reengineering its training program to be more responsive to the needs of its graduate students and faculty. The model for future training within the various departments in the college is being drawn directly from the Rush GITT Project educational format. Although it is too early to determine the final impact of the GITT Project on the restructuring of the College of Health Sciences educational program, it is a promising start on a long-term effort. Success in achieving system change in training and the delivery of care will ultimately require a demonstrative impact on faculty (including non-GITT faculty), program content, and adaptability of the interdisciplinary team training format for use with other population groups and clinical settings within the System.

Barriers to GITT Implementation
Externalities and System Priorities

The greatest challenges of GITT are adapting to factors that affect the entire health care system and that, for the most part, are out of the control of those involved in geriatric education. Issues such as the constantly changing federal and state regulatory environment and regional changes in health care delivery such as the rapid introduction of managed care have a disproportionately strong effect on the speed, direction, and form in which GITT can be introduced.

In two of the Rush GITT Project modules the clinical training settings underwent significant organizational change within 6 months of start-up. This exposed the GITT facilitator, the respective preceptors, and the trainees to several organizational and policy changes that had significant potential to change the GITT implementation process.

Academic Systems and Requirements

Structural and process requirements of the University, as well as multiple discipline-specific rules and regulations, posed significant hurdles to the implementation of the Rush GITT Project. Although we anticipated significant conflicts and differences in the various curricula and new training paradigms that were interwoven in the GITT Project, these issues have not been a significant impediment to implementation.

Of more pressing concern to an efficient implementation and the long-term success of the initiative are the difficulties in scheduling that result from conflicting academic calendars. This problem has led to differences in the composition of teams and the amount of time in which all team members have an opportunity to interact. An additional problem in maximizing the GITT experience is the variability in team members' geriatric backgrounds and clinical strengths and experience. Many members of the GITT teams come with significant clinical geriatric experience while others have minimal experience, with a clear impact on team dynamics. Finally, an especially common problem among the academic partners is the variability in faculty understanding of the health care system and its changes.

Clinical Setting Constraints

Several aspects of the clinical settings contributed to problems in GITT start-up. A fundamental challenge to implementing the Rush GITT has been that not all clinical training settings had functional clinical teams prior to start-up of training. Where new teams had to be developed, interdisciplinary team training was more rudimentary compared to what could be provided in fully operational and experienced team settings. No one model or approach to team training fit all clinical settings perfectly; staff at each setting have made modest variations in the model to ensure that it best fits the needs of the clinicians and clinical setting.

While the Rush GITT Project raised concerns about loss of clinical staff productivity and difficulty in staff and patient scheduling, over the short term these issues have not posed significant problems. On the other hand, change of practice patterns in clinical settings is likely to require a significant effort or adjustment on the part of staff to maintain a smoothly operating educational experience.

Factors that Influence GITT Implementation in Health Care Systems

As GITT is being considered for introduction in integrated health care systems, several primary issues will have an impact on the ease of implementation and long-term viability of the project.

Settings History and Experience

The culture of a health care system, the historic service, and educational milieu will determine the feasibility of implementing GITT and configuration of its specific components. Flexibility of the culture is a particularly relevant attribute and indicator of likely success. Similarly, the willingness of system providers to work with students and work them into the clinical system is an important consideration.

Congruence with Mission of System

To be effective, the GITT Project must share common goals with the overall system. Not only will the GITT implementation process be expedited under a common mission, but the final impact will be far more reaching, effective, and permanent. As health care systems focus on population-based care and improved core competencies, interdisciplinary team training will likely be integral to the mission of the system. In the long term, both lead toward improved consumer satisfaction.

Administrative Support

Without support from the highest levels in the health care system, introducing GITT can be a daunting task. With this support, the introduction of GITT can not only be expedited but also have an immediate and more effective impact. The overall success of the program is very likely to be dependent on short-term and long-term budgetary support from the administration.

Size of Practice Setting/Extent of Initial Implementation

The size of the health care system or the number of units or components within the system involved in the GITT Project help determine how easily it can be implemented. GITT will have a greater likelihood of success in health care systems if introduced as a pilot rather than a systemwide program. Another consideration in implementation is the time frame allowed for start-up and provisions or contingencies for the inevitable problems that arise.

Fit between Academic Institutions and Clinical Settings

The Rush GITT Project has been established in what many would find a unique environment, one in which the University and health care delivery system are organizationally within the same institution. Although this certainly enabled the implementation to proceed efficiently, and in some cases helped overcome specific hurdles, it is not the only reason this GITT Project is off to a strong start. The close collaboration and working relationships between faculty and clinicians are central to this effort. The stronger the relationships or closer the ties between clinicians, faculty, units, or institutions, the greater the chances of success.

The Health Care Environment

External structural changes and fiscal changes in the health care delivery environment are still the fundamental variables affecting the implementation of GITT projects. Even if all other factors are in place, the change in a single external variable can instantly affect the direction and nature of a project. Regardless of the level of planning and commitment to implementing interdisciplinary team training, the best of intentions may quickly unravel as the environment of the health care system shifts.

CONCLUSION: THE FUTURE OF GITT AND HEALTH CARE SYSTEMS—THE SEARCH FOR WHAT WORKS

Tremendous flexibility underlies the apparent ease with which the Rush GITT Project has been introduced to RSH. It takes partners who are willing to be open and to change the status quo. In essence, it helps if change is part of the existing culture. The likelihood of success improves if all the players are involved from the beginning so they will own the implementation. Good communication and open decision making are instrumental to this process. As other integrated health systems implement GITT programs, flexibility, ownership, and good communication will be just as critical for them as it is has been for the Rush Project.

The greatest influences on integrated health systems to implement geriatric interdisciplinary teams and team training successfully are likely to be the same issues driving the creation and maintenance of health care systems overall: customer service, utilization, and cost. As changes occur in health care organizations and vertically integrated organizations become virtually integrated organizations, macroorganizational dynamics will determine the success of GITT. However, despite mergers, joint ventures, collaborations, and affiliations, the resulting systems will still be looking at means to improve their core competencies. This is where the true benefits of GITT Projects are likely to be acknowledged and supported.

Implementing collaborative teams offers numerous benefits to health care systems. Geriatric interdisciplinary teams can:

1. Offer the potential for providing care more efficiently. They can expedite the care process by applying multiple perspectives and collaborative problem solving early and improving the efficient use of patients' time.
2. Maximize resources and facilities in the competitive fiscal environment faced by health care systems, shifting from acute, episodic care management to long-term, chronic care management.
3. Provide a shift to more comprehensive health care management, emphasizing health, prevention, and patient education, rather than a disease model of care.
4. Increase provider satisfaction, especially by creating an atmosphere that supports innovation.
5. Improve care of patients, coordination of their services and needs, and ultimately, consumer satisfaction.

Although the efforts of day-to-day survival and immediate needs of the system often overshadow long-term goals, integration appears to be a requirement for success over the next 5 to 10 years. One component of this integration effort will be the need for a highly trained, flexible set of health care providers who are comfortable working in constantly shifting environments, across levels of care, and with other professionals and management. We know that GITT will have made inroads if professionals are hired to work in health care systems for their interdisciplinary skills and are provided the opportunity and environment to best use these skills in providing care to the elderly. Interdisciplinary team training offers an especially effective way to prepare health care professionals for not only working but excelling in the health care system of the next century.

REFERENCES

Altman, S. H., & Reinhart, U. E. (1996). *Strategic choices for a changing health care system.* Chicago, IL: Health Administration Press.

Bellandi, D. (1996). Growth of health care systems in the U.S. *Modern Healthcare, 26*(40), 40–42.

Campbell, A. (1995). Vertical integration: Synergy or seduction? *Long Range Planning, 28,* 126–128.

Clark, P. G. (1991). Toward a conceptual framework for developing interdisciplinary teams in gerontology: Cognitive and ethical dimensions. *Gerontology & Geriatrics Education, 12,* 79–96.

Clark, P. G., Spence, D. L., & Sheehan, J. L. (1987). Challenges and barriers to interdisciplinary gerontological team training in the academic setting. *Gerontology & Geriatrics Education, 7(3/4),* 93–110.

Cochrane, J. D. (1997). *Health care megatrends 1997.* Lake Arrowhead, CA: Integrated Healthcare Report.

Conrad, D., & Dowling, W. (1990). Vertical integration in health services: Theory and managerial implications. *Health Care Management Review, 15*(4), 9–22.

Conrad, D. A., & Shortell, S. M. (1996). Integrated health systems: Promise and performance. *Frontiers of Health Services Management, 13,* 3–40.

Farrell, M. P., Schmitt, M. H., & Heinemann, G. D. (1988). Organizational environments of health care teams: Impact on team development and implications for consultation. *International Journal of Small Group Research, 4,* 31–53.

Gillies, R. R., Shortell, S. M., & Young, G. (1996). *Best practices in managing organized delivery systems.* Paper presented at the Leading Organizational Transformation Conference. Washington, DC: Management Development and Research Center of the Veterans Administration and the Association for Health Services Research State of the Art.

Goldsmith, J. C. (1996). The illusive logic of integration. *Health Forum Journal, 37*(5), 26–31.

Griffith, J. R. (1996). Managing the transition to integrated health care organizations. *Frontiers in Health Services Management, 12*(4), 4–50.

Health Resources Services Administration. (1995). *A national agenda for geriatric education: White papers.* Washington, DC: U.S. DHHS, Health Resources Services Administration, Bureau of Health Professions.

Kaluzny, A. (1985). Design and management of disciplinary and interdisciplinary groups in health services: Review and critique. *Medical Care Review, 42,* 77–112.

Nash, R., & Parks, J. (1997). *Reassessing the value of vertical integration.* Lake Arrowhead, CA: Integrated Healthcare Report.

Qualls, S. H., & Czirr, R. (1988). Geriatric health teams: Classifying models of professional and team functioning. *Gerontologist, 28,* 372–376.

Robinson, J. C. (1994). The changing boundaries of the American hospital. *Milbank Quarterly, 72,* 259–275.

Shortell, S. M., & Hull, K. E. (1996). The new organization of the health care delivery system. In S. H. Altman & U. E. Reinhart (Eds.), *Strategic choices for a changing health care system.* Chicago, IL: Health Administration Press.

Shortell, S. M., Gillies, R. R., & Devers, K. J. (1995). Reinventing the American hospital. *Milbank Quarterly, 73,* 131–160.

Shortell, S. M., Gillies, R. R., Anderson, D. A., Erickson, K. M., & Mitchell, J. B. (1995). *Remaking health care in America: Building organized delivery systems.* San Francisco: Jossey-Bass.

Shortell, S. M., Gillies, R. R., Anderson, D. A., Mitchell, J. B., & Morgan, K. L. (1993). Creating organized delivery systems: The barriers and facilitators. *Hospital and Health Services Administration, 38,* 447–466.

Starkweather, D. B., & Carman, J. M. (1987). Horizontal and vertical concentrations in the evolution of hospital competition. *Advances in Health Economics and Health Services Research, 7,* 179–194.

Weisbrod, M. R. (1976). Why organization development hasn't worked (so far) in medical centers. *Health Care Management Review, 1*(2), 17–28.

Zeiss, A. M., & Steffen, A. M. (1996). Interdisciplinary health care teams: The basic unit of geriatric care. In L. L. Carstensen, B. A. Edelstein, & L. Dornbrand (Eds.), *The practical handbook of clinical gerontology* (pp. 423–450). Thousand Oaks, CA: Sage.

Zelman, W. A. (1996). *The changing healthcare marketplace.* San Francisco: Jossey-Bass.

CHAPTER 14

Challenges of Rural Sites

Rebecca Hunter

THE NEEDS OF RURAL ELDERLY

Elderly citizens constitute the fastest growing segment of the rural population. The population growth of rural elders is a dramatic trend that has formidable implications for rural systems of care already struggling with limited resources. Older people living in rural areas are more likely than their urban counterparts to be poor, limited in formal education, and to suffer from an undue burden of chronic illness and risk associated with limited access to health care (Bull, 1993). Access to dental care is also limited, as evidenced by dramatic differences in rates of tooth loss and replacement (Bader, Scurria, & Shugars, 1994) in urban and rural dwellers. Barriers to health care access are numerous: Among the barriers most difficult to overcome are poverty, geography, cultural differences, and lack of transportation. Rural residents must often travel great distances to reach a primary care physician or health care center. Public transportation is rare, limited in flexibility, and inconvenient.

There is a strong minority presence in rural areas. In the Southeast, many of the rural elderly are African American or Native American, for whom there are additional personal, cultural, or economic barriers to obtaining health care and to engaging in positive health practices, such as exercising and ceasing smoking. As Rowles (1991) has noted, there is great variation in the degree to which older people in different rural settings accept modern health care values and practices. Their attitudes are tempered by the views of families, neighbors, and clergy, while peer persuasion and community values are powerful sources of influence. Although the media have homogenized American culture, in rural settings cultural differences can greatly influence clarity of communication and subtly influence the outcomes of care.

Currently, one in four of our nation's elders resides in a rural area. The population of the rural elderly 85 years of age and older is expected to triple in the next decade, presenting tremendous challenges in the care of those who are frail. At the same time, our knowledge and use of efficacious interventions to maintain the health and well-being of older rural people are incomplete and fragmented. We know, for instance, that older women in rural areas are more likely to die of breast cancer than women in metropolitan areas, and that they are less likely to be screened for breast cancer (Van Nostrand, 1993). Unfortunately, we don't know why this is the case, or exactly what to do about it. Is this an issue of access to primary care, availability of mammography, health beliefs, provider attitudes and practices, health-seeking behavior, or environmental influences? How can we design and integrate a variety of approaches to address this significant problem? How can rural interdisciplinary team training incorporate sensitive approaches to address this?

As the breast cancer example suggests, rural older persons typically receive less preventive care, although there is evidence that rural hospitals are becoming more active in this area (Hendryx, 1993). The typical participant in health-promotion programs for older adults is still urban, relatively well educated, and already favorably disposed to health-promoting behavior (Simmons et al., 1989).

DELIVERY OF HEALTH CARE
TO THE RURAL ELDERLY

Our understanding of the most effective ways to overcome barriers and to deliver health and health-related care in rural areas is limited. Yawn, Busby, and Yawn (1994) note that medical practice in rural areas is different from that of metropolitan areas. Physicians must respond to a vast array of patient and community problems while lacking the technological and consultative resources of their urban peers. Few have received specialized training to prepare them for the particular challenges of rural practice, including management of large caseloads of elderly patients, stabilization of accident victims, and diagnosis and treatment of psychiatric disorders. Similarly, most are unprepared for the new roles they will be asked to assume, such as nursing home medical director.

A major issue in rural health care is the chronic scarcity of health and health-related professionals. In 1996, for example, 1400 of the nation's 2,100 rural counties were defined as Health Professional Shortage Areas (HPSA) (Human, 1996). The shortage of rural health professionals is especially serious for rural elders, given research linking poor health status to HPSA residence among them (Kohrs & Mainous, 1995). Health care workers, notably in allied health, social work, and psychiatry, may lack a sufficient client base for rural practice (Coward, McLaughlin, Duncan, & Bull, 1994), whereas others, such as physicians, simply gravitate toward the urban settings where they trained and where they will receive greater monetary rewards, enjoy collegial support, and have access to specialty referrals.

Rural health professionals work long hours, have limited peer support, and deliver care that is often compromised by the familiar problems of distance, economics, and understaffed service settings. Data from the American Medical Association (1992) show that rural and urban physicians spend about the same number of hours per week seeing patients, but rural physicians see more patients in the same time period. Although health professionals experience great satisfaction when they play a pivotal role in providing ongoing care and intervene during acute illness, their satisfaction is eroded by bureaucratic complexity, a rapidly expanding information base, and an increasing sense of isolation. Documentation and other paperwork requirements are staggering.

A full continuum of services for elderly persons in rural areas typically is impossible. Moreover, there is a "noticeable lack of geriatric programs, skilled personnel, and resources . . . to treat complex geriatric conditions" (Wallace & Colsher, 1994, p. 109).

Cost is a major consideration; the economic base is fragile, and service settings typically lack working capital.

The delivery of rural long-term care is another area demanding attention. Nursing home care, regardless of setting, is often less than optimal. Among the most significant problems are inappropriate prescribing and use of medications (Beers et al., 1992); high prevalence of mental health problems among residents (Smith, Buckwalter, & Albanese, 1990; Phan & Reifler, 1988); and a host of obstacles to effective care delivery including inadequate staff incentives, high staff turnover, poor preparation for physically and emotionally demanding caregiving roles, and lack of medical staff training in geriatrics.

Long-term care settings in rural areas share the complex problems of their urban counterparts while also struggling with difficulties such as limited resources and geographic isolation that are largely a function of their location. Such difficulties can limit access to medical, psychiatric, and rehabilitative care as well as other specialty care for the long-term care resident. Staff and administration also feel the effects of isolation, frequently lacking support, feedback, and education (Beaulieu & Berry, 1994). Burnout is a significant problem.

The need to improve nursing home care has inspired a variety of strategies. Regulatory incentives and training of front-line caregivers have been extended to rural settings (Smyer, Brandon, & Cohn, 1992); of particular interest is a geriatric mental health training program for rural nursing personnel that Smith and colleagues (1994) developed. Pharmacy consultants now routinely provide oversight to reduce inappropriate medication prescribing and utilization (Beers, Fingold, & Ouslander, 1992), geropsychiatric consultation–liaison teams are in place (Goldman & Klugman, 1990; Sakauye & Camp, 1992), and electronic consultation to nursing homes has been proposed but is not yet widely implemented (Haywood, Francis, Cregler, Freed, & Skorton, 1994). The use of geriatric assessment teams as consultants to nursing homes has received less attention. However, outcomes of a study in which 63 nursing home residents were randomly assigned either to team or to usual care conditions suggest that team assessment has a favorable effect on quality of care (Cavalieri et al., 1993).

Managed care and capitation strategies, including ongoing changes in the Medicare system that threaten areas dependent on Medicare financing, have supplanted the promise of health care reform of the early 1990s. This is a turbulent time for rural health, especially in areas experiencing a proliferation of managed care. Although changes in health care financing have the potential to augment interdisciplinary teamwork and provide more preventive care for rural residents, large health care organizations operating from an urban base may lack information about the needs of rural residents and inadequately address issues important to them, such as lack of transportation. On the other hand, recent innovations such as integrated rural health care networks and telemedicine links to major teaching centers promise to serve as strong sources of support to rural practitioners.

The renewed emphasis on primary care in our health professions schools has attracted more students who profess interest in primary care, geriatric care, and in rural practice. Although this is essential, our institutions must also identify these students earlier in their programs and provide them with experiences to nurture that interest, promote easy access to peers and mentors, and offer appropriate training. Student experiences in rural settings are obviously important as well; the experience of the federally sponsored

Interdisciplinary Rural Training Programs reinforces the premise that such exposure will promote choice of rural practice (Fuller, 1995).

Few rural practitioners have training to cope with the problems of special populations or to deliver interdisciplinary care, both of which are fundamental to the care of vulnerable populations—the very young, the sick or injured, the physically or emotionally disabled, and the very old. The Pew Health Professions Commission (1995) has advanced a more intensive focus on interdisciplinary care and training as a sound strategy for addressing the rising specter of chronic disease, enhancing quality of primary care, and improving practitioner recruitment and retention. Interdisciplinary care is the cornerstone of integrated community systems of care that holistically address the needs of individuals and groups along a full continuum. Interdisciplinary teams offer support for members, thereby reducing isolation and promoting retention. Practical models for addressing the geriatric interdisciplinary training needs of rural practitioners have yet to be fully articulated and widely applied, however.

ESSENTIAL COMPETENCIES FOR RURAL GERIATRIC INTERDISCIPLINARY PRACTICE

Effective geriatric interdisciplinary practice in rural communities requires a broad range of skills and knowledge. Although the importance of competency in clinical geriatrics is obvious, other areas of professional preparation and practice have traditionally received less attention in health professions education. Development of a broad perspective in primary care, one that embraces the health of the community, is crucial. Practitioners in training must also understand the context of rural practice, including cultural, economic, management, and programmatic dimensions. Given the prevailing realities of resource scarcity and problem complexity, both training in interdisciplinary teamwork and preparation for leadership roles are also critical.

Skills in Clinical Geriatrics

By necessity, rural care has almost always been a generalist practice requiring a broad range of clinical skills. The topical areas highlighted throughout this volume are all pertinent to clinical practice in rural areas.

Community-Oriented Primary Care

During this decade, educators have recognized the need for a broad vision of health care that goes beyond the treatment of individuals with particular illnesses. The Pew Health Professions Commission (1995) has been a particularly vocal advocate for an expanded set of competencies in health professional education that include care for the health of the community and strategies for health promotion and disease and disability prevention.

This imperative is rarely more evident than in rural practice settings, where the interface between the patient, the family, and the community is more direct and visible than in urban areas. Practitioners may treat members of three or four generations of a single family and see firsthand the powerful interplay of forces that either facilitate or impede the health of its members. Experienced clinicians understand that poverty, limited education, and cultural differences may defeat the practitioner's interventions if they are ignored. This is not to say that community problems and attitudes have an impact on health and health practices only in rural settings; rather that they may be more discernible in rural settings than in complex urban environments, making clinicians more aware of the limitations of individual approaches.

To date, most health professions education focuses on the patient-clinician dyad with some attention to familial encounters. Clinicians in training rarely learn about the concept of community and how it is pertinent to the health of individuals and populations. Similarly, clinicians in training typically have limited opportunities to learn to collaborate with persons from other disciplines and to participate in experiences that will prepare them to function in integrated delivery systems. Without such preparation, novice practitioners who elect to work in rural settings must undergo considerable on-the-job training before they can deliver effective community-oriented primary care.

Skills in Interdisciplinary Teamwork and Collaboration

The basic skills highlighted throughout this volume are as important to rural practitioners as to their counterparts in urban areas. However, effective interdisciplinary work with older people in rural communities demands a broader perspective than is common in urban settings and skills in teamwork both within and across organizations.

Many different permutations of teams and teamwork exist in rural areas. Teams may be organized for the purpose of health care delivery, service coordination, program management, or problem solving. Teams frequently bridge organizational boundaries. For example, a primary care clinic that lacks needed social work services may recruit team members from local service organizations. Teams may include paraprofessionals, lay health advisors, clergy, and others contingent on the nature of the team and its mission. In addressing the needs of a border community, the University of Arizona employs a teamwork model that includes *promotoras,* lay health workers who serve as a vital link between professional team members and the patient. In defining team membership, front-line caregiver involvement is essential. Nursing assistants, physical therapy assistants, and others are integral to patient care and can make powerful contributions to interdisciplinary teamwork.

Practitioners may be affiliated with several teams. A physician may work collaboratively with a nurse practitioner and pharmacist in the clinic setting, serve on the care planning team of a nursing home, and be a member of an interagency service coordination team targeted at the frail older population. These multiple roles promote communication among participants, which carries over into other activities. Teams also provide a collegial support system to their members. This is one of the best buffers against the professional isolation and burnout that are so common in rural practice.

Although we tend to think of a core team of interdisciplinary professionals who typically work together, sharing some common physical and organizational space, teamwork also may be viewed as a more fluid concept. Teams often reconfigure themselves; persons from additional disciplines, such as speech therapy, are added to a core team on an as needed basis and function as part of the team. Teams may relate to and join with other teams; for example, a primary care team may work with an interagency team about the needs of specific patients or the older community at large. Also, important teamwork activity takes place outside of the traditional team meeting, with technology, such as voice mail, e-mail, and advanced telecommunications, facilitating collaborative communication that is not limited by traditional time and distance constraints.

With the rise of integrated service networks and advanced telecommunications technology, practitioners in multiple sites can engage in virtual teamwork. For example, a physical therapist based in a referral center can conduct a gait assessment on a patient in a remote rural location, joining with a physician, physical therapy assistant, and nurse practitioner in the patient's community to discuss impressions and to develop a plan of intervention jointly. Trainees in remote clinical settings can access academic resources and consultation. These capabilities are of particular importance to rural health care, as they improve patient access to expertise that is not locally available.

In summary, although trainees must learn to function effectively within core teams, they must also develop teamwork skills to enable them to engage in ad hoc teams and evolving virtual teams. This requires social skills and knowledge of team development, organizational structure and mandates of various senior-serving agencies, and strategies for overcoming turf issues.

Understanding the Context of Rural Practice

The context of rural practice is very different from that of the academic health care centers where most health professionals are trained. Intra- and interprofessional relationships in rural settings tend to be less hierarchical, and collaboration is viewed as an effective way of getting things done. Although there is a tendency to overly romanticize rural life, rural communities are recognizable entities with opportunities for personal engagement. Health care practitioners are afforded status as highly valued members of the community and often have opportunities for community service and leadership beyond the health care arena. Patients (or clients) are the practitioners' neighbors, fellow Parent–Teacher Association members, and auto mechanics.

Beyond the personal context of rural practice are innumerable factors that influence the practitioner's capacity to meet the health care needs of older persons. Practitioners must pay attention to disparate belief systems, be aware of costs and effective management, and develop a good repertoire of programmatic solutions.

Diversity of Cultures, Health Beliefs, and Practices

Although the metropolitan practitioner may provide service within a well-defined niche to a relatively homogenous patient population, practitioners in rural communities must be prepared to deal with a highly diverse patient population: young and old, affluent and poor, well-educated and poorly educated, from many ethnic backgrounds, with distinct health care beliefs and practices. An appreciation for cultural diversity and its many implications for health care is therefore essential.

Culture can be defined as "the sum of beliefs, practices, habits, likes, dislikes, norms, customs, rituals, and so forth that we have learned from our families" (Spector, 1991).

In a classic article, Kleinman first articulated the concept of healthcare systems as cultural systems (1978). Elements of a cultural model of a healthcare system include our definitions of health, what we experience as illness, our beliefs about the cause and prevention of illness, how we manage our illness, including selection of treatment and healthcare providers, and how we deal with treatment failure, recurrence, chronic illness, and dying. Kleinman coined the term explanatory model to refer to a person or group's conceptualization of health and illness, including its etiology, diagnosis, pathophysiology, preventive measures, and treatment.

All individuals and cultures have explanatory models of health and illness. Often, health care professionals are indoctrinated into and utilize the biomedical model (Engel, 1977). This model explains disease as abnormal functioning of body organs or systems; disease results from pathogens (e.g., bacteria and viruses), biochemical changes (e.g., hormonal imbalances), and environmental factors (e.g., pesticides). Abnormal genes are fast gaining credence as another major cause. Diagnosis requires identification of the responsible pathogen or process, and treatment necessitates removing (e.g. surgery), destroying (e.g., antibiotics), or modifying (e.g., hormone therapy) the disease-causing agent. Prevention involves avoiding the disease-causing pathogen, agent, or activity (e.g., by washing hands, avoiding smoking). Sanctioned curers are highly trained clinicians who diagnose and treat with scientifically tested agents and procedures.

Although Engel (1977) called for health professions to embrace a new model, the biopsychosocial model, as a more realistic and useable account of the cause and treatment of health and illness, the biomedical component still predominates in the training of physicians, pharmacists, and dentists, and to a lesser extent, nurses. For example, substantive material about nutrition and chemical dependency is only now being introduced into medical school curricula.

Other members of the interdisciplinary team may receive training in, and utilize, different explanatory models. Social workers and psychologists, for example, emphasize psychosocial explanations and treatment for illness, particularly mental illness, although they pay homage to the expertise of their colleagues in biomedicine. Health educators, for whom the community may be the patient, seek behavioral and political explanations for illness. Appreciation for team members' differing perspectives on a particular illness may enrich the diagnosis and treatment of a particular condition. For example, depression in a rural elderly person may be seen as due to a biochemical imbalance, loss of social support, or both.

The older patient, who is also considered to be a member of the interdisciplinary team, may have a very different explanatory model and different health care practices from those of health professionals. Individuals in rural cultures, particularly those who have had less access to modern health care throughout their lives, often use various folk systems of healing in addition to available biomedical personnel and technology. For example, one study found that 76% of patients attending rural primary care clinics (and 70% attending urban clinics) in West Virginia used folk remedies (Cook & Baisden, 1986). Another study in rural Mississippi found that 96% of those surveyed used herbal remedies (Blake, 1984). Patients may seek remedies for incurable ailments, including chronic diseases that are highly prevalent in the elderly, such as arthritis. One study found that 55% of caregivers of Alzheimer's patients tried one or more alternative treatments in efforts to improve patients' memories, with 40% perceiving the remedy to be helpful (Coleman, Fowler, & Williams, 1995).

Another folk healing system used in rural areas is faith healing, often practiced in the context of religious services. In one study of patients attending a family-practice clinic in rural North Carolina (King, Sobal, & DeForge, 1988), 21% reported attending a faith-healing service, 56% reported watching faith healers on television, and 6% reported being healed by faith healers. Twenty-nine percent believed that faith healers can help some people whom physicians cannot, and 34% believed that physicians and faith healers can work together to cure people.

Although these folk health systems do not have official recognition, they are vigorous and persistent and show no signs of dying out (Hufford, 1992), perhaps because they provide a coherent system of meaning for the whole person: body, mind, and spirit.

Patients who use alternative and complementary systems of health care in addition to biomedicine often find themselves as managers of their own team of health providers. Some of these team members may include alternative care providers. For example, in addition to attending a health care clinic, one patient may be visiting a root doctor or herbal specialist. Another may be making regular visits to a chiropractor. Some members of the patient's team may not even know of the existence of certain other members. One study found that 72% of patients visited the offices of alternative care providers without informing their primary care physician (Eisenberg et al., 1993). Common sense tells us that respect for others' explanatory models and health care practices improves communication. Open communication builds mutual trust and cooperation, resulting in better health care.

Different explanatory models also affect self-care and preventive practices. White and Maloney (1990) write of the hard-to-reach Americans—the disadvantaged, minorities, and others—for whom there are personal, cultural, or economic barriers to engagement in positive health practices. In a market research study of these groups, the authors identified a "chasm between awareness and practice" (p. 277), suggesting a limited understanding of relationships between health status and behavior and specific health practices. For example, most participants believed that positive health behavior would decrease risk of acute but not chronic illness; the latter they attributed to heredity and fate.

Well-rounded education of interdisciplinary team members must include information about the powerful and ubiquitous role of belief systems in health behavior. Such training should also include awareness building of team members' own explanatory models, as well as those of various folk health traditions and alternative care providers. In addition, training should include skill building in communication strategies with patients of diverse cultural backgrounds, knowledge of various cultural values and traits, and training in avoiding stereotyping. Rural practitioners should take the time to develop an acquaintance with other providers like the local root doctor, chiropractic physicians, herbalists, and faith healers; this knowledge will promote better coexistence and more culturally appropriate care.

Serving the Underserved and Disadvantaged

Although not all rural citizens are poor, poverty is nonetheless a pervasive problem in many rural communities. Many of the rural elderly live in substandard housing and have extremely limited resources, forcing very difficult choices with consequences for nutritional status, treatment adherence, and socialization. Economic hardship also affects help-seeking and health care practices. For example, cost has been shown to be a deterrent to seeking medical care among rural Southerners (Blazer, Landerman, Fillenbaum, & Horner, 1995). Despite the availability of Medicare and Medicaid, the subjects in the study delayed treatment because of significant out-of-pocket expenses connected with treatment access.

Rural practitioners are acutely aware of the problems of poverty, and they find it frustrating that health-professions students so often come to field experiences with little to no appreciation of the issues. Poverty is frequently associated with limited education, another condition that can complicate the provision of care. Trainees must learn that literacy is not a given, that many off-the-shelf patient educational materials are totally inappropriate for many patients, and that people may go without needed services simply because of the overwhelming complexity of the bureaucracy. Clearly, social workers can play a key role in addressing some of these issues in patient care while educating their fellow team members.

Trainees must be prepared intellectually and emotionally to deal with people of different socioeconomic and educational backgrounds, including those in living in abject poverty. Without preparation, there is a risk that they will be subtly condescending or controlling in their encounters, failing to recognize that although older rural people may be uneducated or poor, they are nonetheless capable, intelligent, and able to shape their own destinies. Recognition of this fact is essential in intervention. Trainees must learn to solve problems with rather than for people.

Trainees are concerned about the plight of the poor and the disenfranchised. They must also be sensitive to the ways in which information about rural communities is communicated, however. Older rural people typically have pride no matter what their circumstances. In one example, local people recoiled from a regional newspaper's depiction of their community as impoverished.

Empowerment is another key concept for trainees to learn. Fostering a sense of competence and enabling the rural elderly to draw on their strengths are essential. Among the key components of the empowerment model are involvement of community stakeholders in the planning process, a fundamental belief in the basic capacity of people to help themselves, and good community organizing (Iutcovich, 1993).

Administering Programs

Like their patients or clients, many rural service settings are economically fragile. Local governments, which offer a safety net of services, may be financially strained; the financial viability of rural hospitals has been threatened for many years. There is, accordingly, a great need in rural health for strong management and close working relationships between administrators and clinicians.

Developing Academic and Clinical Partnerships for Rural Interdisciplinary Training

Partnerships between academic institutions and rural communities seem a logical choice for preparing health professions trainees to address the health and well-being of older persons living in rural areas. The success of such partnerships is clearly dependent on the mutual respect of academicians and community practitioners; the cultivation of sound working relationships among the parties; and effective strategies to overcome the potential barriers of divergent missions, time constraints, and distance. Moreover, academicians must actively seek the good will and support of the rural communities in which training is to take place and learn about the assets and problems of the areas.

Building collaborative relationships and developing training programs require careful attention to the process of planning and implementation and the selection of specific methods. In the past, educational institutions have tended to embrace a parochial view of the training process, focused on the needs of trainees without regard to their impact on service settings and the larger community. True partnerships depend on recognition of advantages of training and mutual shaping of the training agenda, design, and methods. Special attention to the service element of training should provide the greatest benefit to all. Partnerships can (and should) address real problems in rural communities. This is not possible in the traditional tourist model of health-professions education, however, in which trainees spend 1 to 4 weeks on site with little advance preparation other than clinical studies. This is barely enough time to begin to understand the context of rural practice.

Overcoming Differences in Perspectives, Missions, and Values

Health professions training institutions are rarely close to rural clinical sites. Moreover, the two types of institutions are also likely to be separated by differences in mission, perspectives, and values. University faculty vary in their understanding of rural settings and rural people. Faculty typically live comfortable middle-class lives in metropolitan areas. They may or may not have direct personal experience with rural life. Contingent on their experiences, they may cherish romantic stereotypes of rural living, or alternatively, be poorly prepared to deal with the poverty and unfamiliar life experiences of those with very different educational and cultural backgrounds. Similarly, faculty may not fully appreciate the demands of rural practice. To enhance their own effectiveness and promote the understanding that is necessary to program planning, faculty should invest time to understand both the specific practice settings and the rural community in which training is to take place. Exchanges of academic faculty and community practitioners can address these objectives.

Even more than in other areas, in rural settings a distinct tension may exist between the requirements of training and provision of service. Time and money are critical to rural service settings, a fact that is often underappreciated by those in academic settings. Rural service providers carry heavy caseloads, and they must make prudent use of time away from their primary service mission. Moreover, rural settings usually lack working capital and have little, if any, monetary cushion. In the best training partnerships, the academic center allocates funds to participating service settings to compensate staff for their time and to offset the potential loss of revenue.

Historically, health professions training schools and individual departments have retained significant control over training program design and implementation; rural clinical settings have been left trying to meet a plethora of disparate objectives for trainees from different disciplines and institutions. This situation has generated considerable frustration on the part of rural preceptors and, in some cases, alienation. Training institutions must improve coordination of field-based training protocols across disciplines and make them responsive to the needs of the community and practice settings. True partnerships engage the community as collaborator throughout all phases of the training effort, in defining the objectives, exploring pertinent factors, and designing acceptable goals and methods.

Overcoming Barriers of Time and Distance

Modern telecommunications technology is improving rural health care access and has the potential to increase access to training. Available technologies (see chapter 7) are quite sophisticated and include video-conferencing and diagnostic capabilities for radiology, cardiology, and other specialty areas. In a 1995 nationwide survey of rural telemedicine, the Office of Rural Health Policy (1997) ascertained that nearly 30% of rural hospitals were using some real-time telemedicine technology as part of relatively complex networks, averaging 9.3 sites per network. Most of the surveyed programs were new, with substantial start-up and transmission costs and low utilization; systems surviving beyond a demonstration phase reported higher utilization with each year of operation. Limited specialist access was a major issue for the rural communities of the hospitals surveyed: 72% had no dermatologist locally; 62%, no neurologist; 53%, no psychiatrist; and 51%, no oncologist.

Telemedicine is likely to expand in both quantity and range of sessions from the current low utilization base. Although individual diagnostic consults still dominate clinical applications, some networks now use teleclinics. Interdisciplinary team consultations in geriatrics also use this system. Team training applications are also very promising and directly address some of the most pressing problems in rural health training.

Discipline-specific preceptor availability can limit training opportunities; for example, rural communities often lack social workers with a master's degree to provide required supervision to social work students. With telemedicine capabilities, telesupervision of students by faculty at the educational institution becomes a viable option. Telemedicine can also be a vehicle for enhancing involvement of trainees based in remote sites, allowing nontraditional students greater access to faculty, and allowing students on rotation to enjoy joint planning and evaluative time with community preceptors and academic faculty. Students can also "visit" community sites and learn about them well before their actual rotations. Telemedicine can greatly facilitate communication between academic and clinical partners, reducing the need for time-consuming travel.

Lower level technologies also have an important role in overcoming time and distance constraints. E-mail allows a free flow of communication among individuals or groups at the convenience of both senders and recipients.

Preceptor Identification, Development, and Support

There are two significant obstacles to preceptor recruitment in rural areas: high service demands and the limited availability of practitioners in specific disciplines. For example, finding physical therapy preceptors may be difficult; physical therapists tend to be in short supply and those who are in practice are often affiliated with contractual agencies. Practitioner level of educational preparation can also be an issue. Many rural social workers are prepared at the bachelor's level rather than the master's level and therefore are technically ineligible to precept graduate students in social work. Consequently, preceptor recruitment requires considerable effort, a task that Area Health Education Centers, with their knowledge of practitioners in their regions, have performed admirably well. Conferences, which bring together community practitioners and academic personnel, are also good venues for recruitment. Recruitment must take into account the needs of prospective preceptors and the potential benefits of participation in trainees' development. Indeed, many rural practitioners are delighted to forge a teaching alliance with the training institution and to have an important role in preparing trainees for rural practice. They recognize the social merit of this activity as well as the potential personal and professional benefits.

Geriatric Interdisciplinary Team Training (GITT) projects provide an opportunity to move beyond traditional discipline-specific precepting to a team-based model of clinical teaching. Of course, the model must include strong discipline-specific role modeling, but it also permits diffusion of teaching and mentoring responsibilities across all team members. The team-based model has real merit in rural settings when the goals are to teach trainees the context for rural practice as well as interdisciplinary teamwork and geriatric clinical care.

In a 1993 study (Stritter, Beza, Harward, & Hytten, 1993), rural preceptors underscored the importance of consistent liaison with the educational institution, preferably through a personal relationship and regular visitation. Such a relationship allows for discussion, feedback, and reformulation of goals and strategies as needed. Rural preceptors also expressed interest in networking with other preceptors to share knowledge and experiences.

CHALLENGES TO TRAINING IMPLEMENTATION

Trainee Recruitment and Retention

Health manpower initiatives such as the National Health Service Corps have focused on attracting and retaining trainees to rural practice for several decades. Another strategy that has demonstrated value is recruitment and targeted admission of students from rural areas who desire to practice in rural areas (Roberts et al., 1993). A variety of incentives such as loan forgiveness have also been employed as recruiting tools.

Attracting trainees to geriatric practice in rural sites is no easier than at other institutions. In response to a 1996 survey, 41% of 729 health professions students at the University of North Carolina at Chapel Hill indicated that they were not likely to spend a significant portion of their professional time working with older people (Carl & Hunter, 1997). Only 24% of social work students and 24% of entering medical students expected to spend significant professional time with older people; figures for pharmacy (37%), dentistry (42%), and physical therapy (30%) were higher (nursing was not queried), but still below what would be expected based on projections of need and actual practice patterns in primary care.

Given the recruiting challenges for programs with a rural or geriatric focus, identifying prospective rural or geriatric practitioners before admission or early in the orientation process may be helpful. Rural health and geriatrics, often relatively invisible or greatly diffused programs within educational institutions, must organize across schools and departments into visible entities, offering peer and faculty support to students and providing focal points for rural health or aging interests and activities. Interest group sessions, list-serves, interdisciplinary service learning activities, and faculty mentoring can all serve a vital role in student socialization, identity formation, and commitment to rural health and geriatrics (see chapter 4).

Balancing Campus and Community-Based Commitments

Achieving the optimal balance of campus-based and community-based training program activities, including rural experiences, requires considerable thought and effort. Advanced learners seek to maximize experiential learning in clinical settings. Because health professions training institutions are usually located in population centers, traveling distance to rural clinical training sites is almost always a problem.

In the future, increased access to computer-based distance learning and advanced telecommunications technology will enable trainees to be stationed in a remote rural community while still completing coursework and interacting with academic faculty and other trainees on campus and in other settings. Although the basic capabilities for the university without walls exist now, further development of courses, infrastructure, and operational integration must take place before telecommunications can substitute for face-to-face learning in a meaningful way.

The question of how best to configure trainee time on campus and in clinical settings, including rural sites, is daunting. The extent to which preparation for rural practice is part of the mission of a GITT project will be an important factor in resolving this question. The configuration chosen by programs seeking simply to expose trainees to the care of the rural elderly will vary greatly from that chosen by programs whose central mission is preparation for rural practice. I will describe a middle ground position.

For trainees who will ultimately practice in rural communities, the greatest challenge is to provide them with substantive experience in the rural setting. *Substantive* experience constitutes more than just another in a series of uncoordinated rotations. The experience must be of sufficient duration and intensity to allow the trainee to:

- Participate fully in the provision of primary care
- Comprehend the local health care system and the interaction of its components
- Take part in the life of the community
- Provide service of value to the community.

Unfortunately, these goals are likely to conflict with other learning demands in the discipline-specific or interdisciplinary training program. A 3-month block experience may be exceedingly difficult to implement. Nonetheless, it is feasible to enable trainees to engage in a series of activities over the course of several months that facilitate a relationship with a rural community.

A rural practice sequence can be planned to acquaint trainees progressively with rural practice in geriatrics. To implement this approach, early in the program trainees visit the site in which they will ultimately have a block rotation. During the visit, they meet practitioners, have a general orientation to the community, and learn about some of the health and health-related problems confronting elderly citizens in the area. Subsequently, this site and the community in which it is located are the foci for several specific activities.

In campus-based didactic instruction in rural health issues, trainees can work with data from their assigned community, and academic faculty can draw from the community for case-based or problem-focused learning. Trainees who have a degree- or course-related research requirement can conduct that research in the rural community. In addition, trainees can serve on a board, project-planning committee, Total Quality Management team, or in another appropriate service role in their community. These groups typically meet infrequently, perhaps monthly, allowing the trainee to have some ongoing interaction with the community while maintaining involvement in other required training experiences. These assignments promote an understanding of health care management issues and foster leadership and program planning skills.

The partnership between the School of Medicine's Program on Aging at the University of North Carolina and rural practice sites in Northampton and Halifax counties provides this kind of education. Trainees join the Program's geriatric interdisciplinary team to make consultative visits to the rural practice settings either in person or via telemedicine. In this capacity, they have an opportunity to engage in a problem-solving process with interdisciplinary team members from the rural community and to begin to understand some of the constraints and positive aspects of rural practice.

Structuring the Rural Community-Based Experience

Trainees should enter into a community care experience familiar with the community, its assets, and its problems. They have a better background for the field experience and are in a better position to be contributing members of the local team.

Because commuting distances to rural communities are often substantial, residential block placements may be the preferred structure, and of course, offer the distinct advantage of allowing the trainees to fully experience rural life. Nonresidential placements are feasible when commutes are short or budgets permit students to stay overnight in the community, traveling to the site early one day and returning late the next day.

While on site, trainees should participate in local interdisciplinary teams serving older people, clinical care, and community-oriented problem-solving. In the initial orientation period, trainees should meet key staff, such as the receptionist, and learn how they see their roles. Meeting program administrators, learning how they interface with clinical staff, and developing some understanding of financing on the service setting are also important. Also, as part of the orientation, visiting other agencies and patients in their homes and shadowing persons from disciplines other than one's own can be of value.

Geriatric interdisciplinary trainees can participate in block placements individually as their schedules permit or take part as teams of trainees who enter and leave the system at the same time. The latter method offers some efficiencies, particularly for orientation, and is especially adaptable to the community problem-solving component of the experience, permitting trainees to apply their interdisciplinary collaborative skills to a defined problem identified by the community. In one application of this approach, students worked with rural preceptors and the local community to obtain a better grasp of factors leading to complications of diabetes. They developed a teaching module on diabetes care for front-line caregivers and a foot care screening protocol, which they taught to health professionals throughout the community. They also scripted a nutrition video with plans to use people from the community. The opportunity to design projects such as these can greatly enrich clinical experiences and foster the acquisition of skills necessary to practice in rural settings (Williams, Rabiner, & Hunter, 1995).

CONCLUSIONS

Rural areas are in great need of health professionals trained to provide sensitive care, and GITT provides an opportunity to teach more providers the team and geriatrics skills essential to the care of elderly in these communities. The greatest challenge to rural GITT is the creation of clinical experiences that provide meaningful exposure to rural health care. To do this, rural GITT must foster new linkages between remote communities and academic settings, experimentation with new technologies, and creation of innovative educational experiences.

REFERENCES

American Medical Association Center for Health Policy Research. (1992). *Socioeconomic characteristics of medical practice.* Chicago: American Medical Association.

Availability of health care in rural communities: Hearing on Rural Health Issues before the Subcommittee on Health, Committee on Ways and Means, 104th Cong., 2d Sess. (1996), (testimony of J. Human).

Bader, J. D., Scurria, M. S., & Shugars, D. A. (1994). Urban/rural differences in prosthetic dental service rates. *Journal of Rural Health, 10,* 26–30.

Beaulieu, J. E., & Berry, D. E. (1994). *Rural health services: A management perspective.* Ann Arbor, MI: ALPHA Press.

Beers, M. H., Fingold, S. F., & Ouslander, J. G. (1992). A computerized system for identifying and informing physicians about problematic drug use in nursing homes. *Journal of Medical Systems, 16,* 237–245.

Beers, M. H., Ouslander, J. G., Fingold, S. F., Morgenstern, H., Reuben, D. B., Rogers, W., Zeffren, M. J., & Beck, J. C. (1992). Inappropriate medication prescribing in skilled-nursing facilities. *Annals of Internal Medicine, 117,* 685–689.

Blake, H. J. (1984). Doctor can't do me no good: Social concomitants of health care attitudes and practices among elderly blacks in isolated rural populations. In W. Watson (Ed.), *Black folk medicine* (pp. 33–40). New Brunswick, NJ: Transaction.

Blazer, D. G., Landerman, L. R., Fillenbaum, G., & Horner, R. (1995). Health services access and use among older adults in North Carolina: Urban vs rural residents. *American Journal of Public Health, 85,* 1384–1390.

Bull, C. N. (Ed.). (1993). *Aging in rural America.* Newbury Park, CA: Sage.

Carl, L., & Hunter, R. (1997). *Interdisciplinary service learning: Attitudes and experiences of health professions students.* Unpublished manuscript.

Cavalieri, T. A., Chopra, A., Gray-Miceli, D., Shreve, S., Waxman, H., & Forman, L. J. (1993). Geriatric assessment teams in the nursing home: Do they work? *Journal of the American Osteopathic Association, 93,* 1269–1272.

Coleman, L. M., Fowler, L. B., & Williams, M. E. (1995). Use of unproven therapies by people with Alzheimer's disease. *Journal of the American Geriatrics Society, 43,* 747–750.

Cook, C., & Baisden, D. (1986). Ancillary use of folk medicine by patients in primary care clinics in Southwestern West Virginia. *Southern Medical Journal, 79,* 1098–1101.

Coward, R. T., McLaughlin, D. K., Duncan, R. P., & Bull, C. N. (1994). An overview of health and aging in rural America. In R. T. Coward, C. N. Bull, G. Kukulka, & J. M. Galliher (Eds.), *Health services for rural elders* (pp. 1–32). New York: Springer Publishing Co.

Eisenberg, D. M., Kessler, R C., Foster, C., Norlock, F. E., Calkins, D. R., & Delbanco, T. L. (1993). Unconventional medicine in the United States. Prevalence, costs, and patterns of use. *New England Journal of Medicine, 328,* 246–252.

Engel, G. L. (1977). The need for a new medical model. A challenge for biomedicine. *Science, 196,* 129–135.

Fuller, K. (1995). Grant project graduates surveyed on factors influencing job seeking behavior. *Rural route.* Kalamazoo, MI: Western Michigan University.

Goldman, L. S., & Klugman, A. (1990). Psychiatric consultation in a teaching nursing home. *Psychosomatics, 31,* 277–281.

Haywood, L. J., Francis, C. K., Cregler, L. L., Freed, M. D., & Skorton, D. J. (1994). Task force 1: The underserved. *Journal of the American College of Cardiology, 24,* 282–290.

Hendryx, M. S. (1993). Rural hospital health promotion: Programs, methods, resource limitations. *Journal of Community Health, 18,* 241–250.

Hufford, D. J. (1992). Folk medicine in contemporary America. In J. Kirkland, H. Mathews, C. W. Sullivan, III, & K. Baldwin (Eds.), *Herbal and magical medicine. Traditional healing today* (pp. 14–31). Durham, NC: Duke University Press.

Iutcovich, J. M. (1993). Assessing the needs of rural elderly: an empowerment model. *Evaluation and Program Planning, 16,* 95–107.

King, D. E., Sobal, J., & DeForge, B. R. (1988). Family practice patients' experience and beliefs in faith healing. *Journal of Family Practice, 27,* 505–508.

Kleinman, A. (1978). Concepts and a model for the comparison of medical systems as cultural systems. *Social Science and Medicine, 12,* 85–93.

Kohrs, F. P., & Mainous, A. G., III. (1995). The relationship of health professional shortage areas to health status. *Archives of Family Medicine, 4,* 681–685.

Office of Rural Health Policy. (1997). *Exploratory evaluation of rural applications of telemedicine.* Rockville, MD: Office of Rural Health Policy.

Pew Health Professions Commission. (1995). *Critical challenges: Revitalizing the health professions for the twenty-first century.* San Francisco: UCSF Center for the Health Professions.

Phan, T. T., & Reifler, B. V. (1988). Psychiatric disorders among nursing home residents: depression, anxiety, and paranoia. *Clinics in Geriatric Medicine, 4,* 601–612.

Roberts, A., Foster, R., Dennis, M., Davis, L., Well, J., Bodemuller, M. F., & Bailey, C. A. (1993). An approach to training and retaining primary care physicians in rural Appalachia. *Academic Medicine, 68,* 122–125.

Rowles, G. D. (1991). Changing health culture in rural Appalachia: Implications for serving the elderly. *Journal of Aging Services, 5,* 375–389.

Sakauye, K. M., & Camp, C. J. (1992). Introducing psychiatric care into nursing homes. *Gerontologist, 32,* 849–852.

Simmons, J. J., Nelson, E., Roberts, E., Salisbury, Z., Kane-Williams, E., & Benson, L. (1989). A health promotion program: staying healthy after fifty. *Health Education Quarterly, 16,* 461–472.

Smith, M., Buckwalter, K. C., & Albanese, M. (1990). Geropsychiatric education programs: providing skills and understanding. *Journal of Psychosocial Nursing, 28*(12), 8–12.

Smith, M., Buckwalter, K. C., Garland, L., Mitchell, S., Albanese, M., & Kreiter, C. (1994). Evaluation of a geriatric mental health training program for nursing personnel in rural long-term care facilities. *Issues Mental Health Nursing, 15,* 149–168.

Smyer, M., Brandon, D., & Cohn, M. (1992). Improving nursing home care through training and job redesign. *Gerontologist, 32,* 327–333.

Spector, R. E. (1991). *Cultural diversity in health and illness* (3rd ed.) Norwalk, CT: Appleton and Lange.

Stritter, F., Beza, J., Harward, D., & Hytten, K. (1993). *Education for interdisciplinary rural health care: The role of the preceptor.* Rockville, MD: HRSA, Bureau of Health Professions.

Van Nostrand, J. F. (Ed.). (1993). Common beliefs about the rural elderly: What do national data tell us? *Vital Health Statistics.* Hyattsville, MD: National Center for Health Statistics.

Wallace, R. B., & Colsher, P. L. (1994). Improving ambulatory and acute care services for the rural elderly: Current solutions, research, and policy directions. In R. T. Coward, C. N. Bull, G. Kukulka, & J. M. Galliher (Eds.), *Health services for rural elders* (pp. 108–126). New York: Springer Publishing Company.

White, S. L., & Maloney, S. K. (1990). Promoting healthy diets and active lives to hard-to-reach groups: market research study. *Public Health Reports, 105,* 224–231.

Williams, M. E., Rabiner, D. J., & Hunter, R. H. (1995). The interdisciplinary geriatric team evaluation project: A new approach to the delivery of geriatric medicine in geographically remote locations. *North Carolina Medical Journal, 56,* 502–505.

Yawn, B. P., Busby, A., & Yawn, R. A. (Eds.). (1994). *Exploring rural medicine: Current issues and concepts.* Thousand Oaks, CA: Sage.

CHAPTER 15

Planning GITT:
The Academic Setting

Nancy L. Smith and Ernestine Kotthoff-Burrell

The health care system in the United States is undergoing a massive evolution driven by demands from a variety of sources. When health care reform at the federal level slipped away in 1993, the private sector and market forces, usurping state-initiated change, took the lead and have created profound and fundamental change at unprecedented speed.

These changes in the delivery and financing of health care have influenced both the health care work force and the academic health centers whose mission it is to educate health care professionals. It is imperative that the academic health centers reform health care education to align more closely with marketplace requirements for health care professionals. The Geriatric Interdisciplinary Team Training (GITT) model is one of the ways that this educational reform can become reality.

CREATING THE COMMUNITY–ACADEMIC PARTNERSHIP

Linking Practice and Academe

Mutual benefit drives the linkage of practice and academe. For the academic health center, the graduates of its health professions educational programs must meet the needs of the community customers—hospitals, health maintenance organizations, or community health centers among others—that are potential sources of work for the graduate. Although terms such as customer or market are clearly used in the business world, their use by academicians facilitates the linkage and the relationships between practice and academe.

For the GITT clinical partners, working with the academic health centers offers a potential relationship that can guide both the development of health professions curriculum and the clinical experiences of health professions students during their course of study. The graduates of the health-professions programs, then, are more closely aligned to the needs of the marketplace. These partnership models are occurring throughout the country and in a variety of models.

History of Interdisciplinary Efforts at the University of Colorado Health Sciences Center

At the University of Colorado Health Sciences Center (UCHSC), interdisciplinary efforts date to the mid-1980s. The Seniors Clinic at the UCHSC was established in 1985. At that time and for several years thereafter, faculty from the academic programs at UCHSC (medicine, nursing, and dentistry) together with academic faculty from other public and private universities around the state (the University of Colorado at Boulder, the University of Colorado at Colorado Springs, the University of Colorado at Denver, and the University of Denver, a private university) met on a quarterly basis to share information and conduct educational seminars around issues in aging. Subsequently, the UCHSC received federal funding for several interdisciplinary initiatives. For example, the federal Administration on Aging (AOA) funded a Gerontology Training Program for Health Professionals to enhance their awareness of oral health needs in the older adult. The project included dentistry, nursing, social work, and others. This project was followed by the Dental Education for Colorado Hospice Program (1985–1986), the Statewide Plan for Care of the Elderly (1986–1988), the Robert Wood Johnson Foundation-supported GITT Project that trained teams of health professionals from four statewide community hospitals to conduct comprehensive geriatric assessment and provide interdisciplinary geriatric consultation and referral, and a UCHSC Chancellor's Academic Enrichment Award to ascertain the geriatric content in the five health professional programs on the UCHSC campus.

This historic success gave rise to the first award from the Health Resources and Services Administration, Bureau of Health Professions to establish the interdisciplinary Colorado Geriatric Education Center (CGEC). The CGEC initially involved three academic institutions, UCHSC, University of Colorado at Colorado Springs, and Denver University, and seven health professions (medicine, nursing, dentistry, pharmacy, physical therapy, psychology, and social work). The project involved close collaboration with the Colorado Area Health Education System (AHEC) and the National Center for American Indian and Alaska Native Mental Health Research Center, directed by the internationally known Native anthropologist and researcher, Dr. Spero Manson.

The CGEC faculty were successful in introducing new geriatric content into the health professional programs, developing minority aging content, and producing a videotape that demonstrates a method to conduct a culturally competent health interview. The CGEC collaborated with the federally funded Rural Interdisciplinary Team Training Project that was awarded to the Colorado AHEC System.

The CGEC received funding for an additional 3 years in 1993. The gerontology program from yet another public university, the University of Northern Colorado, was added to the list of participating disciplines and institutions. The second cycle of funding built on the successes of earlier collaborative efforts and included liaisons with the mental health professionals throughout the state.

In the spring of 1993, the newly appointed UCHSC Chancellor, Dr. Vincent Fulginnetti, stated his strong commitment to both geriatrics and to interdisciplinary education. In the fall of 1993, Dr. Dennis Jahnigen was recruited to create the new interdisciplinary UCHSC Center on Aging (CA). The CA became the first formal interdisciplinary structure on the UCHSC campus. The administrative structure and the funding for the CA represented a dramatic departure from the usual departmental organization; each of the deans of the respective health professional programs as well as the UCHSC central administration committed funds for the operation. The CA serves as the organizational umbrella for the geriatric clinical, educational, and research activities at UCHSC. It houses the outpatient and inpatient clinical activities, the geriatric consultation service, the geriatric fellowship program, the CGEC, the community outreach activities, and the interdisciplinary geriatric research.

The CA faculty is comprised of geriatricians, gerontologic nurse practitioners, social workers, doctors of pharmacy, dentists, clinical psychologists, dietitians, and clinical registered nurses. The interdisciplinary program team provides direct patient health care services in the Senior's Clinic at University Hospital as well as clinical education for health professions students and medical residents.

Interdisciplinary geriatric activities have continued to expand. The National Center for American Indian and Alaska Native Mental Health Research received funding from AOA in 1994 to establish one of two national resource centers for Native Elders. The new Native Elder Health Care Resource Center has worked collaboratively with the interdisciplinary faculty from the CA to produce four monographs on common health problems in Native American elderly. The modules address diabetes, depression, cancer, and alcohol abuse in Native American populations.

Creating GITT at an Academic Center

The interdisciplinary team in the Center on Aging provided the core members for the GITT Steering Committee. In addition, Dr. Jahnigen recruited community-based partners for this unique endeavor. The community-based clinical partners each have geriatric interdisciplinary teams practicing in their agencies, and students enrolled in the GITT course rotate through these clinical settings. Table 15.1 lists the current partners in the GITT Project.

The members of the GITT Steering Committee began meeting approximately 9 months before implementing the first course. They held monthly meetings to foster a sense of team among the committee members and to develop the curriculum and the syllabi for the course offerings. The monthly meetings were held from 5:30 to 8:00 P.M. on a mutually agreed on evening to facilitate attendance by representative of the clinical partners. A light dinner was offered because most members were coming directly from work. Meeting locations were also rotated among the partners. This rotation served several purposes (a) it gave equal focus to clinical partners, (b) members on the committee had opportunity to visit sites, and (c) it enhanced the learning potential for trainees at the clinical settings.

The committee functioned by having individual members or subgroups work between meetings and bring draft products back to the group for review. Examples of some of these projects included discipline-specific prerequisite knowledge and skills for guiding potential students, a pretest and a posttest, recruitment brochures, and course syllabus.

Each of the Steering Committee members provided discipline-specific didactic content during course implementation. Members were also responsible for visiting trainees at the clinical settings.

TABLE 15.1 Colorado GITT Project Partners

UCHSC School of Dentistry
UCHSC School of Medicine
UCHSC School of Nursing
UCHSC School of Pharmacy
University of Denver Graduate School of Social Work
Kaiser Permanente
UCHSC Center on Aging
Colorado Geriatric Education Center
Total Long-Term Care
Geriatric Medicine Associates
Denver Department of Veterans Affairs Hospital
University of Denver College of Law
Columbia Senior Health Care Center
Colorado Access

FACING THE INTERDISCIPLINARY ACADEMIC CHALLENGES

The challenges facing the GITT Steering Committee to implement the course, "Geriatric Interdisciplinary Teams in a Managed Care Setting," were common to many interdisciplinary efforts. The Committee made many accommodations to reconcile differences across agencies to create an interdisciplinary course that would be both attractive to potential learners and based on learner-centered teaching strategies. They identified three primary areas that required special collaboration for resolution: (a) scheduling of course offerings; (b) academic credit for courses; and (c) tuition collection and revenue assignment.

Scheduling of Course Offerings

The challenge was not only to find a schedule that would be possible across all of the clinical settings and the individual curricula, but one that would entice potential students. After much discussion of potential alternatives, the committee developed an initial format. For the first offering of the course, a Friday evening/Saturday session followed by two Saturday sessions scheduled a month apart were scheduled. This timing did not interfere with any of the previously scheduled courses for any of the programs and also allowed participation by faculty both from within the universities and from clinical settings.

For the first Friday evening session, the Center on Aging served pizza. During the Saturday sessions, coffee and bagels were available, and students frequently went to lunch together for informal socializing across disciplines. Food proved to be a great facilitator of learning and participation.

Academic Credit

At least one academic unit or school must review, approve, and list a course before the University can offer it. Because the course coordinator was a faculty member in the School of Nursing, the Committee decided to list the course within that school and cross-list it with other schools as a graduate-level interdisciplinary course offering. There were two separate listings: one for the didactic portion and one for the practicum. Students registered for the course with the School of Nursing.

In addition, the courses were approved by the appropriate committees in the Graduate School of Social Work at the University of Denver. This allowed learners from the University of Denver to register for the course on their campus.

Like many health professions educational programs, curricula and degree plans for individual students were fairly fixed on admission. Potential learners did not require additional academic credits; GITT faculty had to recruit them. The Steering Committee developed a marketing brochure that was distributed across the appropriate programs. In addition, a faculty representative personally visited targeted classes of learners to recruit participants. Chapter 4 describes recruitment strategies in more detail.

Tuition Collection and Revenue Assignment

Tuition patterns were as variable across programs as schedules were. In some cases, students paid tuition at a per credit hour rate, in others, students paid a flat annual tuition for enrollment in their professional programs. For the first offering of the course, the Committee negotiated that tuition be collected and assigned to the school and university in which registration occurred, and obtained agency approval for this agreement from the appropriate authority. On the UCHSC campus, tuition for the course was not collected from dental or pharmacy students because these students pay an annual tuition that is preset regardless of the specific courses taken. Students from the School of Nursing paid tuition per credit hour at the regular graduate course rate. Revenues remained within the School of Nursing. Students from the Graduate School of Social Work registered for the course and paid tuition directly to the University of Denver at their tuition rates. Revenues also remained at the University of Denver.

It is anticipated that these arrangements will remain flexible and subject to renegotiation. For example, in the future, there might be participants who work in one of the clinical settings or who are just taking the courses for professional development. How and where these participants might register and how their tuition revenues will be assigned would need review. In addition, future negotiations might create a more direct relationship between faculty assigned to teach in the program and the return of tuition revenue to their academic appointment or employing clinical partner.

BENEFITS OF THE COMMUNITY– ACADEMIC PARTNERSHIP

There are many strengths to an interdisciplinary community–academic partnership. The Pew Health Professions Commission in *Health Professions Education for the Future: Schools in Service to the Nation,* was a landmark publication urging and defining educational reform for health professionals (O'Neil, 1993). That document also called for the "realignment and recasting of relationships" (p. 17) and suggested that educational institutions:

- Develop a commitment to becoming a service organization,
- Focus on serving the needs of the emerging health care system,
- Bring creativity to the identification of new partnerships,
- Understand their work within the context of public need,
- Approach this task from a generalist-interdisciplinary orientation (pp. 17–18).

The GITT Project is realigning and recasting the relationships with a new model of the community–academic partnership. Clinical partners are sitting at the curricular/programmatic table as equals in decision making. They bring their unique insights, currency in the private practice arena, innovative practice models, managed care experience, and individual areas of expertise to the development, implementation, and evaluation of the project.

Clinical-Setting Benefits

Health professionals working at the clinical settings have the opportunity to apply for volunteer clinical faculty appointments in the appropriate school. The specific advantages to this vary according to the location of appointment, but typically include access to library and data base searches and participation in selected faculty events. Many preceptors appreciate recognition for their work with students by having an academic title that may be included on the Curriculum vitae—even without financial remuneration. In addition, the clinical setting has the potential to become an official University affiliate, which is viewed as an award of distinction, pride, and demonstration of clinical excellence.

Academe

Academicians have been frequently criticized for their distance from the real world of clinical practice and the managed care environment. Sitting at the same table with staff from clinical settings offers the opportunity to build bridges of understanding and mutual commitment toward the common goals of improving patient care for the elderly and the education of future health care professionals. There are new clinical opportunities for students and potential postgraduate employment opportunities, as well.

By mentoring trainees at clinical settings, academic faculty gain exposure to innovative models of health care delivery in the managed care marketplace. In addition, some faculty have had multiple queries from clinical setting personnel regarding other educational programs at the University. Informal recruitment of potential students to the University at large and increased community visibility of University faculty are significant benefits.

Joint Collaborative Benefits

These community–academic partnerships offer opportunities for innovative practice model development, professional development, faculty practice sites, research opportunities, and consultation. Expertise from both settings can be shared to improve the environment, knowledge, and skills of health professionals without regard to the primary place of employment. For example, University faculty give lectures at the clinical settings to agency staff, and clinical experts from these settings have shared their expertise in University classrooms.

SUMMARY

The Association of Academic Health Centers published *The U.S. Health Workforce: Power, Politics, and Policy* (Osterweis, McLaughlin, Manasse, & Hopper, 1996) to address the changing demands of the health care system and the subsequent changes in the health care workforce and cited interdisciplinary care teams as one model of tomorrow's health care system (p. 179). The GITT Project is one model that incorporates the recommendations for the future education of health care professionals.

GITT has explored both the challenges and benefits of the community-academic partnerships. The creation, implementation, and careful evaluation of these partnerships have the potential to revolutionize the way in which health professions students are educated. The feedback and excitement from the trainees and the clinical partners are positive. These partnerships are possible and are mutually beneficial.

REFERENCES

O'Neil, E. H. (1993). *Health professions education for the future: Schools in service to the nation.* San Francisco: Pew Health Professions Commission.

Osterweis, M., McLaughlin, C. J., Manasse, H. R., & Hopper, C. L. (Eds.). (1996). *The U.S. health workforce: Power, politics, and policy.* Washington, DC: Association of Academic Health Centers.

Epilogue

Madeline H. Schmitt

Even though much has been written about teams in health care over the past several decades, I find this book and the Geriatric Interdisciplinary Team Training (GITT) Program that inspires it truly exciting. As is noted in the opening chapters, interdisciplinary health care teams are not a new phenomenon, especially in geriatric health care. The field of geriatrics has been interdisciplinary since its inception, and teams have been featured consistently in the writing about geriatric health care delivery. Books about teamwork in health care also are not a new phenomenon; there have been many good ones written over the years, particularly on the subject of team dynamics, whose content is still relevant to the current enterprise (e.g., Brill, 1976; Ducanis & Golin, 1979; Eichhorn, 1973; Leathard, 1994; Siegler & Whitney, 1994; Soothill, Mackay, & Webb, 1995; Walby, Greenwell, Mackay, & Soothill, 1994; Wise, Beckhard, Rubin, & Kyte, 1974). So what about this project and this book generates my enthusiastic response?

First, the project is timely. The GITT Program that the Hartford Foundation has undertaken is a truly important and ambitious one at a critical time in the history of health care for older persons. There are more older persons than ever needing care, and that number is rapidly increasing. What we know about normal aging and disease processes in older persons is expanding at a rapid rate. The health care needs of older persons are more complex and individualized. We know they often require the resources of many disciplines for effective and efficient care. In the United States, however, much of the health care delivered to older people has been either institutionally based or focused on efforts to keep people out of institutions. For the most part, what we know about geriatric health care teams comes from study of teams in institutions. We know much less about how to educate professionals to deliver interdisciplinary care in primary care settings. In the 1990s, health care reform has meant that most health care is being deinstitutionalized. The changes toward managed care and integrated delivery systems challenge us to become better prepared to work together, as clinicians and as educators, to meet the needs of older persons in the community and in primary health care settings just as these settings are undergoing enormous changes toward managed care and integrated delivery systems.

It is precisely this set of challenges that The Hartford Foundation in collaboration with the New York University Resource Center and the eight national GITT implementation projects have taken on: to develop curricula for and educate a new generation of health professionals in core disciplines who will work in interdisciplinary teams to meet the primary health care needs of older persons; and to reshape how educational institutions educate health professions students for future clinical practice. The process offers participating clinical caregivers the opportunity to learn how to enhance the quality and sophistication of the care they deliver to older persons. The Program participants' enthusiastic commitment to meet these challenges pours out into the pages of this book.

Not only are the timeliness and scope impressive, but the design of the project is rigorous and is highly likely to generate meaningful outcomes. First, commitment of the Project personnel is high. Only proposals from clinical and academic settings willing to be partnered in these geriatric educational efforts were considered. At each setting, buy-in from the top administrators in both settings is assured, as is the involvement of the three core disciplines: medicine, nursing, and social work. Fortunately, many settings have found ways to involve in their training proposals additional health care disciplines whose roles are critical in the health care of older persons.

Equally important has been the collaboration of the eight implementation sites and the Resource Center in developing core curricular components. The three components—knowledge and skills in geriatrics, in interdisciplinary teams, and in current health care systems—are all essential elements of educational preparation for future practice. The projects represent diverse academic-clinical partnerships and community care settings. The commitment to implement the curriculum across these diverse settings is another impressive feature of the GITT Project. The set of goals undertaken in the GITT Program are important, but we do not know if they can be achieved across these diverse settings. The diversity of initiatives, along with the efforts to tailor the initiatives at each site, maximizes the likelihood that a core interdisciplinary curriculum will be identified. By capitalizing on the unique and diverse resources of their clinical and academic settings, the project teams will be able to develop an array of specific curricular resource materials, as well as a variety of ways of disseminating those materials to a national audience. In addition, we can learn more about how to shift our educational experiences to a community context. Unlike parallel and competing learning agendas that overwhelm community settings, integrated interdisciplinary learning will enable the provision of efficient and improved education in community sites.

The Resource Center, the core measures, and the national evaluation team will help the grantees to articulate what they have learned, and they will guarantee that nationally we will all benefit from this knowledge.

Another distinguishing feature of this Program is the integration of new quality improvement technologies. The new technologies provide concrete means through which teams can set goals, create feedback loops to assess their own processes and productivity, and thereby learn and grow in capability. Experimentation with Continuous Quality Improvement at some of the GITT settings will offer opportunities to discover how these technologies can enhance the learning team in education and practice.

In chapter 3 of this book, Ruth Ann Tsukuda notes that interdisciplinary educational initiatives and innovative practice have been hard to separate historically. Although the GITT Program's goals are primarily educational and curricular, in their implementation they cannot help but have an impact on the nature of clinical practice for older persons in the settings where they are operationalized. As Joann Castle says in chapter 6, "The change we propose is not a surface change. It is far reaching and fundamental. It affects the way clinicians practice and the way administrators organize a clinic . . . It is a transformation in thinking about our work." To the extent that clinical practice in these settings is reshaped by the Program to be more of an interdisciplinary team effort, especially through the role modeling of preceptor teams, clinicians and practice settings will also be changed in ways that are likely to benefit older people. I anticipate that these experiences will raise a whole new set of questions and initiatives about how to demonstrate these benefits in consumer satisfaction, care quality, and cost savings in rural settings, integrated delivery system settings, and managed care settings. Research into the costs and effectiveness of team delivery of care has been slow to develop, especially in primary care contexts.

In chapter 7, the authors explore existing and emerging technologies for interdisciplinary education. The authors in this chapter and in other chapters raise exciting possibilities about what sites will be able to teach us about the costs and benefits of these technologies, not only for instruction, but also for the improvement of interdisciplinary practice. We know that open communication is a necessary component of effective interdisciplinary care. Perhaps the new technologies will contribute in novel and important ways to the improvement of team communication processes.

Because of the scope and sophistication of this project, we may gain new insights into old issues of interdisciplinary education and practice as they emerge in new practice contexts. For example, on the educational side, authors of these chapters frequently refer to the problems of integrating conflicting schedules across professional schools to allow for the interdisciplinary education of physicians, nurses, and social workers. This scheduling impasse is an old problem that educational institutions must solve if they are going to meet the challenges of preparing disciplines for the realities of interdisciplinary clinical practice. We need to move beyond the practice of doing interdisciplinary education in the cracks and spaces of discipline-based educational programs. I hope that the GITT Program will generate new insights into this old problem.

Another old issue from the practice perspective has to do with the role of the physician in team delivery of care. As physicians become salaried employees of integrated and managed health care delivery systems, how will their responsibility and accountability for care be reshaped? How will their roles and function on teams change? What kind of impact will changes in the physician role have on other health professionals? What kind of impact will changes in the physician role have on other health professionals' responsibility and accountability? Legal issues are inherent in these sorts of questions and have been hinted at in several chapters. Similar questions might be raised about the reshaping of some basic ethical considerations. For example, team delivery of care creates serious dilemmas with the confidentiality norms around the patient-provider relationship.

As noted in the beginning of this Epilogue, although there are numerous books available on health care teams, none has been written about a national interdisciplinary team demonstration program as a work in progress. If we want interdisciplinary teams to be a part of primary care for older persons, it is critical that we learn how to create academic-community partnerships for interdisciplinary education in the context of changing health delivery systems. Many of us teach and practice in institutions where community-focused interdisciplinary educational initiatives are just beginning, not only in geriatrics but in other areas. The principles articulated in this book for the creation of interdisciplinary academic-community practice initiatives are generally applicable. I am grateful that the Hartford Foundation, Resource Center, and project sites have not waited until the end of the Program to convey what they have learned to date. They have already engaged me in the Program and collectively they have raised my expectations and enthusiasm for what is to come.

REFERENCES

Brill, N. I. (1976). *Team work: Working together in the human services.* Philadelphia: Lippincott.

Ducanis, A. J., & Golin, A K. (1979). *The interdisciplinary health care team: A handbook.* Germantown, MD: Aspen.

Eichhorn, S. F. (1973). *Becoming: The actualization of individual differences in five student health teams.* Bronx, NY: Institute for Health Team Development.

Leathard, A. (Ed). (1994). *Going inter-professional: Working together for health and welfare.* London: Routledge.

Siegler E. L., & Whitney, F. W. (Eds). (1994). *Nurse–physician collaboration: Care of adults and the elderly.* New York: Springer Publishing Co.

Soothill, K., Mackay, L, & Webb, C. (1995). *Interprofessional relations in health care.* London: Edward Arnold.

Walby, S., Greenwell, J. Mackay, L., & Soothill, K. (1994). *Medicine and nursing professions in a changing health service.* London: Sage.

Wise, H., Beckhard, R., Rubin, I., & Kyte, A. L. (1974). *Making health teams work.* Cambridge: Ballinger.

Appendixes

Section I: Houston GITT Curriculum*†

BACKGROUND

The overall goal of the Houston Geriatric Interdisciplinary Team Training (HGITT) Project is to foster effective, comprehensive geriatric care by preparing health professionals to use teamwork in meeting diverse patient needs in a range of settings. The HGITT Project has developed a multiinstitutional education and training model for trainees from seven academic programs housed in three institutions.

The participating academic programs include:

- Baylor College of Medicine: Internal Medicine, Family Medicine, Psychiatry, and Physician Assistant Programs
- University of Texas Houston Health Science Center School of Nursing
- University of Houston Graduate School of Social Work
- University of Houston College of Pharmacy

As noted in Table A.1, each participating academic program has existing didactic content in geriatrics/gerontology and each program (except pharmacy) has at least one required clinical rotation in geriatrics.

ORGANIZATION OF CURRICULUM

Core Learning Objectives

The geriatric team training curriculum is designed around core learning objectives for the essential knowledge, skills, and attitudes required for team care of geriatric patients and families. Because trainees will differ in their exposure to didactic and clinical learning, they will differ in their achievement of the learning objectives.

---

* Curriculum created by Baylor College of Medicine Huffington Center on Aging in collaboration with: University of Texas Houston Health Science Center School of Nursing, University of Houston Graduate School of Social Work, University of Houston College of Pharmacy, Harris County Hospital District, Kelsey–Seybold Clinic, MacGregor Medical Association, The Hospice at the Texas Medical Center, Houston Veterans Affairs Medical Center Geriatrics and Extended Care Service, and Houston Veterans Affairs Medical Center Geropsychiatry Unit.

† *Note.* From *Houston GITT Planning Year Curriculum,* by GITT Resource Center, Division of Nursing, New York University, 1996, New York: GITT Resource Center. Copyright 1996 by GITT Resource Center. Reprinted by permission.

TABLE A.1   Geriatric Training in the Houston GITT Curriculum

	Overall Program Time	Clinical Geriatric Training
Advanced Practice Nurses (University of Texas)	The five-semester full-time Master's program for both Geriatric and Adult Nurse Practitioner students includes didactic courses, clinical hours associated with courses, and a clinical preceptorship of 400 hours.	Clinical hours in geriatrics go with each didactic course. The preceptorship of 400 hours is done in rotations of approximately 150 hours at one site.
Family Medicine Residents (Baylor College of Medicine)	Three years of full-time training including required conferences and seminars on geriatric topics.	Two months of geriatrics required. Ambulatory Care and Long-Term Care Electives available.
Internal Medicine Residents (Baylor College of Medicine)	Three years of full-time training including required conferences and seminars on geriatric topics.	Minimum of 1 month of geriatrics required. Elective in Managed Care (1 month)
Psychiatry Residents (Baylor College of Medicine)	Three years of full-time training including required conferences and seminars on geriatric topics.	Minimum of 1 month of inpatient geriatrics required and 3 to 6 months part-time geriatric outpatient care required.
Social Workers (University of Houston)	The Master's program is two academic years with students choosing one of five concentrations for their second year (Gerontology and Health are two of the five).	Each student chooses a practicum of 450–675 hours in second year—usually 2–3 days per week in one site.
Pharmacists (University of Houston)	Pharm.D. program—2 years.	Students choose a 6-week rotation in geriatrics or pediatrics in year 2.
Physician Assistants (Baylor College of Medicine)	Twenty-seven–month graduate program (13-month didactic; 14-month clinical).	Two-month required geriatric medicine rotation in final 6 months of program.

Note. From *Houston GITT Curriculum Planning Year,* by GITT Resource Center, Division of Nursing, New York University, 1996, New York: GITT Resource Center. Copyright 1996 by GITT Resource Center. Reprinted by permission.

Upon successful completion of the GITT didactic and clinical experiences trainees should be able to:

1. Describe concepts of a geriatric interdisciplinary team approach and differentiate it from other care models.
2. Identify the different training attitudes and philosophies that distinguish professional subcultures.
3. Identify the unique capabilities of different disciplines required for particular geriatric problems.

4. Articulate the roles of patient, family, and community in caring for the older adult.
5. Recognize the dynamic process of leadership within a team and demonstrate appropriate leadership roles.
6. Recognize cultural, gender, age, ethnic, racial, and socioeconomic barriers that may affect communication and exchange among providers, patients, their families, and communities.
7. Identify how diverse styles of communication contribute to team function.
8. Communicate effectively with other team members, patients, family members, and community representatives.
9. Demonstrate role negotiation skills and effective involvement of other team members in patient care.
10. Determine treatment and management goals with other team members and the patient and describe methods that maximize outcome evaluation in geriatric interdisciplinary team care.
11. Demonstrate an ability to adapt behavior to changing team dynamics, patient care demands, or both.
12. Demonstrate cultural competency in interactions with team members, patients, and their families.
13. Demonstrate skills at resolving problems between team members.
14. Demonstrate a collaborative spirit by showing respect and support for other members' skills in providing patient care.

The philosophy and approach of HGITT are to introduce team training content early and often into the education and training of each participating discipline through creating new didactic and practicum experiences. As illustrated in the two examples in Table A.2, each discipline has an individual sequence of when didactic and practicum experiences are offered within the degree plan. The specific didactic offerings are described in the Didactic Component Section, and Practicum Learning is also explained.

Didactic Component of the Curriculum

Each academic program has been modified to include team training content, although the breadth and depth of the didactic menu for each discipline varies. One benefit of this model is that all trainees in a program have some basic exposure to teamwork concepts. HGITT trainees participate in didactic instruction through required and elective courses, conferences, workshops, and use of both text and computer-based resources. Trainees in each academic discipline except internal medicine have exposure to content addressing objectives 1 through 5 prior to beginning a practicum experience. Table A.3 lists the proposed menu for each discipline, indicating the total amount of didactic content that HGITT trainees will receive through the various formats.

Didactic Resources and Evaluation

The syllabus for each didactic offering includes required readings from a master bibliography, and participating faculty utilize lecture materials, handouts, and other appropriate

TABLE A.2   GITT Didactic and Practicum Experiences

	Advanced Practice Nursing	
	Year 1 of GNP Program	Year 2 of GNP Program
Didactic	Issues in Aging course (6 hrs) Healthy Aging course (3 hrs)	Geriatric Interdisciplinary Team Training (15 hrs) Didactic with preceptorship (8–24 hrs)
Practicum	Clinical Hours (8–16 hours/week for 8–10 weeks)	Preceptorship (32–40 hours/week for 4–12 weeks)

	Family Medicine		
	Year 1	Year 2	Year 3
Didactic	6 Noon conferences (6 hrs) 2 Interdisciplinary (8 hrs) half-day seminars	6 Noon conferences 2 Interdisciplinary half-day seminars	6 Noon conferences 2 Interdisciplinary half-day seminars
Practicum		Required geriatric outpatient rotation (1 month full-time)	Comprehensive geriatric outpatient elective (2 months part-time)

GNP, geriatric nurse practitioner.

learning activities from a team training resource manual, for example, experiential exercises, case studies, and self and team assessment tools. A key resource for all didactic offerings is the HGITT Trainee Manual. This manual includes readings, handouts, and case-based materials addressing key knowledge areas: roles, training and philosophy of interdisciplinary team members, interdisciplinary team development, communication; leadership, conflict resolution, cultural diversity, as well as a tool for observing teams.

The HGITT Trainee Manual will eventually be developed into a self-paced learning module on interdisciplinary teamwork. In addition to the other material previously identified, there will be pretest and posttest materials enabling the trainee to demonstrate increased understanding of the geriatric competencies of other disciplines and team dynamics. Ultimately, the manual will be developed into a hypertext product.

The methods of evaluation utilized for each didactic offering vary depending on the audience and course content. However, in addition to relevant core measures, we have paid attention to trainee satisfaction as well as self-assessment and perceived acquisition of knowledge and skills. The semester credit courses use some common case studies for written analysis by students, and the learning modules include pretest and posttest questions.

The following listing of didactic offerings illustrates the range of academic opportunities, but it is not comprehensive.

Single Discipline Courses, Seminars, Lectures (Selected Examples)

1. Social Work Practice in Interdisciplinary Health Care Settings: This annual semester-long course for second-year social work students addresses the diverse practice skills needed to function as a professional social worker in interdisciplinary health care

TABLE A.3 Didactic Menu for Each Discipline

Academic program	Didactic hours—all trainees[1]	Didactic hours—GITT trainees[2]	Single-discipline courses/ lectures/ seminars	Interdisciplinary course/lectures/ workshops	Self-guided instructional module
Advanced Practice Nursing	32	32–48	X	X	
Family Medicine	14-24	14–24	X	X	
Internal Medicine[3]	9	9	X		X
Social Work	6	11–60	X	X	
Pharmacy[3]	6	18–22	X		X
Physician Assistant Program	22	22		X	
Psychiatry	10	18–26	X		X

[1] This column reports the total hours each student enrolled in the degree program will receive through required coursework and seminars as identified in the adjacent columns and described previously.

[2] This column reports the hours all GITT trainees in a discipline will receive, including the minimum of 2 hours of didactic instruction that occurs each week in the clinical practicum. In some cases this is the same as the column for all trainees because GITT participation is 100% of the degree program. Ranges reflect electives or additional seminars taken beyond the required courses and lectures.

[3] These GITT Trainees will be required to complete the module; however, others may use this resource in conjunction with another course or seminar.

settings. This course includes theoretical frameworks for interdisciplinary practice, teamwork, group roles, group processes in teams, models for collaboration, the context for collaborative practice, case studies, case assessment methods, strategies for integrating diversity in teamwork efforts, decision making to affect discrimination in resource allocation, and ethical and moral issues in teamwork and service delivery.

2. Gerontology Interdisciplinary Team Training Seminar for Geriatric Nursing Students: This required semester-long clinical course combines didactic seminar learning with 45 hours of clinical time within a GITT clinical site and is designed to prepare students to implement roles in advanced practice nursing as a member or leader of an interdisciplinary team. Topics addressed include principles of teamwork, group process and team skills, conflict management, role differentiation/negotiation, communication principles, and professional roles. The precepted clinical experience provides the opportunity to work effectively as a member of an interdisciplinary health care team providing comprehensive care to older adults in a range of settings.

3. Family Medicine and Internal Medicine Noon Conferences: The core series of required noon conferences for residents in all 3 years incorporates an interdisciplinary approach to core geriatric topics and one on interdisciplinary teamwork. Hour-long interactive presentations are done by professionals of other disciplines illustrating their contributions to geriatric care.

Interdisciplinary Courses and Seminars (Selected Examples)

1. Issues in Aging: (required for all advanced practice nursing, gerontological social work, and physician assistant students). This semester-long interinstitutional survey course examines normal age- and disease-related processes from a biopsychosocial

perspective. The impact of the environment on the aging person is examined, including the familial and societal forces that most effect the elderly. Course faculty come from multiple disciplines, and formal lectures present the background training, skills, and roles of various disciplines. Trainees in nursing, social work, and physician assistant programs work in small interdisciplinary teams using problem-based learning to analyze a geriatric case study. The team learning experience associated with the Issues in Aging course is intended to stimulate an interdisciplinary analysis of a problem being experienced by an older person and expose individual students to the parameters of interdisciplinary team function.

2. Interdisciplinary Team Training Seminars: (family medicine, nursing, social work) Twice a year, a series of three noon conferences and a half-day seminar are dedicated to teaching geriatric interdisciplinary team knowledge and practice skills. Initially the seminar will utilize paper cases; ultimately, standardized patients or actual clinic patients will be involved. The training facilities in the Family Practice Center have videotaping capabilities for observing patient-clinician interactions. Family medicine residents will form training teams with trainees from pharmacy, social work, or nursing and, with the geriatric patient's consent, the patient–clinician interaction will be videotaped. This videotape can be played for other trainees assembled to observe the team or saved to be reviewed at a later date.

FACILITATED INTERDISCIPLINARY TEAM LEARNING IN PRACTICUM SETTINGS

Trainees in each discipline complete a defined and supervised clinical practicum in a project clinical site generally following some exposure to formal team training instruction in required courses or conferences as outlined above. The practicum-based didactic content addresses learning objectives 8 through 14, with an emphasis on skill development. Trainees in many of the academic programs (nursing, medicine, psychiatry, pharmacy, and physician assistant) have clinical learning opportunities in both a managed care Medicare-risk program as well as a public (Houston Veterans Affairs Medical Center, Harris County) or fee-for-service settings. The practicum experience varies in length according to the trainee: internal and family medicine (1 month); advanced practice nursing (2 months); social work (8 months part-time); pharmacy (6 weeks); physician assistant (8 weeks); and psychiatry (3 months). Trainees have clinical preceptors in their respective disciplines; although not all seven disciplines are active at each site, the experiences will share the following five fundamentals:

1. Orientation to GITT and the Clinical Site: Each trainee receives a standard packet of material about the clinical site geriatric training and team learning including an operations orientation packet defining clinician roles, operating teams, and settings at that site; team development materials; and readings.

2. A clinical preceptor responsible for the trainee's overall discipline-specific and team training learning and a team learning facilitator who is either a clinician at the site or a project-based geriatric faculty member are on site. The role of the team-learning

facilitator is to work with the clinical preceptors at the site to implement the explicit team-learning activities.

3. There is a defined plan of educational activities for trainees of each discipline to achieve designated knowledge and skill objectives for geriatric interdisciplinary team care. This will include:

a. Team-building exercises
b. Tools for self-assessment of communication styles and approaches to conflict (Meyers Briggs/ Strength Deployment Inventory)
c. Observation of established clinical teams (debriefing with site facilitator)
d. Participation in a functioning interdisciplinary health care team and opportunities under supervision to contribute to patient care
e. Participation in interdisciplinary rounds and patient/family conferences
f. Structured educational activities for trainees (lectures, group exercises, case presentations)

4. There are methods for trainee self-assessment, team self-assessment, and trainee evaluation.

5. A geriatric syllabus and other relevant print and audio-visual materials are available to all disciplines at each clinical site.

CURRICULUM BIBLIOGRAPHY

Casto, R. M., Julia, M. C., Platt, L. J., Harbaugh, G. L., Waugaman, W. R., Thompson, A., Jost, T. S., Bope, E. T., Williams, T., & Lee, D. B. (1994). *Interprofessional care and collaborative practice.* Pacific Grove, CA: Brooks/Cole.

Clark, P. G. (1991). Toward a conceptual framework for developing interdisciplinary teams in gerontology: Cognitive and ethical dimensions. *Gerontology & Geriatrics Education, 12,* 79–96.

Drinka, T. J. K. (1991). Development and maintenance of an interdisciplinary health care team: A case study. *Gerontology & Geriatrics Education, 12,* 111–127.

Drinka, T. J. K., & Streim, J. (1994). Case studies from purgatory: Maladaptive behavior within geriatric health care teams. *Gerontologist, 34,* 541–547.

Ducanis, A. J., & Golin, A. K. (1978). *Interdisciplinary health care teams: A handbook.* Germantown, MD: Aspen Systems Corporation.

Fagin, C. M. (1992). Collaboration between nurses and physicians: No longer a choice. *Academic Medicine, 67*(5), 91–99.

Francis, D. & Young, B. V. (1979). *Improving work groups: A practical manual for team building.* San Diego, CA: University Associates.

Geist, P. (1994). Negotiating cultural understanding in health care communication. In L. A. Samovar & R. E. Porter (Eds.), *Intercultural communication: A reader* (7th ed.) Belmont, MA: Wadsworth.

Geriatric Health Institute (1995). *Caring for the older adult: The team approach.* (Available from Susan L. Schrader, Ph.D, Project Director, 4201 South Oxbow Ave., Sioux Falls, SD 57106).

Ham, R. J., & Sloane, P. D. (1992). *Primary care geriatrics: A case-based approach.* St. Louis, MO: Mosby-Year Book.

Mears, P. (1994). *Healthcare teams: Building continuous quality improvement.* Delray Beach, FL: St. Lucie Press.

Nahemow, L., & Pousada, L. (1983). *Geriatric diagnostics: A case study approach.* New York: Springer Publishing Co.

Pesznecker, B. L., & Paquin, R. (1982). Implementation of interdisciplinary team practice in home health of geriatric clients. *Journal of Gerontological Nursing, 8,* 504–508.

Pew Health Professions Commission. (1995). *Critical challenges: Revitalizing the health professions for the twenty-first century.* San Francisco: Author.

Pew Health Professions Commission and California Primary Care Consortium. (1995). *Interdisciplinary collaborative teams in primary care: A model curriculum and resource guide.* San Francisco: Pew Health Professions Commission.

Ryan, E. B., with the AGHE Study Section on Interdisciplinary Education. (1994). *Brief bibliography: Interdisciplinary education/teamwork in gerontology and geriatrics.* Washington, DC: Association for Gerontology in Higher Education.

Satin, D. G. (1994). *The clinical care of the aged person: An interdisciplinary perspective.* New York: Oxford University Press.

Scholtes, P. R. (1988). *The team handbook: How to use teams to improve quality.* (Available from P. R. Scholtes, P. O. Box 5445, Madison, WI 53705-0445).

Smoyak, S. A. (1986). Problems in interprofessional relations. In J. E. Steel (Ed.), *Issues in collaborative practice.* Orlando, FL: Grune and Stratton.

Snyder, J. (Ed). (1990). *Interdisciplinary health care teams: Proceedings of the Twelfth Annual Conference.* Indianapolis, IN: School of Allied Health Sciences, Indiana University School of Medicine.

Snyder, J. (Ed). (1991). *Interdisciplinary health care teams: Proceedings of the Thirteenth Annual Conference.* Indianapolis, IN: School of Allied Health Sciences, Indiana University School of Medicine.

Stritter, F. (1993). *Education for interdisciplinary rural health care: Program director's resource manual,* and *Education for interdisciplinary rural health care: The role of the preceptor.* (Available from the School of Education and Medicine, University of North Carolina, CB#7530, 322 MacNider Building, Chapel Hill, NC 27599-7530).

Ulschak, F. (1983). *Human resource development.* Reston, VA: Reston Publishing Co.

Ulschak, F. (1988). *Creating the future of health care education.* Chicago: American Hospital Publishing.

Ulschak, F., & Snowantle, S. (1995). *Team architecture: The manager's guide to designing effective work training.* (Available from the Foundation of the American College of Health Care Executives, Health Administration Press).

University of Colorado Health Sciences Center. (1995). *Interdisciplinary rural teams training project resource manual.* Boulder, CO: The Colorado Area Health Education Center.

University of New Mexico. (1993). *Tool kit for interdisciplinary training grant programs.* Unpublished manuscript.

Waite, M., Harker, J., & Messerman, L. (1994) Interdisciplinary team training and diversity: problems, concepts and strategies. *Gerontology & Geriatrics Education, 15,* 65–82.

Woodcock, M., & Francis, D. (1994). *Teambuilding strategy.* Brookfield, VT: Gower.

Zeiss, A. M., & Steffen, A. M. (1996). Interdisciplinary health care teams: The basic unit of geriatric care. In L. L. Carstensen, B. A. Edelstein, & L. Dornbrand (Eds.), *The practical handbook of clinical gerontology.* Thousand Oaks, CA: Sage.

HGITT TRAINEE BIBLIOGRAPHY BY TOPIC

Interdisciplinary Training—General Information

Pew Health Professions Commission and California Primary Care Consortium. (1995). *Interdisciplinary collaborative teams in primary care: A model curriculum and resource guide.* San Francisco: Pew Health Professions Commission.

Interdisciplinary Team Members

Abramson, J., & Mizrahi, T. (1986). Strategies for enhancing collaboration between social workers and physicians. *Social Work in Health Care, 12,* 1–21.

Clark, P. G. (1994). Social, professional, and educational values on the interdisciplinary team: Implications for gerontological and geriatric education. *Educational Gerontology, 20,* 35–51.

Dane, B. O., & Simon, B. L. (1991). Resident guests: Social workers in host settings. *Social Worker, 36,* 208–213.

Goldstein, M. K. (1989). Physicians and teams. *Geriatric Medicine Annual: 1989,* pp. 256–275.

Lister, L. (1982). Role training for interdisciplinary health teams. *Health and Social Work, 7,* 19–25.

Poole, D. L. (1995). Partnerships buffer and strengthen. *National Association of Social Workers, 20,* 2–4.

Prescott, P. A., & Bowen, S. A. (1985). Physician–nurse relationships. *Annals of Internal Medicine, 103,* 127–133.

Robinson, J. D., Stewart, R. B., & Curry, R. W. (1982). The pharmacist as a member of the primary care team: Experience in a university-based program. *Postgraduate Medicine, 71,* 97–102.

Interdisciplinary Team Development

Billups, J. O. (1987) Interprofessional team process. *Theory Into Practice, 26,* 146–152.

Campbell, L. J., & Cole, K. D. (1987). Geriatric Assessment Teams. *Clinics in Geriatric Medicine, 3,* 99–110.

Drinka, T. J. (1994). Interdisciplinary geriatric teams: Approaches to conflict as indicators of potential to model teamwork. *Educational Gerontology, 20,* 87–108.

Julia, M. C., & Thompson, A. (1994). Essential elements of interprofessional teamwork: Task and maintenance functions. In R. M. Casto, M. C. Julia, L. J. Platt, G. L. Harbaugh, W. R. Waugaman, A. Thompson, T. S. Jost, E. T. Bope, T. Williams, & D. B. Lee (Eds.), *Interprofessional care and collaborative practice* (pp. 43–57). Pacific Grove, CA: Brooks/Cole.

Moulder, P. A., Staal, A. M., & Grant, M. (1988). Making the interdisciplinary team work. *Rehabilitation Nursing, 13,* 338–339.

Tsukuda, R. A. (1989). Interdisciplinary collaboration: Teamwork in geriatrics. In W. H. Green (Ed.), *Management of the frail elderly by the health care team.* St. Louis, MO: W. H. Green.

Ulschak, F. (1983). *Human resource development* (pp. 104–109, 137–143). Reston, VA: Reston Publishing.

Wertheimer, D. S., & Kleinman, L. S. (1990). A model for interdisciplinary discharge planning in a university hospital. *Gerontologist, 30,* 837–840.

Zeiss, A. M., & Steffen, A. M. (1996). Interdisciplinary health care teams: The basic unit of geriatric care. In L. L. Carstensen, B. A. Edelstein, & L. Dornbrand. (Eds.), *The practical handbook of clinical gerontology.* Thousand Oaks, CA: Sage.

Communication

Clark, P. G. (1995). Quality of life, values, and teamwork in geriatric care: Do we communicate what we mean? *Gerontologist, 35,* 402–411.

Pew Health Professions Commission and California Primary Care Consortium (1995). *Interdisciplinary collaborative teams in primary care: A model curriculum and resource guide* (pp. 36–40, 48–48). San Francisco: Pew Health Professions Commission.

Cultural Diversity

Kirchmeyer, C., & Cohen, A. (1992). Multicultural groups: Their performance and reactions with constructive conflict. *Group and Organization Management, 43,* 153–170.

Pachter, L. M. (1994). Culture and clinical care: Folk illness beliefs and behaviors and their implications for health care delivery. *Journal of the American Medical Association, 271,* 690–694.

Putsch, R. W. (1985). Cross-cultural communication: The case of interpreters in health care. *Journal of the American Medical Association, 254,* 3344–3348.

CURRICULUM RESOURCES

Experiential Exercises

Team Building

1. Nahemow & Pousado–Hospital Case, Sophie Milkiewcz
2. Nahemow & Pousado–Rehab. Case #5, Anthony D'Angelo (Clinical & Didactic)
3. Pesznecker & Paquin–Case Study, Mr. L.
4. Pew–Learning Exercises for Students (Clinical & Didactic)
5. Satin–An Interdisciplinary Case Conference
6. Scholtes–Disruptive Group Behavior (Clinical & Didactic)
7. Scholtes–Information Hunt: A Preliminary Look at a Process
8. Scholtes–The Responsibility Matrix (Didactic)
9. Snyder (13th)–Agreement Building: A Syncretistic Approach to Negotiating (Didactic)
10. University of New Mexico (1991)–Case 100: "The Family that Wheezes Together"

Communication

1. Francis & Young–Team Communications (Clinical)
2. Scholtes–Warm Ups, Chapter 7 (Clinical)

Multicultural Issues

1. Nahemow & Pousado–Community Case #10: Chao-Kuang Peng (Didactic)
2. Nahemow & Pousado–Community Case #13: Nauela Cuevas (Didactic)
3. University of Colorado HSC–Appendix 3: Identifying the Value Differences (Didactic)
4. University of Colorado HSC–Appendix 4: Cultural Introductions (Didactic)

Evaluating Team Outcomes

1. Scholtes–Exercise 10: Advanced (Clinical)
2. Scholtes–Exercise 10: Observing Group Process 2–5 (Clinical)
3. Ulschak & Snowantle–Feedback: An Exercise

Section II: Great Lakes GITT Curriculum*

WEEK 1: THE GITT ORIENTATION WORKSHOP

All participants—nursing students, social work students, medical residents, facilitating practitioners, and program faculty—from both Cleveland and Detroit convene at the same place and time for a 2-day seminar designed to:

1. Introduce the GITT program and its principal goals and objectives
2. Establish the major themes for the program: Specifically, the five domains covered by the curriculum—interdisciplinary teamwork, care of elders, culture and communications, continual improvement, and managed care; of these, interdisciplinary teamwork will be the principal focus
3. Orient all participants to the general structure of the curriculum, the specific activities they will be involved in, and the program schedule
4. Orient participants to their respective roles and responsibilities within the program and inform them of our general performance expectations
5. Allow each participant to complete a focused self-assessment of his or her own learning needs and to draft a personal learning plan for the remainder of the program
6. Provide initial bonding experiences for learning team members (nursing student, social work student, medical resident, practitioner–facilitator) and establish formal learning partnerships between individual teams from each city
7. Allow each team to identify an integrated work project—a collaborative effort to learn enough about one particular aspect of interdisciplinary teamwork to be able to return to the larger group at the end of the program and teach others about it
8. Provide initial training in the use of techniques to conduct effective meetings
9. Allow distribution of core program materials and instruction in using the program syllabus and study guide
10. Provide hands-on training in the use of specific electronic media (see below), which will be used to support communications between all participants and learning sites (see Table A.4 and A.5)

Note. From Great Lakes GITT Planning Year Curriculum, by GITT Resource Center, Division of Nursing, New York University, 1996, New York: GITT Resource Center. Copyright 1996 by GITT Resource Center. Reprinted by permission.

TABLE A.4 Curriculum for Introductory Workshop for Great Lakes GITT Interdisciplinary Teamwork for the Care of Older Patients and Their Families

Objectives	Content (topics)	Teaching methods faculty/time frame	Evaluation
ID learning teams: On completion of the Introductory Workshop, the participants will be able to:			
1. Discuss the use of team care to provide health services for older persons.	Definition of teams Types of teams When to form a team Values, attitudes and expectations about teams	Faculty: N. Wadsworth Readings (assigned beforehand) & discussion In-class team discussions using team values/expectations exercises	Learner self-assessment (1 hr.)
2. Describe the history and underlying philosophy of teamwork in caring for older adults.	(a) history of teamwork in geriatric care (b) philosophy of teamwork in geriatric care		
3. Relate the differences between multidisciplinary and interdisciplinary teamwork in caring for older adults and their families.	Definitions of interdisciplinary and multidisciplinary	(90 min.)	
4. Demonstrate the ability to use teamwork structures and processes.	7-step meeting process Team roles Ladder of Inference Dialogue techniques Giving and receiving feedback	Faculty: S. Moore, N. Wadsworth, M. B. Tupper Group practice exercises—team roles in class (45 min)	Team self-analysis using specified criteria
5. Describe features and functions of a learning team.	Mental models Use of experimental cycles for improvement of team functioning	Faculty: S. Moore Storyboard examples (45 min)	

TABLE A.4 *(Continued)*

Objectives	Content (topics)	Teaching methods faculty/time frame	Evaluation
6. Develop a first learning team goal/project.		In-class team meetings using structured agenda on team learning goal/project with facilitators present In-class discussion of process of using a structured instrument (2 hrs)	Analysis of team goals/projects
Cultural & communication issues			
1. Describe how culture affects a team member's own perspective, values and beliefs, including barriers to understanding communication they have experienced with people from other cultures or ethnic groups	(a) Definition of cultural terms (b) Understanding cultural stereotypes (c) Cultural self-awareness (d) Communicating with persons from other cultures	Faculty: P. Anderson, C. Hyduk, N. Wadsworth, E. Duffy Readings, lecture & discussion Videotaped scenario of patient situation (1.5 hr)	Discussion of video example using specified criteria
Clinical process improvement			
1. Describe the concept of quality and value applied to health care, in particular, the interdependence of four dimension: clinical quality, functional status, client satisfaction against need, and total costs	(a) Clinical quality (b) Functional status (c) Satisfaction/need expectation (d) Understanding cost	Faculty: L. Seriguchi Readings, lecture, & group discussion; group exercise; case study	
2. Examine the meaning and significance of "customer focus" for health care professionals and health care institutions, including	(a) Identification of all customer groups (b) Diversity of needs (c) Organization commitment to customer	Readings & group discussion Group exercise on customer needs Group work on organization's mission, values	

(cont.)

TABLE A.4   Curriculum for Introductory Workshop for Great Lakes GITT Interdisciplinary Teamwork for the Care of Older Patients and Their Families *(Continued)*

Objectives	Content (topics)	Teaching methods faculty/time frame	Evaluation
identification of the needs and expectations of customer groups		(45 min)	
Technology to support learning teams			
1. Demonstrate use of the communication information systems to be used among team members and across team learning sites	Technology to facilitate learning and team communication: (a) E-mail software (b) WEB site for this project (c) Interactive videos (d) "Interactive patient"	Faculty: P. Whitehouse Demonstration with return demonstrations (45 min)	Successful return demonstrations
Geriatrics in the managed care environment			
1. Describe common geriatric health & social problems and and management strategies	(a) Common social problems of older persons and their families (b) Common health problems of older persons and their families	Faculty: A. Early, J. Wisniewski, B. Zarowitz Introduction to interdisciplinary case-study approach using the "interactive patient"	Assessment of team outcomes on case method study
2. Explain the fundamental relationship between cost-reduction and quality improvement in health care	Quality and value in health care	Readings & group discussion	
3. Describe practical methods for adapting team function to a managed care environment	Examples of successful interdisciplinary teamwork in managed care organizations	Readings & discussion	Workshop evaluation (30 min)
4. Describe the key determinants of interdisciplinary team success in managed care settings	Determinants of team success in managed care organizations	(2.5 hr)	

TABLE A.5 Curriculum for Field Teamwork Experience for Great Lakes GITT Interdisciplinary Teamwork for the Care of Older Patients and Their Families

Objectives	Content (topics)	Teaching methods (time frame)	Evaluation[*]
Team skills: On completion of a 8-month field teamwork experience, the participants will be able to:			
1. Demonstrate use of techniques for team building and decision-making	Team-building activities Team decision-making techniques Team techniques to support patient outcomes	Readings & activities from Learning Guide Experiential group building exercises (4 1-hr group learning sessions with facilitator)	Team self-analysis using specified criteria Minute Paper
2. Demonstrate the ability to participate in and lead teams	7-step meeting process Team roles/tasks	Weekly practice of team member and team leader roles during team meetings	Team self-analysis
3. Demonstrate the ability to give and receive constructive feedback	Principles of giving and receiving constructive feedback	Weekly practice during team meetings	Team self-analysis using specified criteria
4. Use dialogue techniques in team communication	Ladder of inference Dialogue techniques	Readings from Learning Guide Group practice exercises Weekly practice during team meetings	Feedback from facilitator
5. Demonstrate use of interpersonal skills that are useful in managing conflict	Types of differences Interpersonal skills to manage conflict Establishment of team ground rules for managing conflict	Readings & activities from Learning Guide Group discussion (2 1-hr group learning sessions with facilitator)	Minute Paper Team self-analysis using specified criteria
Interdisciplinary work:			
1. In their work with the interdisciplinary team, analyze the contributions of each discipline and culture	Interdisciplinary versus multidisciplinary approaches When interdisciplinary teams are most effective	Readings & discussion from Learning Guide	Team self-evaluations using specified criteria

(cont.)

TABLE A.5 Curriculum for Field Teamwork Experience for Great Lakes GITT Interdisciplinary Teamwork for the Care of Older Patients and Their Families (*Continued*)

Objectives	Content (topics)	Teaching methods (time frame)	Evaluation[*]
to the group project, evaluate the success of these efforts, and identify ways to improve collaborative efforts			
2. Revises opinions and decisions based on consideration of contribution of other disciplines and cultural groups.	(a) Active listening to opinions of others (b) Techniques to obtain opinions of all members of the team	Practice in weekly team meetings	Feedback from facilitator Team self-evaluation of decisions made
3. Incorporate patients and families as members of the team	(a) Assessing patient and family readiness for team involvement (b) Techniques for successful inclusion of patients and families in team meetings	Readings & group discussions Videotape examples Participates in family meetings (2 1-hr learning sessions)	Evaluation of behavior in teams by facilitator using specified criteria Videotape analysis using specified criteria
Learning teams:			
1. Design and conduct experimental cycles to improve interdisciplinary teamwork	(a) Rapid cycles for learning (b) Mental models (c) Assessment of team functional level & use of group techniques (d) Identify opportunities for improvement in team's functioning (e) PDCA cycles (Plan-Do-Check-Act) (f) Evaluate improvements the team has made or plans to make in its functioning	Clinical teams do team functioning improvement process projects Team storyboard Facilitator assistance in team improvement process	Number and type of learning cycles Report by team of lessons learned from learning cycle Team self-analysis using specified criteria

TABLE A.5 *(Continued)*

Objectives	Content (topics)	Teaching methods (time frame)	Evaluation[*]
Cultural and communication issues:			
1. Demonstrate selected communication skills and describe their impact on the satisfaction of the older patient and family	(a) Principles of communication (b) Communication styles; verbal and nonverbal (c) Barriers to provider/patient communication	Readings & small-group discussions from Learning Guides	Team self-analysis using specified criteria Facilitator feedback
2. Evaluate existing team and individual communication skills, style of communication and readiness for change.	(a) Inventory of communication skills (b) Disciplinary jargon (c) Importance of team communication to team effectiveness	Small-group discussions Video & role play of provider and patient interactions using "interactive patient"	Team self-analysis Facilitator feedback
3. Use cultural information elicited from patients/ families in the selection of intervention and treatment approaches that are most appropriate for the patient/ family's socio-cultural circumstances	(a) Concepts of health and illness (b) Cultural beliefs related to self-care and healing practices (c) Potential barriers to the formal health care delivery system (d) Patient-driven care processes developed through patient communication	Readings & small-group exercises centered around the patient information collected	Team self-assessment using specified criteria including data collected from patient outcomes
4. Demonstrate the consideration of ethical dilemmas in the care of older persons in team decision making	(a) Ethics as a decision-making process in long-term care (b) Autonomy of the caregiver vs. the patient (c) Limits to self-determination (d) Direct vs. delegated autonomy	Readings & discussions of videotaped case studies Guest speakers (2–3 1-hr learning sessions with facilitator) First Class self-instructional materials	Presentations of decision-making processes

(cont.)

TABLE A.5 Curriculum for Field Teamwork Experience for Great Lakes GITT Interdisciplinary Teamwork for the Care of Older Patients and Their Families (*Continued*)

Objectives	Content (topics)	Teaching methods (ime frame)	Evaluation[*]
	(e) Issues of reciprocity (f) End-of-life care (g) Advance directives (h) Informed consent; refusal of treatment		
Clinical process improvement			
1. Describe the historical background of approaches to quality assessment and improvement in health care—for example, regulatory legislative and voluntary approaches—including both successes and failures	(a) History of concept of quality (b) Regulations (e.g., JCAHO) (c) Current efforts to improve (e.g., HEDIS)	Readings & discussion (1 1-hr learning session)	
2. Demonstrate use of the continuous quality improvement process	(a) Use of process analysis tools, e.g., flow charts and Pareto diagrams (b) Data collection methods for measurements and improvement (c) Use of statistical tools such as control charts (d) PDCA cycles (e) Group work for effective CQI	Readings & discussion from Learning Guide Team learning project throughout field experience Personal Improvement Workbooks	Storyboard analysis of CQI project using specified criteria
3. Demonstrate the use of patient management information systems team and communication technology	(a) Patient management systems (b) Learning systems, searches (c) Communication networks	Readings & discussion Practice using for team projects and patient care (3 1-hr learning sessions)	Self-assessment

TABLE A.5 *(Continued)*

Objectives	Content (topics)	Teaching methods (time frame)	Evaluation[*]
Managed care:			
1. Explain the structural elements and evolutionary history of Managed Care Organizations (MCOs)	Evolution of corporate medicine Functional definitions of managed care Taxonomy of MCOs Overview of the managed care 'industry'	Lecture discussion Readings from study guide Structured journalizing by learners	
2. Explain the fundamental economics and finances of MCOs	Capitation economics Medicare risk contracting Restrictions of choice Effects on patient and provider behavior	Care discussion Readings & discussion	
3. Describe MCO approaches to conserving resources and reducing cost	Rationale for utilization control systems How MCO costs break down Approaches to reducing hospital costs Approaches to reducing ambulatory costs Special considerations for older populations	Readings & discussion from Learning Guide	
4. Describe MCO approaches to assuring and improving quality	Quality & value in health care Relationship to cost containment Evolution of quality assurance in health care Current popular approaches	Readings & discussion from Learning Guide	Self-assessment
5. Discuss the fundamental ethical issues in managed care	Autonomy, beneficence, and justice as core issues The virtuous provider The virtuous MCO	Readings & discussion from Learning Guide	Facilitator feedback

(cont.)

TABLE A.5   Curriculum for Field Teamwork Experience for Great Lakes GITT Interdisciplinary Teamwork for the Care of Older Patients and Their Families *(Continued)*

Objectives	Content (topics)	Teaching methods (time frame)	Evaluation[*]
6. Describe team opportunities and lessons for success in MCOs	Examples of successful interdisciplinary teamwork in MCOs Interdisciplinary population management Organizational barriers and opportunities Determinants of team success in MCOs	Readings & discussion from Learning Guide	Facilitator feedback

Care of elders:

Objectives	Content (topics)	Teaching methods (time frame)	Evaluation[*]
1. Describe changes that occur with aging including physical, psychosocial, and functional	(a) Physical changes (b) Functional changes (c) Psychosocial changes	Readings: 1. Kane, R., Ouslander, J., & Abrass, I. D. (1994). *Essentials of clinical geriatrics,* (3rd ed., Chp. 1). New York: McGraw Hill. 2. Articles	Participation in group discussion and case studies
2. Identify clinical implications of the aging process	Clinical implications of aging 1. physical 2. functional 3. psychosocial	Case studies	Self-evaluation
3. Identify common ethical issues	Common ethical issues (a) Advanced directives and living wills (b) Competency (c) Informed consent (d) Refusal of treatment (e) Resource allocation	Case studies Group discussion Readings: 1. Selected articles 2. Kane, R., Ouslander, J., & Abrass, I. D. (1994). (Chp. 18). *Essentials of clinical geriatrics.* New York: McGraw-Hill.	Participation in discussion for each ethical issue Self-evaluation

TABLE A.5 *(Continued)*

Objectives	Content (topics)	Teaching methods (time frame)	Evaluation[*]

4. Identify different approaches to assessing elderly persons and their support system's capacity for care	(a) Physical functioning, i.e., ADL, IADL
	(b) Mental status
	(c) Social functioning
		Readings:
		  Kane et al. (1994). (pp. 44–79).
		Activities:
		  Team activity at clinical site:
		  As a team, complete a physical and mental and social functioning assessment (3 hr)
			Self-evaluation

5. Identify common geriatric health problems and their management strategies	Common health problems and management strategies (a) urinary incontinence (b) falls (c) cognitive impairment (d) immobility (e) inadequate nutrition	Readings 1. Kane et al. (1994). (Chp. 5, 4–12, selected sections).	Participation in group discussion Self-evaluation

[*] Course evaluation will also include participants', faculty, and facilitator evaluation of the course objectives and methods.

Major Activities During the GITT Orientation Workshop

Foundation of Learning Teams and Creation of Team Partnerships

Individual participants meet their assigned team members, including facilitators, and spend time getting acquainted before formal instructional activities begin. Bonding continues as the newly formed teams work together on specific exercises built into the 2-day agenda (see below). Each team is also be asked to select a partner team from the other city (Cleveland or Detroit). These partners collaborate in the completion of an integrated work project (see below) or other joint learning activity.

Presentation of an Interactive Narrative

This establishes the major themes for the program, illustrates the linkages between the major curricular domains, and serves as a focusing device for the self-assessment process and creation of personal learning agendas.

We tell a story in which we follow the experiences of two or three sets of elderly individuals and their friends and families over the course of a year. We begin by introducing the first pair of characters in our drama—a middle-class elderly couple (the Wilsons) with a specific set of health problems and social circumstances—and follow their adventures as they decide to enroll in a Medicare-risk contract, a decision that moves them out of the care stream with their regular physician (a practitioner in a traditional indemnity network) and into an integrated (and managed) health care system. As the Wilsons experience some of the more common health and social problems of older people, they initially receive care under a multidisciplinary paradigm and suffer some setbacks and missed opportunities as a consequence.

Later in the story, the Wilsons move under the care of an interdisciplinary team, and their subsequent experiences are used to highlight the major features and advantages of such care, as well as some of its difficulties. The story itself, a sort of rolling case study, provides many opportunities to go off on tangents to explore the background stories of other characters in the drama, the professionals working in traditional multidisciplinary clinics, interdisciplinary team members, the people running the health maintenance organization (HMO) and delivery system, and so on. Short didactic tangents appear, as well: "By the way, just what is this risk-contract the Wilsons just signed up for? Well, Medicare risk contracting is a program first established in...and so forth." The story of the Wilsons ends when Mrs. Wilson suffers a massive and severely debilitating stroke, and Mr. Wilson and the interdisciplinary team members are faced with some difficult decisions regarding her care during the final part of her life.

As the Wilsons progress through the healthcare system, they encounter fellow travelers in the persons of their next-door-neighbor, Mr. Cavender, a down-and-out, medically frail old man, alone in the world and rapidly deteriorating; the Clarkstons, an extended minority family of very limited means, whose matriarch is chronically and severely ill; as well as some others. Each has an individual storyline, into which we can detour when it intersects the story of the Wilsons, or return to once the Wilson story is concluded.

All events described in these storylines are based on actual cases and situations, drawn from the experiences of our faculty and cleaned up and composited to facilitate instruction.

Shaggy-dog tales are extremely long and very detailed stories, generally built around comparatively weak jokes. The real pleasure of the experience resides in the recitation of the detail and anticipation of the punchline. Our shaggy-dog narrative technique uses the detail to impart information relevant to each of our major curricular domains and replaces the joke with important lessons and messages regarding interdisciplinary team care for the older persons. The story device holds the audience's attention, and also allows members to participate: "Okay, so now we find that the HMO is telling Mr. Wilson he can no longer see his previous doctor for care. Why would they do that? Are they trying to upset him? What do you think is going on here?"

The stories of the Wilsons, the Clarkstons, Mr. Cavender, and all the other characters in the drama are told jointly by project faculty from both cities, working from a detailed and rehearsed script (an example of interdisciplinary teaching). There are one or two narrators to present the main storylines and a Greek chorus of faculty content experts to handle the tangential background material. The script and storyline reunite and integrate the core content of each of the major learning domains, and this approach is intended to highlight the connections between interdisciplinary team care, communications skills, cultural considerations, health care improvement, managed care, and so on. We believe integration of material from the five domains is essential to the success of the orientation workshop. Approximately 4 to 6 hours are needed to complete the tale, but it is broken up into segments (acts) and interspersed with the activities described below.

This instructional method, which to the best of our knowledge is not in widespread use, is one of the principal instructional approaches used in the HFHS Managed Care College's 1996–1997 curriculum. The prototype, One Year In the Life of an HMO Family, has already been used successfully for multiple audiences.

Structured Self-Assessment and Development of Personal and Group Learning Agendas

At selected points in our narrative and at other times during the orientation session, we pause the activity in progress and ask learners to reflect on a short series of questions that will help them focus on their own learning needs. For example, on concluding the act or chapter in the story of the Wilsons in which they decide to enroll in a Medicare risk program, we might ask learners to rate their own level of agreement with the following statements:

- I can clearly explain the basics of traditional Medicare insurance coverage.
- I can clearly explain the basics elements of Medicare risk programs.
- I can clearly explain the major considerations people commonly make when choosing health insurance coverage.
- I am well-prepared to discuss the choice of health insurance coverage with my own patients.

Later, when Mr. Wilson "falls through the cracks" in a traditional multidisciplinary care clinic, and is rescued from his predicament by an interdisciplinary care team, we might pause the story again and assess learners' agreement with the following:

- I can clearly explain the major differences between multidisciplinary care and interdisciplinary care.
- I can clearly explain the major advantages interdisciplinary team care has over multidisciplinary approaches.
- I can clearly identify the steps needed to establish an effective interdisciplinary care team.
- I am ready to participate as a fully effective member of an interdisciplinary care team.

A tangent to this particular act is exposition of the background story of how the interdisciplinary care team that eventually assumed responsibility for the Wilsons' care came into existence, including some of the major problems and obstacles they faced. We model it on the actual history of existing interdisciplinary teams.

Participants record their responses on a worksheet. During the second day of the orientation seminar, they are given time to review their worksheets, reflect on their answers, and write their own core learning agendas for the duration of the GITT program. They use a standardized format do this. In addition, each learning team convenes to share the results of their individual assessments and individual learning objectives and draws on them to draft a set of learning goals and objectives for the group as a whole.

Assigning Integrated Work Projects

Once individual team members have drafted their personal learning agendas and selected a set of learning goals and objectives for the entire team, they are told that each team is also responsible for designing and completing an integrated work project. The project helps them explore selected aspects of interdisciplinary team care in depth, work together as a team to produce a tangible product, and allows them to share what they have learned with other participants in the program. Project options might include writing a research paper about an important dimension of team care; observing, analyzing, and commenting on the growth and development of their own team (a team-journal approach); or tracking and reporting on the experiences of a particular patient or group of patients within their own practices. At the end of the program year, those who select either of the latter two options may translate their work into the narrative instructional format described earlier and use it for their final presentation to the group.

Introduction of Essential Meeting Skills

Drafting group-learning goals, objectives, and work projects gives nascent interdisciplinary teams their first opportunity to work together toward a common end. These exercises are used to introduce them formally to techniques for conducting effective meetings. They will be instructed in these techniques before each of the exercises described above and debriefed afterward. The interdisciplinary team workgroup has recommended for this purpose the use of an explicit 7-step process for managing meetings and group discussions.

Instruction in Electronic Communications

Electronic communications are the principal means of keeping participants engaged and on track once they return to their respective cities, institutions, and worksites. We have considered three possible platforms: Virtual Campus, the automated teleconferencing system used at CWRU for educational purposes; a GITT website; and Lotus Notes®, the groupware platform presently in use within the Group Practice Improvement Network. The latter two have the advantages of a visual user interface and data transmission capabilities.

We recommend the use of a single platform: Using two or all three would probably result in confusion and miscommunication, requiring participants to log in regularly to them all in order not to miss something important. We provide hands-on training in a special computer lab during the orientation workshop.

Review of Program Schedule and Site-Based Learning Activities

On completion of the orientation workshop, participants return to their respective worksites for the duration of the program. Learning at the worksites is guided in three ways:

1. *Facilitators:* They are responsible for monitoring and fostering the growth of desirable skills and behaviors within their assigned teams. Facilitators are coached most closely by GITT Project members who have joined the interdisciplinary teams workgroup, but also receive input from the continual improvement, culture and communications, care of the elderly, and managed care groups.

2. *Syllabus and study guide:* This is the student-learners' bible, containing a week-by-week schedule of learning activities, including assigned readings, problem sets, group exercises, and similar activities. A think-and-do book for adult learners, the syllabus and study guide also prompts learners to call Virtual Campus or log on through Lotus Notes to hear the latest news about the program; find tips for completing exercises, problem sets, and work projects; and participate in special teleconferencing activities, such as presentation and discussion of special case studies. Each of the five curriculum domain workgroups has developed study guide material for each week of the program.

3. *Electronic communications:* This is the principal means by which faculty responsible for each of the five learning domains transmits essential new information and instructions to learners. Teleconferencing capabilities allow learners to communicate with each other between sites as needed, and we encourage such communication wherever we are able. Distance learning approaches are becoming more prevalent and are in routine use by several master's degree programs in health administration, a few medical schools, and other university-based programs.

The final portion of the Orientation Workshop orients learning teams to the use of the syllabus and study guide and establishes the general weekly schedule of activities for the rest of the program.

WEEKS 2–39: EXPERIENTIAL LEARNING THROUGH GITT

On completion of the orientation workshop, learners return to their respective institutions and worksites and do most of their learning in the company of their own team members and practitioner–facilitators. Three-member student teams join practitioners/ facilitators at separate clinical worksites to spend approximately 4 hours each week involved in direct patient care and 1 hour meeting to discuss their learning experiences, work on their assignments, and practice team skills.

Each week, learners are prompted by their facilitators and the syllabus & study guide to do one or more of the following:

1. Complete assigned readings from each of the major curriculum domains
2. Complete written practice problems, group discussion exercises related to the readings, or both
3. Review an instructional videotape
4. Fill in another section of the weekly learning diary included in their study guide
5. Continue work on their team's integrated work project
6. Use our preferred electronic forum to participate in special learning activities or receive new information

Where our curriculum requires didactic lectures, we distribute videotapes to individual learning teams or try set up a live videoconference.

A standard two-semester academic year (i.e., about 9–10 continuous months) is required to accomplish all major objectives identified for each of the major learning domains.

WEEK 40: GITT SHARED LEARNING SEMINAR

The wrap-up session reunites all participants in the program for a 1½ or 2 day seminar that includes:

1. Formal presentation of integrated work projects and lessons learned in doing them
2. Group discussions of the major issues and lessons learned in interdisciplinary team care and the care of older people using learners' journals as the principal basis for discussion
3. Presentation of a new interactive narrative, this time built around the actual experiences of GITT learners and the patients they cared for and presented by the student-learners, rather than the faculty
4. Focus group activities designed to solicit recommendations for improving the GITT learning experience for the next group of participants.

Section III: Minnesota GITT— Complex Case #9—Betsy Jones*

Mrs. Jones was referred to a geriatric ambulatory clinic by her primary care physician, who was leaving the community. She is 76, Caucasian, divorced for many years, and lives in a two-bedroom, subsidized, handicapped accessible apartment with her 43-year-old daughter, who is currently unemployed, and her 13-year-old granddaughter. Mrs. Jones states that she depends on her daughter and is satisfied with their relationship, although they disagree at times on the best way to raise her granddaughter. She has a high school education and worked as a legal secretary until her retirement. She states she drank her way out of many jobs. She quit drinking when she had a stroke 11 years ago. She has been wheelchair-bound since then, and currently uses a motorized wheelchair. She has been treated for depression with fluoxetine since her stroke and is also taking acetaminophen/oxycodone three times a day for pain control. Mrs. Jones comes alone to clinic visits using Metro Mobility. The team told Mrs. Jones that her daughter was welcome to accompany her to the clinic, however, a brief phone conversation with the daughter led the team to believe she was not interested in coming in because "my mother never follows doctor's orders anyway."

At the initial visit to the Senior Clinic, Mrs. Jones said she wanted help with the following problems: a loss of bladder control (she complains that she has had to start wearing incontinence pads because she usually has a sudden urge to urinate and then it's already too late to get into the bathroom; she denies pain or burning with urination); sleep problems (she goes to bed at 11 P.M., but complains that her mind keeps going and going at night; she sometimes has wild dreams; she's fearful of people breaking into the apartment at the subsidized complex where she lives; she rarely leaves her apartment, watches TV in her wheelchair most of the day, and usually takes a morning and an afternoon nap to make up for lost sleep); and trouble getting around (daughter has back problems and can't help much with transferring; patient has had several falls in past year while attempting independent transferring, has pain in both hips and in knees that improves with use of pain medications, is just generally weaker since she's been in the wheelchair).

Other data obtained during the history include dietary intake of approximately one pot of coffee per day; she smokes 2 packs of cigarettes per day.

---

*Note. From *University of Minnesota Planning Your Curriculum,* by GITT Resource Center, Division of Nursing, New York University, 1996, New York: GITT Resource Center. Copyright 1996 by GITT Resource Center.

Medications

1. Fluoxetine 20 mg every day
2. Acetaminophen/oxycodone 1 every 4–6 hr as needed (but she takes 1 three times a day)
3. HCTZ/triamterene 1 capsule every day
4. Folate 1 mg every day
5. Extra strength aspirin with caffeine at bedtime

On Examination

She is an obese, older female who appears somewhat jittery and nervous; height = 5′3″, weight = 175 lbs., afebrile, blood pressure = 145/80, pulse = 72, respirations = 16. Only positive findings are as follows:

- Some areas of redness and excoriation on buttocks, no measurable open areas.
- Musculoskeletal: Knees are enlarged bilaterally, no increased warmth, mild flexion contractures at right knee and hip, otherwise range of motion of extremities is good.
- Neurologic: General decreased strength of upper and lower extremities. Right side is somewhat weaker than left. Is unable to stand up without assistance. Cannot demonstrate walking more than 2 steps with the assistance of two people. Didn't bring walker to clinic because she hasn't used it in a long time.
- Mental status: Scores 25 of 30 on Mini-Mental State Examination (MMSE); has difficulty copying figures, misses two points on calculations, gets 2 of 3 words on recall, and misses 1 orientation question (date).

Task

1. Identify a main problem and goal for Mrs. Jones
2. Develop a care plan to achieve this goal
3. Identify two to three specific issues for team consultation

Note, for this assignment:

- You are to independently examine this case—you should not consult with other student/learner team members
- You are strongly encouraged to consult with your discipline-specific mentor at the clinic
- You are strongly encouraged to consult with at least one other mentor of another discipline at the clinic

FACULTY INFORMATION ONLY

Objective for this Case

Students should recognize that previous health care providers plans likely did not consider the patient's values or goals, leading to noncompliance. The team should recognize that the patient and family are an essential part of the team and take care to negotiate a plan of care with the patient. The team will need to determine what the patient is willing to do and how she would hope to reach those goals. It is most important that all students are able to identify the need to make joint plans and goals with the patient and daughter.

Additional Faculty Information

Overarching concerns from the interdisciplinary perspective:

1. Difficulty maintaining independence due to multiple factors:
   - limited mobility, obesity, fatigue and incontinence
   - mental health issues
   - poor family dynamics
   - lack of motivation on the part of the patient
2. Goal of keeping patient in the community by improving above problems.

Interdisciplinary Plan of Care (may include the following; this is not meant to be an exhaustive list)

Medical

Impairment: History of stroke; extent of stroke ill-defined. She has been in a wheelchair since the event. Physical exam suggests right lower extremity weakness/paralysis. She was able to take several steps.
Disability: Impaired mobility.
Intervention: Physical therapy consult for increased exercise endurance and transfer training. This should also help to define the extent of the physical impairment related to the stroke. Obtain further history regarding activities of daily living and instrumental activities of daily living.

Impairment: Knee and hip pain. Again, this is somewhat ill-defined in the case history. Pain improved with pain medication. A list of previously attempted interventions is not given, nor is there a very detailed pain history (quality, quantity, relieving/aggravating factors, radiation of pain, course of illness).
Disability: Likely contributes to her immobility and weakness.
Intervention: Avoid narcotic pain relievers, especially given her history of substance abuse. Discontinue extra-strength aspirin and taper or discontinue acetaminophen/oxycodone; Switch to 650 to 1000 mg acetaminophen three to four times daily.

Impairment: Urinary incontinence; history suggests a combination of both urge incontinence with a functional component. The fact that she has the urge to void would suggest that the stroke has not caused a neurogenic problem. No comment regarding loss of urine with activities (i.e., stress). The learners should recognize that HCTZ/triamterene is probably contributing to the incontinence.

Disability: Incontinence.
Intervention: Evaluate need for the diuretic. Have the patient start on a scheduled toileting plan. A trial of ditropan may be warranted, but both the nurse practitioner and physician should recognize that this alone will not solve the functional problems of transferring to the toilet.

Occupational therapy consult for a home visit to check on the placement of bars near the toilet and make recommendations for the use of a bedside commode during the night.

Impairment: Falls likely related to her functional impairment (weakness/paralysis). The falls do raise one's concern regarding safety.
Disability: Safety concerns.
Intervention: Physical therapy consult as above, consider Life Line (emergency response notification system).

Impairment: Borderline cognitive impairment (MMSE 25/30) with no specific mention of concern regarding memory from patient or family.
Disability: Many if loss progresses.
Intervention: Consider evaluation of reversible causes (complete blood count; syphilis test, thyroid-stimulating hormone, electrolyte imbalance), repeat MMSE over time.

Impairment: Insomnia, again not described well, she has difficulty falling asleep because mind keeps going. She is sedentary and naps during the day. Caffeine intake is moderate. The causes are multiple: age related, unrelieved pain, caffeine intake, poor sleep hygiene, and depression. Fluoxetine is a stimulating antidepressant with a long half-life (2–3 days). It can cause bad dreams and sleep problems. Aspirin with caffeine is not a good choice for a bedtime pain medication.
Disability: Poor sleep will have an adverse effect on almost all aspects of daily life.
Intervention: Consider changing antidepressants. Control pain if present. Discuss age related sleep changes so that patient is realistic regarding sleep. The gerontological nurse practitioner student should also recommend nursing interventions to improve sleep including reducing daytime napping, increasing daytime activities, reducing time spent in bed.

Emotional

Impairment: History of depression; from the history we are told that she has been treated for depression since the stroke, however, we are not given anything about previous psychiatric history. Difficulty sleeping is noted. Television seems to be her major source of entertainment. We don't know if she rarely leaves her apartment because of fear or lack of interest. On physical examination, affect is nervous.
Disability: Depression will have an adverse effect on almost all aspects of daily life.
Intervention: Consider changing her antidepressant for the reasons discussed above. The team needs to take a much more detailed history and explore the client's social/recreational needs and interest.

Social

Impairment: Dysfunctional family dynamics. There does not really seem to be enough in the history to say much about the family dynamics.

Intervention: Determine social history and, in particular, family dynamics. What are goals and needs for the family unit? How do they interact with each other? What is impact of client's addiction on family? Explore possibility of family conference that would involve problem solving and goals setting for each member about care plan, contracting, and monitoring.

Environmental

Impairment: Dangerous neighborhood and the patient worries about crime in her subsidized housing complex.

Disability: May be contributing to her isolation and depression.

Intervention: Explore the reality of the patient's fears.

Impairment: Decreased mobility.

Intervention: Occupational therapy evaluation for assistive devices that will aid the client in performing daily activities.

Economic

Impairment: Low-income status, and one may assume that the patient is dependent on a fixed low income.

Intervention: Need for financial assessment. Does patient qualify for medical assistance? Explore problem of unemployment. Can family be linked to further resources?

Section I: Core Measures for the GITT Program

The John A. Hartford Foundation
Geriatric Interdisciplinary Team Training Program (GITT)
DEMOGRAPHIC QUESTIONNAIRE: TRAINEE VERSION

Instructions:
* Your answers are confidential and will be reported only in grouped data.
* Use a dark blue or black pen (not pencil) to complete questionnaire.
* Print in capital letters as shown.

| A | B | C | D | E | F | G | H | I | J | K | L | M | N | O | P | Q | R | S | T | U | V | W | X | Y | Z |

* Unless otherwise instructed, choose only one response to each question/statement.
* Fill in bubbles completely as shown.   correct wrong wrong
* Do not fold or staple the pages.
* Make no stray marks on the questionnaire.

ID [ ][ ][ ][ ][ ]   Project ID [ ][ ]   Today's Date [ ][ ] / [ ][ ] / [ ][ ]
                                                          MONTH   DAY   YEAR
FIRST LETTER of last name plus
LAST 4 DIGITS of Social Security No.   Clinical Setting ID [ ][ ][ ][ ]

What is your student status?   ○ Full Time   TDEMO1
                                ○ Part Time
                                ○ Other -specify [ ][ ][ ][ ][ ][ ][ ][ ][ ][ ]   TDEMO1A

Enrolled in?   ○ Academic Degree Program   TDEMO2
                ○ Residency Program
                ○ Other -specify [ ][ ][ ][ ][ ][ ][ ][ ][ ][ ]   TDEMO2A

If you have worked for pay, how many years
have you worked predominantly with older patients   - in geriatrics? [ ][ ]   TDEMO3
(please respond to each)
                                                     - with teams? [ ][ ]   TDEMO4

Have you ever received any formal training in gerontology or geriatrics
before this team training program?   ○ Yes   ○ No   TDEMO5

What formal training in gerontology or geriatrics have you completed? (Mark all that apply) TDEMO6

- ◯ ANA Gerontological certification exam
- ◯ Certificate of added qualification in geriatrics
- ◯ Bachelors Degree in Geriatrics/Gerontology
- ◯ Masters Degree in Geriatrics/Gerontology
- ◯ Minor in Geriatrics/Gerontology
- ◯ Conferences, Workshops, Continuing Education
- ◯ None
- ◯ Certificate Program in Geriatrics/Gerontology
- ◯ Geriatric Education Center Programs
- ◯ Individual Course(s) in Geriatrics/Gerontology
- ◯ Geriatrics Rotation
- ◯ Other - specify

TDEMO6AA

Have you ever received any team training before this program?   ◯ Yes   ◯ No   TDEMO7

If yes, about how many hours?   TDEMO7A

If you hold a job, what is your primary place of employment?   TDEMO8

- ◯ Ambulatory Care/Outpatient Clinic
- ◯ Government (Non VA)
- ◯ Government (VA)
- ◯ Group Medical Practice
- ◯ Home Care
- ◯ Hospice
- ◯ Hospital
- ◯ Individual Medical Practice
- ◯ Medical School
- ◯ Nursing Home
- ◯ Nursing School
- ◯ Other Health Professions Schools
- ◯ School of Public Health
- ◯ School of Social Work
- ◯ Other - specify

TDEMO8A

Are you currently working in a managed health care organization?   ◯ Yes   ◯ No   TDEMO9

What degrees/certifications do you currently hold? (Mark all that apply)   TDEMO10

- ◯ B.A.
- ◯ B.S.
- ◯ B.S.N.
- ◯ B.S.W.
- ◯ R.N.
- ◯ CNP
- ◯ CNS
- ◯ M.A.
- ◯ M.S.
- ◯ M.S.N.
- ◯ M.S.W.
- ◯ M.Ed.
- ◯ M.P.H.
- ◯ M.D.
- ◯ Ph.D.
- ◯ Ed.D.
- ◯ D.P.H.
- ◯ D.S.W.
- ◯ D.N.Sc / N.D.
- ◯ D.Pharm.
- ◯ D.D.S.
- ◯ Psy.D.
- ◯ Other - specify

TDEM10AA

In what degree programs are you currently enrolled? (Mark all that apply). Indicate the year you are currently in for each program.

- ○ CNP
- ○ CNS
- ○ D.Pharm.
- ○ D.S.W.
- ○ Ed.D.
- ○ M.A.
- ○ M.D. (Resident)
- ○ M.D. (Student)

- ○ M.P.H.
- ○ M.S.
- ○ M.S.N.
- ○ M.S.W.
- ○ Ph.D.
- ○ Post-Doctorate
- ○ Psy.D.
- ○ Other - specify

TDEMO11

TDM11PPP

What is your gender? ○ Female ○ Male

TDEMO12

What is your date of birth? [ ] [ ] / [ ] [ ] / [ ] [ ]

MONTH   DAY   YEAR

TDEMO13

What is your race?

- ○ White/Caucasian
- ○ Black/African American
- ○ Black/Non-African American
- ○ Asian/Pacific Islander
- ○ Native American/Alaskan Native
- ○ Other - specify

TDEMO14

TDEMO14A

Are you of Latino descent? ○ Yes ○ No

TDEMO15

If yes, what is your country of origin?

- ○ Puerto Rico
- ○ Mexico
- ○ Cuba
- ○ Dominican Republic
- ○ Other-specify

TDEMO15A

TDEM15AA

The John A. Hartford Foundation
Geriatric Interdisciplinary Team Training Program (GITT)
TRAINEE ENTRY QUESTIONNAIRE

Instructions:
* Your answers are confidential and will be reported only in grouped data.
* Use a dark blue or black pen (not pencil) to complete questionnaire.
* Print in capital letters as shown.

| A | B | C | D | E | F | G | H | I | J | K | L | M | N | O | P | Q | R | S | T | U | V | W | X | Y | Z |

* Unless otherwise instructed, choose only one response to each question/statement.
* Fill in bubbles completely as shown.   correct   wrong   wrong
* Do not fold or staple the pages.
* Make no stray marks on the questionnaire.

ID [ ][ ][ ][ ][ ]

FIRST LETTER of last name plus
LAST 4 DIGITS of Social Security No.

Project ID [ ][ ]

Clinical Setting ID [ ][ ][ ][ ]

Today's Date [ ][ ] / [ ][ ] / [ ][ ]
                MONTH   DAY   YEAR

This is the ○ 1st ○ 2nd ○ 3rd ○ 4th ○ 5th ○ 6th or more time I have completed this questionnaire

Please indicate your trainee status:

○ Student Trainee (includes medical residents)

○ Staff Trainee (GITT is NOT part of a degree requirement)

○ Other -specify [ ][ ][ ][ ][ ][ ][ ][ ][ ][ ][ ]

We would like to know about your attitudes toward interdisciplinary health care teams and the team approach to care.   By interdisciplinary health care team, we mean three or more health professionals (e.g., nurse, physician, social worker) who work together and meet regularly to plan and coordinate treatment for a specific patient population.[1]

"IN MY OPINION":

	Strongly Disagree	Moderately Disagree	Somewhat Disagree	Somewhat Agree	Moderately Agree	Strongly Agree	
1. Working in teams unnecessarily complicates things most of the time	①	②	③	④	⑤	⑥	A1
2. The team approach improves the quality of care to patients	①	②	③	④	⑤	⑥	A2
3. Team meetings foster communication among team members from different disciplines	①	②	③	④	⑤	⑥	A3
4. Physicians have the right to alter patient care plans developed by the team	①	②	③	④	⑤	⑥	A4
5. Patients receiving team care are more likely than other patients to be treated as whole persons	①	②	③	④	⑤	⑥	A5
6. A team's primary purpose is to assist physicians in achieving treatment goals for patients	①	②	③	④	⑤	⑥	A6
7. Working on a team keeps most health professionals enthusiastic and interested in their jobs	①	②	③	④	⑤	⑥	A7

"IN MY OPINION":

	Strongly Disagree	Moderately Disagree	Somewhat Disagree	Somewhat Agree	Moderately Agree	Strongly Agree	
8. Patients are less satisfied with their care when it is provided by a team	①	②	③	④	⑤	⑥	A8
9. Developing a patient care plan with other team members avoids errors in delivering care	①	②	③	④	⑤	⑥	A9
10. When developing interdisciplinary patient care plans, much time is wasted translating jargon from other disciplines	①	②	③	④	⑤	⑥	A10
11. Health professionals working on teams are more responsive than others to the emotional and financial needs of patients	①	②	③	④	⑤	⑥	A11
12. Developing an interdisciplinary patient care plan is excessively time consuming	①	②	③	④	⑤	⑥	A12
13. The physician should not always have the final word in decisions made by health care teams	①	②	③	④	⑤	⑥	A13
14. The give and take among team members help them make better patient care decisions	①	②	③	④	⑤	⑥	A14
15. In most instances, the time required for team meetings could be better spent in other ways	①	②	③	④	⑤	⑥	A15
16. The physician has the ultimate legal responsibility for decisions made by the team	①	②	③	④	⑤	⑥	A16
17. Hospital patients who receive team care are better prepared for discharge than other patients	①	②	③	④	⑤	⑥	A17
18. Physicians are natural team leaders	①	②	③	④	⑤	⑥	A18
19. The team approach makes the delivery of care more efficient	①	②	③	④	⑤	⑥	A19
20. The team approach permits health professionals to meet the needs of family caregivers as well as patients	①	②	③	④	⑤	⑥	A20
21. Having to report observations to the team helps team members better understand the work of other health professionals	①	②	③	④	⑤	⑥	A21

Please rate your ability to carry out each of the following tasks at this point in your training using a five-point scale.[2]

	Poor	Fair	Good	Very Good	Excellent	
22. Function effectively in an interdisciplinary team	①	②	③	④	⑤	TSS1
23. Treat geriatric team members as colleagues	①	②	③	④	⑤	TSS2
24. Identify contributions to patient care that different disciplines can offer	①	②	③	④	⑤	TSS3
25. Apply your knowledge of geriatric principles for the care of older persons in a team care setting	①	②	③	④	⑤	TSS4
26. Ensure that patient/family preferences/goals are considered when developing the team's care plan	①	②	③	④	⑤	TSS5

Please rate your ability to carry out each of the following tasks at this point in your training using a five-point scale.

	Poor	Fair	Good	Very Good	Excellent	
27. Handle disagreements effectively	①	②	③	④	⑤	TSS6
28. Strengthen cooperation among disciplines	①	②	③	④	⑤	TSS7
29. Carry out responsibilities specific to your discipline's role on a team	①	②	③	④	⑤	TSS8
30. Address clinical issues succinctly in interdisciplinary meetings	①	②	③	④	⑤	TSS9
31. Participate actively at team meetings	①	②	③	④	⑤	TSS10
32. Develop an interdisciplinary care plan	①	②	③	④	⑤	TSS11
33. Adjust your care to support the team goals	①	②	③	④	⑤	TSS12
34. Develop intervention strategies that help patients attain goals	①	②	③	④	⑤	TSS13
35. Raise appropriate issues at team meetings	①	②	③	④	⑤	TSS14
36. Recognize when the team is not functioning well	①	②	③	④	⑤	TSS15
37. Intervene effectively to improve team functioning	①	②	③	④	⑤	TSS16
38. Help draw out team members who are not participating actively in meetings	①	②	③	④	⑤	TSS17

Please rate your attitude, at this point in your training, using a five-point scale.

	Poor	Fair	Good	Very Good	Excellent	
39. Toward other disciplines working in the team setting	①	②	③	④	⑤	TSS18
40. Towards providing care to the elderly	①	②	③	④	⑤	TSS19
41. About practicing in a team care environment	①	②	③	④	⑤	TSS20

	Not at all				Extensively	
42. To what extent do you anticipate an emphasis in geriatrics in your career?	①	②	③	④	⑤	B1

	Negatively		Neutral		Positively	
43. When choosing (looking) for your next position, how will the opportunity to participate in an interdisciplinary team influence your decision?	①	②	③	④	⑤	B2

	Not Important				Very Important	
44. To what extent do you believe that your ability to work in an interdisciplinary team will contribute to your professional success?	①	②	③	④	⑤	B3

	Highly Unlikely				Highly Likely	
45. What is thle likelihood that you will seek additional training in team care after completing this program?	①	②	③	④	⑤	B4

	Highly Unlikely				Highly Likely	
46. What is the likelihood that you will seek additional training in geriatrics after completing this program?	①	②	③	④	⑤	B5

The John A. Hartford Foundation
Geriatric Interdisciplinary Team Training Program (GITT)
TRAINEE EXIT QUESTIONNAIRE

Instructions:
* Your answers are confidential and will be reported only in grouped data.
* Use a dark blue or black pen (not pencil) to complete questionnaire.
* Print in capital letters as shown.

| A | B | C | D | E | F | G | H | I | J | K | L | M | N | O | P | Q | R | S | T | U | V | W | X | Y | Z |

* Unless otherwise instructed, choose only one response to each question/statement.
* Fill in bubbles completely as shown.   correct wrong wrong
* Do not fold or staple the pages.
* Make no stray marks on the questionnaire.

ID   [ ][ ][ ][ ][ ]

FIRST LETTER of last name plus
LAST 4 DIGITS of Social Security No.

Project ID   [ ][ ]

Clinical Setting ID   [ ][ ][ ][ ]

Today's Date   [ ][ ] / [ ][ ] / [ ][ ]
      MONTH   DAY   YEAR

This is the ◯ 1st ◯ 2nd ◯ 3rd ◯ 4th ◯ 5th ◯ 6th or more time I have completed this questionnaire

Please indicate your trainee status:

◯ Student Trainee (includes medical residents)

◯ Staff Trainee (GITT is NOT part of a degree requirement)

◯ Other -specify [ ][ ][ ][ ][ ][ ][ ][ ][ ][ ][ ]

We would like to know about your attitudes toward interdisciplinary health care teams and the team approach to care. By interdisciplinary health care team, we mean three or more health professionals (e.g., nurse, physician, social worker) who work together and meet regularly to plan and coordinate treatment for a specific patient population.[1]

"IN MY OPINION":

	Strongly Disagree	Moderately Disagree	Somewhat Disagree	Somewhat Agree	Moderately Agree	Strongly Agree	
1. Working in teams unnecessarily complicates things most of the time	①	②	③	④	⑤	⑥	A1
2. The team approach improves the quality of care to patients	①	②	③	④	⑤	⑥	A2
3. Team meetings foster communication among team members from different disciplines	①	②	③	④	⑤	⑥	A3
4. Physicians have the right to alter patient care plans developed by the team	①	②	③	④	⑤	⑥	A4
5. Patients receiving team care are more likely than other patients to be treated as whole persons	①	②	③	④	⑤	⑥	A5
6. A team's primary purpose is to assist physicians in achieving treatment goals for patients	①	②	③	④	⑤	⑥	A6
7. Working on a team keeps most health professionals enthusiastic and interested in their jobs	①	②	③	④	⑤	⑥	A7

IN MY OPINION":	Strongly Disagree	Moderately Disagree	Somewhat Disagree	Somewhat Agree	Moderately Agree	Strongly Agree	
8. Patients are less satisfied with their care when it is provided by a team	①	②	③	④	⑤	⑥	A8
9. Developing a patient care plan with other team members avoids errors in delivering care	①	②	③	④	⑤	⑥	A9
10. When developing interdisciplinary patient care plans, much time is wasted translating jargon from other disciplines	①	②	③	④	⑤	⑥	A10
11. Health professionals working on teams are more responsive than others to the emotional and financial needs of patients	①	②	③	④	⑤	⑥	A11
12. Developing an interdisciplinary patient care plan is excessively time consuming	①	②	③	④	⑤	⑥	A12
13. The physician should not always have the final word in decisions made by health care teams	①	②	③	④	⑤	⑥	A13
14. The give and take among team members help them make better patient care decisions	①	②	③	④	⑤	⑥	A14
15. In most instances, the time required for team meetings could be better spent in other ways	①	②	③	④	⑤	⑥	A15
16. The physician has the ultimate legal responsibility for decisions made by the team	①	②	③	④	⑤	⑥	A16
17. Hospital patients who receive team care are better prepared for discharge than other patients	①	②	③	④	⑤	⑥	A17
18. Physicians are natural team leaders	①	②	③	④	⑤	⑥	A18
19. The team approach makes the delivery of care more efficient	①	②	③	④	⑤	⑥	A19
20. The team approach permits health professionals to meet the needs of family caregivers as well as patients	①	②	③	④	⑤	⑥	A20
21. Having to report observations to the team helps team members better understand the work of other health professionals	①	②	③	④	⑤	⑥	A21

Please rate your ability to carry out each of the following tasks at this point in your training using a five-point scale. [2]

	Poor	Fair	Good	Very Good	Excellent	
22. Function effectively in an interdisciplinary team	①	②	③	④	⑤	TSS1
23. Treat geriatric team members as colleagues	①	②	③	④	⑤	TSS2
24. Identify contributions to patient care that different disciplines can offer	①	②	③	④	⑤	TSS3
25. Apply your knowledge of geriatric principles for the care of older persons in a team care setting	①	②	③	④	⑤	TSS4
26. Ensure that patient/family preferences/goals are considered when developing the team's care plan	①	②	③	④	⑤	TSS5

[2] Hepburn, Tsukuda, and Fasser (1996), Team Skills Scale, all rights reserved

Please rate your ability to carry out each of the following tasks at this point in your training using a five-point scale.

	Poor	Fair	Good	Very Good	Excellent	
27. Handle disagreements effectively	①	②	③	④	⑤	TSS6
28. Strengthen cooperation among disciplines	①	②	③	④	⑤	TSS7
29. Carry out responsibilities specific to your discipline's role on a team	①	②	③	④	⑤	TSS8
30. Address clinical issues succinctly in interdisciplinary meetings	①	②	③	④	⑤	TSS9
31. Participate actively at team meetings	①	②	③	④	⑤	TSS10
32. Develop an interdisciplinary care plan	①	②	③	④	⑤	TSS11
33. Adjust your care to support the team goals	①	②	③	④	⑤	TSS12
34. Develop intervention strategies that help patients attain goals	①	②	③	④	⑤	TSS13
35. Raise appropriate issues at team meetings	①	②	③	④	⑤	TSS14
36. Recognize when the team is not functioning well	①	②	③	④	⑤	TSS15
37. Intervene effectively to improve team functioning	①	②	③	④	⑤	TSS16
38. Help draw out team members who are not participating actively in meetings	①	②	③	④	⑤	TSS17

Please rate your attitude, at this point in your training, using a five-point scale.

	Poor	Fair	Good	Very Good	Excellent	
39. Toward other disciplines working in the team setting	①	②	③	④	⑤	TSS18
40. Towards providing care to the elderly	①	②	③	④	⑤	TSS19
41. About practicing in a team care environment	①	②	③	④	⑤	TSS20

	Not at all				Extensively	
42. To what extent do you anticipate an emphasis in geriatrics in your career?	①	②	③	④	⑤	B1

	Negatively		Neutral		Positively	
43. When choosing (looking) for your next position, how will the opportunity to participate in an interdisciplinary team influence your decision?	①	②	③	④	⑤	B2

	Not Important				Very Important	
44. To what extent do you believe that your ability to work in an interdisciplinary team will contribute to your professional success?	①	②	③	④	⑤	B3

	Highly Unlikely				Highly Likely	
45. What is thle likelihood that you will seek additional training in team care after completing this program?	①	②	③	④	⑤	B4

	Highly Unlikely				Highly Likely	
46. What is the likelihood that you will seek additional training in geriatrics after completing this program?	①	②	③	④	⑤	B5

Please indicate your level of agreement or disagreement with the following statements:

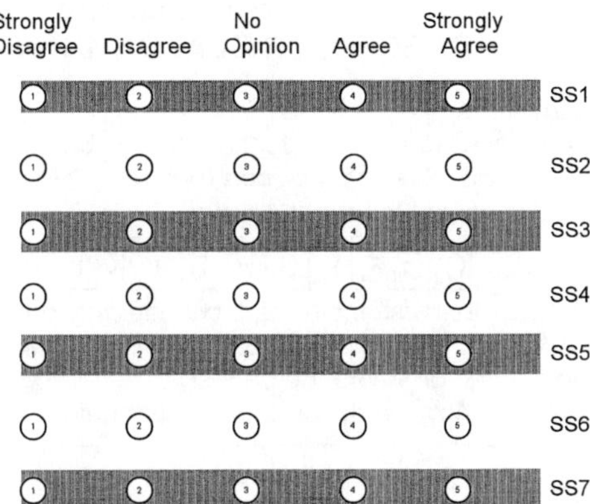

	Strongly Disagree	Disagree	No Opinion	Agree	Strongly Agree	
47. My personal objectives for this training have been achieved	①	②	③	④	⑤	SS1
48. I would recommend this training to other students	①	②	③	④	⑤	SS2
49. The time devoted to this experience was well spent and worthwhile	①	②	③	④	⑤	SS3
50. This experience added to my knowledge of geriatrics	①	②	③	④	⑤	SS4
51. As a result of this experience, I feel more confident with geriatric patients	①	②	③	④	⑤	SS5
52. This experience added to my knowledge of teams	①	②	③	④	⑤	SS6
53. As a result of this experience, I feel more confident working as part of an interdisciplinary team	①	②	③	④	⑤	SS7

The John A. Hartford Foundation
Geriatric Interdisciplinary Team Training Program (GITT)
PRECEPTOR EVALUATION OF TRAINEE'S TEAM SKILLS

Instructions:
* Your answers are confidential and will be reported only in grouped data.
* Use a dark blue or black pen (not pencil) to complete questionnaire.
* Print in capital letters as shown.

| A | B | C | D | E | F | G | H | I | J | K | L | M | N | O | P | Q | R | S | T | U | V | W | X | Y | Z |

* Unless otherwise instructed, choose only one response to each question/statement.
* Fill in bubbles completely as shown.   correct   wrong   wrong
* Do not fold or staple the pages.
* Make no stray marks on the questionnaire.

Preceptor ID

FIRST LETTER of last name plus
LAST 4 DIGITS of Social Security No.

Project ID

Clinical Setting ID

Trainee ID

FIRST LETTER of last name plus
LAST 4 DIGITS of Social Security No.

Today's Date

MONTH   DAY   YEAR

Please rate the above-named trainee's ability to carry out each of the following tasks using a six-point scale. [1]

	Poor	Fair	Good	Very Good	Excellent	Unable to Evaluate	
1. Function effectively in an interdisciplinary team	①	②	③	④	⑤	⑥	PES1
2. Treat geriatric team members as colleagues	①	②	③	④	⑤	⑥	PES2
3. Identify contributions to patient care that different disciplines can offer	①	②	③	④	⑤	⑥	PES3
4. Apply their knowledge of geriatric principles for the care of older persons in a team care setting	①	②	③	④	⑤	⑥	PES4
5. Ensure that patient/family preferences/goals are considered when developing the team's care plan	①	②	③	④	⑤	⑥	PES5
6. Handle disagreements effectively	①	②	③	④	⑤	⑥	PES6
7. Strengthen cooperation among disciplines	①	②	③	④	⑤	⑥	PES7
8. Carry out responsibilities specific to their discipline's role on a team	①	②	③	④	⑤	⑥	PES8

	Poor	Fair	Good	Very Good	Excellent	Unable to Evaluate	
9. Address clinical issues succinctly in interdisciplinary meetings	①	②	③	④	⑤	⑥	PES9
10. Participate actively at team meetings	①	②	③	④	⑤	⑥	PES10
11. Develop an interdisciplinary care plan	①	②	③	④	⑤	⑥	PES11
12. Adjust care to support the team goals	①	②	③	④	⑤	⑥	PES12
13. Develop intervention strategies that help patients attain goals	①	②	③	④	⑤	⑥	PES13
14. Raise appropriate issues at team meetings	①	②	③	④	⑤	⑥	PES14
15. Recognize when the team is not functioning well	①	②	③	④	⑤	⑥	PES15
16. Intervene effectively to improve team functioning	①	②	③	④	⑤	⑥	PES16
17. Help draw out team members who are not participating actively in meetings	①	②	③	④	⑤	⑥	PES17

Please rate the trainee's attitude using the following six-point scale:

	Poor	Fair	Good	Very Good	Excellent	Unable to Evaluate	
18. Toward other disciplines working in the team setting	①	②	③	④	⑤	⑥	PES18
19. Towards providing care to the elderly	①	②	③	④	⑤	⑥	PES19
20. About practicing in a team care environment	①	②	③	④	⑤	⑥	PES20

The John A. Hartford Foundation
Geriatric Interdisciplinary Team Training Program (GITT)
DEMOGRAPHIC QUESTIONNAIRE: PRECEPTOR VERSION

Instructions:
* Your answers are confidential and will be reported only in grouped data.
* Use a dark blue or black pen (not pencil) to complete questionnaire.
* Print in capital letters as shown.

| A | B | C | D | E | F | G | H | I | J | K | L | M | N | O | P | Q | R | S | T | U | V | W | X | Y | Z |

* Unless otherwise instructed, choose only one response to each question/statement.
* Fill in bubbles completely as shown.   correct   wrong   wrong
* Do not fold or staple the pages.
* Make no stray marks on the questionnaire.

ID [ ][ ][ ][ ][ ]   Project ID [ ][ ]   Today's Date [ ][ ] / [ ][ ] / [ ][ ]
MONTH   DAY   YEAR

FIRST LETTER of last name plus
LAST 4 DIGITS of Social Security No.

Clinical Setting ID [ ][ ][ ][ ]

Are you currently a preceptor for GITT Students?   ◯ Yes   ◯ No   P1

What is your primary field?   P2

◯ Dentistry   ◯ Pastoral Care

◯ Geriatrics   ◯ Pharmacy

◯ Gerontology   ◯ Psychology

◯ Health Administration   ◯ Public Health

◯ Medicine   ◯ Physical Therapy

◯ Nursing   ◯ Social Work

◯ Occupation Therapy   ◯ Other- specify [ ][ ][ ][ ][ ][ ][ ][ ][ ]   P2A

What are your areas of speciality?
(Mark all that apply)   P3

◯ Administration/Management   ◯ Emergency Room   ◯ Primary Care

◯ Ambulatory Care   ◯ Ethics   ◯ Public Health

◯ Cardiology   ◯ Geriatrics   ◯ Psychiatric/Mental Health

◯ Case Management   ◯ Gerontology   ◯ Rehabilitation

◯ Clinical Research   ◯ Home Care   ◯ Substance Abuse

◯ Community Health   ◯ Long Term Care   ◯ Women's Health

◯ Counseling   ◯ Neurology   ◯ None at this time

◯ Critical Care   ◯ Oncology   ◯ Other - specify   P3AA

[ ][ ][ ][ ][ ][ ][ ][ ][ ]

What degrees/certifications do you currently hold? (Mark all that apply) — P4

- ○ B.A.
- ○ B.S.
- ○ B.S.N.
- ○ B.S.W.
- ○ R.N.
- ○ CNP
- ○ CNS
- ○ M.A.

- ○ M.S.
- ○ M.S.N.
- ○ M.S.W.
- ○ M.Ed.
- ○ M.P.H.
- ○ M.D.
- ○ Ph.D.
- ○ Ed.D.

- ○ D.P.H.
- ○ D.S.W.
- ○ D.N.Sc / N.D.
- ○ D.Pharm.
- ○ D.D.S.
- ○ Psy.D.
- ○ Other – specify

P4AA [ ][ ][ ][ ][ ][ ][ ][ ][ ][ ][ ]

Have you ever received any formal training in gerontology or geriatrics before this team training program? ○ Yes   ○ No — P5

What formal training in gerontology or geriatrics have you completed? (Mark all that apply) — P6

- ○ ANA Gerontological certification exam
- ○ Certificate of added qualification in geriatrics
- ○ Bachelors Degree in Geriatrics/Gerontology
- ○ Masters Degree in Geriatrics/Gerontology
- ○ Minor in Geriatrics/Gerontology
- ○ Conferences, Workshops, Continuing Education
- ○ None

- ○ Certificate Program in Geriatrics/Gerontology
- ○ Geriatrics Rotation
- ○ Geriatric Education Center Programs
- ○ Individual Course(s) in Geriatrics/Gerontology
- ○ Other – specify

P6AA [ ][ ][ ][ ][ ][ ][ ][ ][ ][ ][ ]

Have you ever received any team training before this program? ○ Yes   ○ No — P7

If yes, about how many hours? [ ][ ][ ] — P7A

What is your primary place of employment? — P8

- ○ Ambulatory Care/Outpatient Clinic
- ○ Government (Non VA)
- ○ Government (VA)
- ○ Group Medical Practice
- ○ Home Care
- ○ Hospice
- ○ Hospital
- ○ Individual Medial Practice

- ○ Medical School
- ○ Nursing Home
- ○ Nursing School
- ○ Other Health Professions Schools
- ○ School of Public Health
- ○ School of Social Work
- ○ Other – specify

P8A [ ][ ][ ][ ][ ][ ][ ][ ][ ][ ][ ]

What is your primary role?

- ○ Academic Administration
- ○ Clinical Administration
- ○ Consultant
- ○ Education
- ○ Patient Care

- ○ Policy Analyst/Planner
- ○ Quality Assurance
- ○ Research
- ○ None
- ○ Other - specify

P9

P9A

Are you currently working in an organization providing health care services to managed care (HMO, PPO, POS) enrollees?

○ Yes   ○ No   P10

What were your former places of employment?
(Mark all that apply)

- ○ Ambulatory Care/Outpatient Clinic
- ○ Government (Non VA)
- ○ Government (VA)
- ○ Group Medical Practice
- ○ Health Maintenance Organization
- ○ Home Care
- ○ Hospice
- ○ Hospital

- ○ Individual Medical Practice
- ○ Medical School
- ○ Nursing Home
- ○ Nursing School
- ○ Other Health Professions Schools
- ○ School of Public Health
- ○ School of Social Work
- ○ Other - specify

P11

P11AA

List all licenses and certifications you hold or have held
(Enter category, not license numbers, e.g. GERIATRIC NURSE PRAC).

Current?

○ Yes   ○ No   P12

○ Yes   ○ No   P13

What is your gender?   ○ Female   ○ Male   What is your date of birth?

P14   P15   MONTH / DAY / YEAR

What is your race?

- ○ White/Caucasian
- ○ Black/African American
- ○ Black/Non-African American
- ○ Asian/Pacific Islander
- ○ Native American/Alaskan Native
- ○ Other - specify

P16

P16A

Are you of Latino descent?   ○ Yes   ○ No   P17

If yes, what is your country of origin?

- ○ Puerto Rico   ○ Mexico
- ○ Cuba   ○ Dominican Republic
- ○ Other-specify

P17A

The John A. Hartford Foundation
Geriatric Interdisciplinary Team Training Program (GITT)
DEMOGRAPHIC QUESTIONNAIRE: STAFF VERSION

Instructions:
* Your answers are confidential and will be reported only in grouped data.
* Use a dark blue or black pen (not pencil) to complete questionnaire.
* Print in capital letters as shown.

| A | B | C | D | E | F | G | H | I | J | K | L | M | N | O | P | Q | R | S | T | U | V | W | X | Y | Z |

* Unless otherwise instructed, choose only one response to each question/statement.
* Fill in bubbles completely as shown.
* Do not fold or staple the pages.
* Make no stray marks on the questionnaire.

correct   wrong   wrong

ID ☐☐☐☐☐
FIRST LETTER of last name plus
LAST 4 DIGITS of Social Security No.

Project ID ☐☐

Clinical Setting ID ☐☐☐☐

Today's Date ☐☐ / ☐☐ / ☐☐
MONTH   DAY   YEAR

Are you currently a preceptor for GITT Students?   ○ Yes   ○ No   S1

What is your primary field?   S2

- ○ Dentistry
- ○ Geriatrics
- ○ Gerontology
- ○ Health Administration
- ○ Medicine
- ○ Nursing
- ○ Occupation Therapy
- ○ Pastoral Care
- ○ Pharmacy
- ○ Psychology
- ○ Public Health
- ○ Physical Therapy
- ○ Social Work
- ○ Other- specify ☐☐☐☐☐☐☐☐☐   S2A

What are your areas of speciality? (Mark all that apply)   S3

- ○ Administration/Management
- ○ Ambulatory Care
- ○ Cardiology
- ○ Case Management
- ○ Clinical Research
- ○ Community Health
- ○ Counseling
- ○ Critical Care
- ○ Emergency Room
- ○ Ethics
- ○ Geriatrics
- ○ Gerontology
- ○ Home Care
- ○ Long Term Care
- ○ Neurology
- ○ Oncology
- ○ Primary Care
- ○ Public Health
- ○ Psychiatric/Mental Health
- ○ Rehabilitation
- ○ Substance Abuse
- ○ Women's Health
- ○ None at this time
- ○ Other - specify

S3AA ☐☐☐☐☐☐☐☐☐☐

What degrees/certifications do you currently hold? (Mark all that apply)   **S4**

- ○ B.A.
- ○ B.S.
- ○ B.S.N.
- ○ B.S.W.
- ○ R.N.
- ○ CNP
- ○ CNS
- ○ M.A.

- ○ M.S.
- ○ M.S.N.
- ○ M.S.W.
- ○ M.Ed.
- ○ M.P.H.
- ○ M.D.
- ○ Ph.D.
- ○ Ed.D.

- ○ D.P.H.
- ○ D.S.W.
- ○ D.N.Sc / N.D.
- ○ D.Pharm.
- ○ D.D.S.
- ○ Psy.D.
- ○ Other – specify

S4AA

Have you ever received any formal training in gerontology or geriatrics before this team training program?   ○ Yes   ○ No   **S5**

What formal training in gerontology or geriatrics have you completed? (Mark all that apply)   **S6**

- ○ ANA Gerontological certification exam
- ○ Certificate of added qualification in geriatrics
- ○ Bachelors Degree in Geriatrics/Gerontology
- ○ Masters Degree in Geriatrics/Gerontology
- ○ Minor in Geriatrics/Gerontology
- ○ Conferences, Workshops, Continuing Education
- ○ None

- ○ Certificate Program in Geriatrics/Gerontology
- ○ Geriatrics Rotation
- ○ Geriatric Education Center Programs
- ○ Individual Course(s) in Geriatrics/Gerontology
- ○ Other – specify

S6AA

Have you ever received any team training before this program?   ○ Yes   ○ No   **S7**

If yes, about how many hours?   **S7A**

What is your primary place of employment?   **S8**

- ○ Ambulatory Care/Outpatient Clinic
- ○ Government (Non VA)
- ○ Government (VA)
- ○ Group Medical Practice
- ○ Home Care
- ○ Hospice
- ○ Hospital
- ○ Individual Medial Practice

- ○ Medical School
- ○ Nursing Home
- ○ Nursing School
- ○ Other Health Professions Schools
- ○ School of Public Health
- ○ School of Social Work
- ○ Other – specify

S8A

What is your primary role?

- ◯ Academic Administration
- ◯ Clinical Administration
- ◯ Consultant
- ◯ Education
- ◯ Patient Care

- ◯ Policy Analyst/Planner
- ◯ Quality Assurance
- ◯ Research
- ◯ None
- ◯ Other - specify

S9

S9A

Are you currently working in an organization providing health care services to managed care (HMO, PPO, POS) enrollees?   ◯ Yes   ◯ No   S10

What were your former places of employment?
(Mark all that apply)

- ◯ Ambulatory Care/Outpatient Clinic
- ◯ Government (Non VA)
- ◯ Government (VA)
- ◯ Group Medical Practice
- ◯ Health Maintenance Organization
- ◯ Home Care
- ◯ Hospice
- ◯ Hospital

- ◯ Individual Medical Practice
- ◯ Medical School
- ◯ Nursing Home
- ◯ Nursing School
- ◯ Other Health Professions Schools
- ◯ School of Public Health
- ◯ School of Social Work
- ◯ Other - specify

S11

S11AA

List all licenses and certifications you hold or have held
(Enter category, not license numbers, e.g. GERIATRIC NURSE PRAC).

Current?

◯ Yes   ◯ No   S12

◯ Yes   ◯ No   S13

What is your gender?   ◯ Female   ◯ Male   What is your date of birth?   ___ / ___ / ___
S14   S15   MONTH   DAY   YEAR

What is your race?

- ◯ White/Caucasian
- ◯ Black/African American
- ◯ Black/Non-African American
- ◯ Asian/Pacific Islander
- ◯ Native American/Alaskan Native
- ◯ Other - specify

S16

S16A

Are you of Latino descent?   ◯ Yes   ◯ No   S17

If yes, what is your country of origin?

- ◯ Puerto Rico   ◯ Mexico
- ◯ Cuba   ◯ Dominican Republic
- ◯ Other-specify

S17A

Section II: Glossary of Terms

Academic Faculty: Faculty at an academic partner(s).

Academic Partner: An academic institution involved in a GITT program—an academic partner may bring more than one college, school, or department to the table.

Academic Program: A degree-granting program offered by an academic partner—each discipline (e.g., medicine) may offer more than one academic program (e.g., internal medicine and primary care).

Class: A method of disseminating the traditional, discipline-specific (or cross-listed) curriculum at an academic partner (e.g., classes, seminars, noon conferences, etc.).

Clinical Partner: An operator of one or more patient-care facilities involved in the GITT project—the clinical partner may be operated by the academic partner or joined to it by an affiliation agreement and may itself bring more than one clinical setting to the table.

Clinical Setting: A patient-care site operated by or in affiliation with a clinical partner—this is where the practicum experience takes place.

Clinical Staff: Nonacademic practitioners paid by the clinical setting to care for patients—sometimes called professional staff.

Curriculum: For the purposes of GITT, an umbrella term encompassing both classes (above) and the GITT didactic (below) and as distinguished from the GITT practicum (below).

Degree Program: For the purposes of the trainee log and the preceptor log (defined below), degree program is broken down into five categories: 1 = Social Work; 2 = Medical; 3 = Nursing; 4 = Pharmacy; 5 = Other.

(A more exhaustive degree program listing is found on the survey measures. As the purpose of the logs is to quickly track and summarize data, we do not want an exhaustive list, rather, categories.)

Didactic: Interdisciplinary course work instruction as part of GITT—may include readings, workshops, lectures, conferences, seminars, etc.

GITT Program: A combination of the didactic and practicum.

GITT Trainee: A trainee from a GITT-eligible academic program who is participating or has participated in the GITT program.

Practicum: For a GITT trainee, the experience of participation in or observation of the clinical team at a clinical setting caring for the older patients.

Preceptor: A person responsible for supervising or evaluating individual GITT trainees in the context of their disciplinary needs or coordinator of team activities for GITT trainees from all disciplines.

Primary Preceptor: The preceptor most familiar with the trainee's performance on the GITT site's learning objectives.

Project: One of the eight awards or unfunded planning year projects where the GITT Program is being implemented and core measures are being collected.

Trainee: Any health-professions student in any of the participating academic programs, not necessarily eligible for or enrolled in the GITT program.

Index

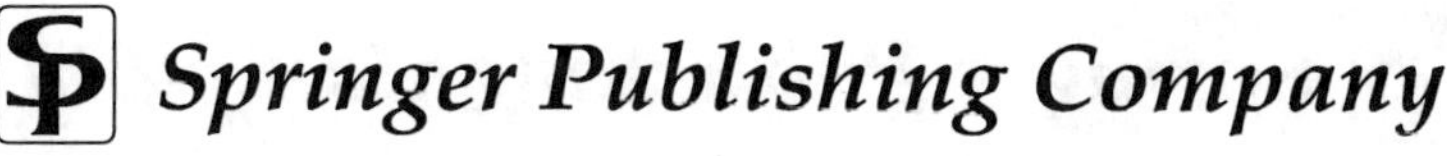

Geriatric Home Health Care
The Collaboration of Physicians, Nurses, and Social Workers

Philip W. Brickner, MD, **F. Russell Kellogg**, MD,
Anthony J. Lechich, MD, **Roberta Lipsman**, MSSW,
Linda K. Scharer, MUP, Editors

Drawing on more than 20 years of work in geriatric home health care, the editors of this book share their experiences in creating and managing home care programs for the frail aged. They have compiled information from diverse disciplines, including medicine, nursing, gerontology, and social services. In addition to in-depth coverage of important clinical issues such as functional ability, mental health, and disease and accident prevention, the book focuses on critical programmatic issues including:

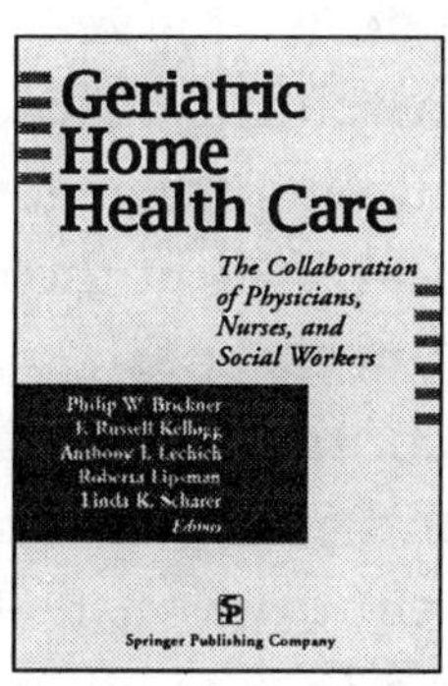

- the use of professional physician, nurse, and social worker teams
- paraprofessional and family supports
- ethical issues and strategies about making choices in life support decisions
- methods for bringing students into this field of care

Furthermore, the editors include analyses of four long-term home health care programs, each with a substantial history of success in working through administrative, financial, and bureaucratic problems. This book should be required reading for all health professionals working with the elderly in long-term home health care settings.

1996   320pp   0-8261-9450-8   hardcover

536 Broadway, New York, NY 10012-3955 • (212) 431-4370 • Fax (212) 941-7842